Health Informatics

This series is directed to healthcare professionals leading the transformation of healthcare by using information and knowledge. For over 20 years, Health Informatics has offered a broad range of titles: some address specific professions such as nursing, medicine, and health administration; others cover special areas of practice such as trauma and radiology; still other books in the series focus on interdisciplinary issues, such as the computer based patient record, electronic health records, and networked healthcare systems. Editors and authors, eminent experts in their fields, offer their accounts of innovations in health informatics. Increasingly, these accounts go beyond hardware and software to address the role of information in influencing the transformation of healthcare delivery systems around the world. The series also increasingly focuses on the users of the information and systems: the organizational, behavioral, and societal changes that accompany the diffusion of information technology in health services environments.

Developments in healthcare delivery are constant; in recent years, bioinformatics has emerged as a new field in health informatics to support emerging and ongoing developments in molecular biology. At the same time, further evolution of the field of health informatics is reflected in the introduction of concepts at the macro or health systems delivery level with major national initiatives related to electronic health records (EHR), data standards, and public health informatics.

These changes will continue to shape health services in the twenty-first century. By making full and creative use of the technology to tame data and to transform information, Health Informatics will foster the development and use of new knowledge in healthcare.

More information about this series at http://www.springer.com/series/1114

Eta S. Berner
Editor

Clinical Decision Support Systems

Theory and Practice

Third Edition

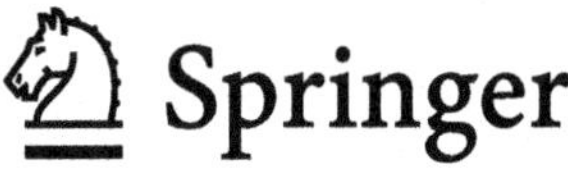

Editor
Eta S. Berner
School of Health Professions
Department of Health Services Administration
and Department of Medical Education
School of Medicine
University of Alabama at Birmingham
Birmingham, AL, USA

ISSN 1431-1917 ISSN 2197-3741 (electronic)
Health Informatics
ISBN 978-3-319-31911-7 ISBN 978-3-319-31913-1 (eBook)
DOI 10.1007/978-3-319-31913-1

Library of Congress Control Number: 2016945364

1st edition: Springer Science + Business media NewYork 1999
2nd edition: Springer Verlag NewYork 2007

Printed on acid-free paper

This Springer imprint is published by Springer Nature
The registered company is Springer International Publishing AG Switzerland

Preface

When the first edition of Clinical Decision Support Systems was published in 1999, I began the preface with the statement, "We are at the beginning of a new era in the application of computer-based decision support for medicine." Usually such statements in hindsight seem unduly optimistic, but if we look at the landscape of healthcare information technology today, that assessment appears to be surprisingly accurate. Shortly after the book was published, the first of several landmark reports from the Institute of Medicine on the quality of health care led to greater awareness of the role these systems can play in improving patient safety and healthcare quality. The second edition was published in 2007, a time when there was increased governmental, research and commercial interest in clinical decision support systems (CDSS), but predated the HITECH Act, which accelerated the use of electronic health records and incentivized the incorporation of CDSS into clinical practice in the US. This third edition of Clinical Decision Support Systems: Theory and Practice is being published at a time when electronic health records are being routinely used in clinical practice, and clinical decision support systems are seeing more use as well.

The purpose of this book is to provide an overview of the background and state-of-the-art of CDSS. Throughout this book we use CDSS to refer to both the singular and plural (system and systems). A persistent theme is that CDSS have enormous potential to transform health care, but developers, evaluators, and users of these tools need to be aware of the design and implementation issues that must be addressed for that potential to be realized as these systems continue to evolve. This book is designed to be (1) a resource on clinical decision support systems for informatics specialists; (2) a textbook for teachers or students in health or medical informatics training programs; and (3) a comprehensive introduction for clinicians, with or without expertise in the applications of computers in medicine, who are interested in learning about current developments in computer-based clinical decision support systems.

The book includes chapters by nationally recognized experts on the design, evaluation and application of these systems. This edition includes updates of chapters in the previous editions, as well as seven entirely new chapters. The first chapter introduces the topics that are explored in depth in later chapters. Chapters 2 and 3 describe the design foundations behind the decision support tools used today. While there is some overlap in the concepts addressed in these chapters, they each have unique foci. Chapter 2 focuses primarily on the mathematical foundations of the knowledge-based systems. Chapter 3 focuses on systems based on pattern recognition and advanced data mining approaches. Chapter 4 includes a detailed discussion of usability principles for CDSS. Chapter 5 discusses newer models for CDSS architecture and Chap. 6 addresses issues in the development and implementation of CDSS. Chapter 7 examines the impact of government regulations on the use of CDSS. Chapters 8 and 9 discuss the legal, ethical, and evaluation issues that must be addressed when these systems are actively used in health care. Chapters 10, 11, and 12 provide examples of specific types of CDSS. CDSS for patients are described in Chap. 10. Chapter 11 addresses diagnostic decision support systems and sets this development in the context of the process of physician, not just computer, diagnosis. Chapter 12 illustrates the application of CDSS to the growing field of genomic medicine. The last three chapters focus on the applications of these systems in clinical practice. The authors of these chapters are from institutions that not only have a strong history of deployment of these systems, but also have performed the research and evaluation studies that provide perspective for others who are considering the use of these tools within the commercial systems that are increasingly incorporating CDSS.

This book represents an effort, not just by the editor or the individual chapter authors, but by many others who have provided assistance to them. We are grateful for the support and encouragement of Grant Weston and Joni Fraser from Springer. The Agency for Healthcare Research and Quality, the National Library of Medicine, and other NIH institutes have provided much appreciated support for my own and many of the chapter authors' research on CDSS. Finally, I want to express my gratitude to the many colleagues who have been collaborators on my research activities in clinical decision support systems over the past 30 years.

Birmingham, AL, USA Eta S. Berner, Ed.D., F.A.C.M.I., F.H.I.M.S.S.

Contents

1 **Overview of Clinical Decision Support Systems** 1
Eta S. Berner and Tonya J. La Lande

2 **Mathematical Foundations of Decision Support Systems** 19
S. Andrew Spooner

3 **Data Mining and Clinical Decision Support Systems** 45
Bunyamin Ozaydin, J. Michael Hardin, and David C. Chhieng

4 **Usability and Clinical Decision Support** 69
Yang Gong and Hong Kang

5 **Newer Architectures for Clinical Decision Support** 87
Salvador Rodriguez-Loya and Kensaku Kawamoto

6 **Best Practices for Implementation of Clinical Decision Support** 99
Richard N. Shiffman

7 **Impact of National Policies on the Use of Clinical Decision Support** 111
Jacob M. Reider

8 **Ethical and Legal Issues in Decision Support** 131
Kenneth W. Goodman

9 **Evaluation of Clinical Decision Support** 147
David F. Lobach

10 **Decision Support for Patients** 163
Holly B. Jimison and Christine M. Gordon

11 **Diagnostic Decision Support Systems** 181
Randolph A. Miller

12 Use of Clinical Decision Support to Tailor Drug Therapy Based on Genomics 209
Joshua C. Denny, Laura K. Wiley, and Josh F. Peterson

13 Clinical Decision Support: The Experience at Brigham and Women's Hospital/Partners HealthCare 227
Paul Varghese, Adam Wright, Jan Marie Andersen, Eileen I. Yoshida, and David W. Bates

14 Clinical Decision Support at Intermountain Healthcare 245
Peter J. Haug, Reed M. Gardner, R. Scott Evans, Beatriz H. Rocha, and Roberto A. Rocha

15 Decision Support During Inpatient Care Provider Order Entry: Vanderbilt's WizOrder Experience 275
Randolph A. Miller, Lemuel Russell Waitman, and S. Trent Rosenbloom

Index 311

Contributors

Jan Marie Andersen, M.A. Clinical and Quality Analysis, Information Systems, Partners HealthCare System, Inc., Wellesley, MA, USA

Division of General Internal Medicine and Primary Care, Brigham and Women's Hospital, Boston, MA, USA

David W. Bates, M.D., M.Sc. Clinical and Quality Analysis, Information Systems, Partners HealthCare System, Inc., Wellesley, MA, USA

Division of General Internal Medicine and Primary Care, Brigham and Women's Hospital, Boston, MA, USA

Department of Medicine, Harvard Medical School, Boston, MA, USA

Eta S. Berner, Ed.D., F.A.C.M.I., F.H.I.M.S.S. School of Health Professions, Department of Health Services Administration and Department of Medical Education, School of Medicine, University of Alabama at Birmingham, Birmingham, AL, USA

David C. Chhieng, M.D., M.B.A., M.S.H.I., M.S.E.M. Pathology, Mount Sinai Health System, New York, NY, USA

Joshua C. Denny, M.D., M.S. Biomedical Informatics and Medicine, Vanderbilt University Medical Center, Nashville, TN, USA

R. Scott Evans, B.S., M.S., Ph.D. Department of Medical Informatics, Intermountain Healthcare, Salt Lake City, UT, USA

Reed M. Gardner, Ph.D. Department of Biomedical Informatics, University of Utah, Salt Lake City, UT, USA

Yang Gong, M.D., Ph.D. School of Biomedical Informatics, University of Texas Health Science Center at Houston, Houston, TX, USA

Kenneth W. Goodman, Ph.D. Institute for Bioethics and Health Policy, University of Miami Miller School of Medicine, Miami, FL, USA

Christine M. Gordon, M.P.H. College of Computer and Information Science, Bouvé College of Health Sciences, Northeastern University, Boston, MA, USA

J. Michael Hardin, Ph.D. Academic Affairs, Samford University, Birmingham, AL, USA

Peter J. Haug, M.D. Department of Medical Informatics, Intermountain Healthcare, Murray, UT, USA

Holly B. Jimison, Ph.D. College of Computer and Information Science, Bouvé College of Health Sciences, Northeastern University, Boston, MA, USA

Hong Kang, Ph.D. Postdoctoral Fellow of UTHealth Innovation in Cancer Prevention Research Training Program, University of Texas Health Science Center at Houston, Houston, TX, USA

Kensaku Kawamoto, M.D., Ph.D., M.H.S. Biomedical Informatics, University of Utah, Salt Lake City, UT, USA

Tonya J. La Lande, M.S.H.I. Information Services, Carolinas HealthCare System, Charlotte, NC, USA

David F. Lobach, M.D., Ph.D., M.S., F.A.C.M.I. Klesis Healthcare, Durham, NC, USA

Community and Family Medicine, Duke University Medical Center, Durham, NC, USA

Randolph A. Miller, M.D. Department of Biomedical Informatics, Vanderbilt University Medical Center, Nashville, TN, USA

Bunyamin Ozaydin, Ph.D. School of Health Professions, Department of Health Services Administration, University of Alabama at Birmingham, Birmingham, AL, USA

Josh F. Peterson, M.D., M.P.H. Biomedical Informatics and Medicine, Vanderbilt University Medical Center, Nashville, TN, USA

Jacob M. Reider, M.D., F.A.A.F.P. Department of Family and Community Medicine, Albany Medical College, Albany, NY, USA

Beatriz H. Rocha, M.D., Ph.D. Division of General Internal Medicine and Primary Care, Department of Medicine, Brigham and Women's Hospital, Information Systems, Partners HealthCare System Inc., Harvard Medical School, Wellesley, MA, USA

Roberto A. Rocha, M.D., Ph.D. Division of General Internal Medicine and Primary Care, Department of Medicine, Brigham and Women's Hospital, Partners eCare, Partners HealthCare System Inc., Harvard Medical School, Wellesley, MA, USA

Salvador Rodriguez-Loya, Ph.D. Biomedical Informatics, University of Utah, Salt Lake City, UT, USA

S. Trent Rosenbloom, M.D., M.P.H. Department of Biomedical Informatics, Vanderbilt University Medical Center, Nashville, TN, USA

Richard N. Shiffman, M.D., M.C.I.S. Yale School of Medicine, New Haven, CT, USA

S. Andrew Spooner, M.D., M.S. Cincinnati Children's Hospital Medical Center, Cincinnati, OH, USA

Paul Varghese, M.D. Clinical and Quality Analysis, Information Systems, Partners HealthCare System, Inc., Wellesley, MA, USA

Division of General Internal Medicine and Primary Care, Brigham and Women's Hospital, Boston, MA, USA

Department of Medicine, Harvard Medical School, Boston, MA, USA

Lemuel Russell Waitman, Ph.D. Internal Medicine, University of Kansas Medical Center, Kansas City, KS, USA

Laura K. Wiley, M.S., Ph.D. Department of Biomedical Informatics, Vanderbilt University Medical Center, Nashville, TN, USA

Adam Wright, M.S., Ph.D. Clinical and Quality Analysis, Information Systems, Partners HealthCare System, Inc., Wellesley, MA, USA

Division of General Internal Medicine and Primary Care, Brigham and Women's Hospital, Boston, MA, USA

Department of Medicine, Harvard Medical School, Boston, MA, USA

Eileen I. Yoshida, B.Sc.Phm., M.B.A. Partners eCare, Partners Healthcare System Inc., Wellesley, MA, USA

Chapter 1
Overview of Clinical Decision Support Systems

Eta S. Berner and Tonya J. La Lande

Abstract Clinical decision support systems (CDSS) are computer systems designed to impact clinician decision making about individual patients at the point in time that these decisions are made. With the increased focus on the prevention of medical errors that has occurred since the publication of the landmark Institute of Medicine report, To Err Is Human, CDSS have been a key element of systems' approaches to improving patient safety and the quality of care and have been a key requirement for "meaningful use" of electronic health records (EHRs). This chapter will provide an overview of clinical decision support systems, summarize current data on the use and impact of clinical decision support systems in practice, and will provide guidelines for users to consider as these systems are incorporated in commercial systems, and implemented outside the research and development settings. The other chapters in this book will explore these issues in more depth.

Keywords Clinical decision support • Knowledge-based systems • Implementation • Knowledge maintenance • Healthcare quality • Safety

Clinical decision support systems (CDSS) are computer systems designed to impact clinician decision making about individual patients at the point in time that these decisions are made. With the increased focus on the prevention of medical errors that has occurred since the publication of the landmark Institute of Medicine report,

---

This chapter is an updated version of Chap. 36 in Ball MJ, Weaver C, Kiel J (eds.). Healthcare Information Management Systems, Third Edition, New York: Springer-Verlag, 2004, 463–477, with permission of Springer.

E.S. Berner, Ed.D. (✉)
School of Health Professions, Department of Health Services Administration
and Department of Medical Education, School of Medicine,
University of Alabama at Birmingham, 1705 University Blvd. Room 590 J,
Birmingham, AL 35294-1212, USA
e-mail: eberner@uab.edu

T.J. La Lande, M.S.H.I.
Information Services, Carolinas HealthCare System,
801 S. McDowell Street, Charlotte, NC 28204, USA
e-mail: tonya.lalande@carolinashealthcare.org

E.S. Berner (ed.), *Clinical Decision Support Systems*, Health Informatics,
DOI 10.1007/978-3-319-31913-1_1

To Err Is Human, computer-based physician order entry (CPOE) systems, coupled with CDSS, have been proposed as a key element of systems' approaches to improving patient safety and the quality of care [1–4]. In addition, CDSS have been a key requirement for "meaningful use" of electronic health records (EHRs) as defined by the Centers for Medicare and Medicaid Services (CMS) [5] and will become even more important with the growth of new models of care that are arising as a result of the passage of the Affordable Care Act (see also Chap. 7) [6]. If used properly, CDSS have the potential to change the way medicine has been taught and practiced. This chapter will provide an overview of clinical decision support systems, summarize current data on the use and impact of clinical decision support systems in practice, and will provide guidelines for users to consider as these systems are incorporated in commercial systems, and implemented outside the research and development settings. The other chapters in this book will explore these issues in more depth.

1.1 Types of Clinical Decision Support Systems

There are a variety of systems that can potentially support clinical decisions. Even Medline and similar healthcare literature databases can support clinical decisions. Decision support systems have been incorporated in healthcare information systems for a long time, but in the past these systems usually have supported retrospective analyses of financial and administrative data [7, 8]. Recently, sophisticated analytic approaches have been proposed for similar retrospective analyses of both administrative and clinical data (see Chap. 3 for more details on data mining approaches to CDSS) [9, 10]. Although these retrospective approaches can be used to develop guidelines, critical pathways, or protocols to guide decision making at the point of care, such retrospective analyses are not usually considered to be CDSS. These distinctions are important because vendors often will advertise that their product includes decision support capabilities, but that may refer to the retrospective type of systems, not those designed to assist clinicians at the point of care. CDSS have been developed over the last 50 years and many of them have been used as stand-alone systems or part of noncommercial homegrown EHR systems (see Chaps. 13, 14, and 15). However, as the interest has increased in CDSS, more EHR vendors have begun to incorporate these types of systems, or at least the capability to include them [11].

Metzger and her colleagues [12, 13] have described CDSS using several dimensions. According to their framework, CDSS differ among themselves in the timing at which they provide support (before, during, or after the clinical decision is made) and how active or passive the support is, that is, whether the CDSS actively provides alerts or passively responds to physician input or patient-specific information. Finally, CDSS vary in how easy they are for busy clinicians to access [12].

Osheroff and colleagues have developed a taxonomy of different types of clinical decision support that broadens the definition to include knowledge bases, order sets, and other ways of supporting clinical care in addition to alerts and reminders [14].

Another categorization scheme for CDSS is whether they are knowledge-based systems, or non-knowledge-based systems that employ machine learning and other statistical pattern recognition approaches. Chapter 2 discusses the mathematical foundations of the knowledge-based systems, and Chap. 3 addresses the foundations of the statistical pattern recognition type of CDSS. In this overview, we will focus on the knowledge-based systems, and discuss some examples of other approaches, as well.

1.1.1 Knowledge-Based Clinical Decision Support Systems

Many of today's knowledge-based CDSS arose out of earlier expert systems research, where the aim was to build a computer program that could simulate human thinking [15, 16]. Medicine was considered a good domain in which these concepts could be applied. Beginning in the 1970s and 1980s, the developers of these systems began to adapt them so that they could be used more easily to support real-life patient care processes [17, 18]. Many of the earliest systems were diagnostic decision support systems, which are discussed in Chap. 11. The intent of these CDSS was no longer to simulate an expert's decision making, but to assist the clinician in his or her own decision making. The system was expected to provide information for the user, rather than to come up with "the answer," as was the goal of earlier expert systems [19]. The user was expected to filter that information and to discard erroneous or useless information, also to be active and to interact with the system, rather than just be a passive recipient of the output. This focus on the interaction of the user with the system is important in setting appropriate expectations for the way the system will be used.

There are three parts to most CDSS. These parts are the knowledge base, the inference or reasoning engine, and a mechanism to communicate with the user [20]. As Spooner explains in Chap. 2, the knowledge base consists of compiled information that is often, but not always, in the form of if–then rules. An example of an if–then rule might be, for instance, IF a new order is placed for a particular blood test that tends to change very slowly, AND IF that blood test was ordered within the previous 48 h, THEN alert the physician. In this case, the rule is designed to prevent duplicate test ordering. Other types of knowledge bases might include probabilistic associations of signs and symptoms with diagnoses, or known drug–drug, drug-allergy, or drug–food interactions.

The second part of the CDSS is called the inference engine or reasoning mechanism, which contains the formulas for combining the rules or associations in the knowledge base with actual patient data.

Finally, there has to be a communication mechanism, a way of getting the patient data into the system and getting the output of the system to the user who will make the actual decision. In some stand-alone systems, the patient data need to be entered directly by the user. In most of the CDSS incorporated into electronic health records, which is the majority of CDSS today, the data are already in electronic form in the EHR, where they were originally entered by the clinician, or they may have come from laboratory, pharmacy, or other systems. Output to the clinician may come in the form of a recommendation or alert at the time of order entry, or, if the alert was triggered after the initial order was entered, systems of email and wireless notification have been employed [21, 22].

CDSS have been developed to assist with a variety of decisions. The example of the IF-THEN rule described above was for a system designed to provide support for laboratory test ordering. Diagnostic decision support systems have been developed to provide a suggested list of potential diagnoses to the users. The system might start with the patient's signs and symptoms, entered either by the clinician directly or imported from the EHR. The decision support system's knowledge base contains information about diseases and their signs and symptoms. The inference engine maps the patient's signs and symptoms to those diseases and might suggest some diagnoses for the clinicians to consider. These systems generally do not generate only a single diagnosis, but usually generate a set of diagnoses based on the available information. Because the clinician often knows more about the patient than can be put into the computer, the clinician will be able to eliminate some of the choices. Most of the diagnostic systems have been stand-alone systems, but researchers at Vanderbilt University incorporated a diagnostic system that runs in the background, taking its information from the data already in the EHR [23]. This system was incorporated into the McKesson Horizon Clinicals™ system. The use of CDSS at Vanderbilt is described in detail in Chap. 15.

Other systems can provide support for medication orders, a major cause of medical errors [1, 24]. The input for the system might be the patient's laboratory test results for the blood level of a prescribed medication. The knowledge base might contain values for therapeutic and toxic blood concentrations of the medication and rules on what to do when a toxic level of the medication is reached. If the medication level was too high, the output might be an alert to the physician [24]. There are CDSS that are part of computerized provider order entry (CPOE) systems that take a new medication order and the patient's current medications as input, the knowledge base might include a drug database and the output would be an alert about drug interactions so that the physician could change the order. Similarly, input might be a physician's therapy plan, where the knowledge base would contain local protocols or nationally accepted treatment guidelines, and the output might be a critique of the plan compared to the guidelines [25]. Some hospitals that have implemented these systems allow the user to override the critique or suggestions, but often the users are required to justify why they are overriding it. The structure of the CDSS knowledge base will differ depending on the source of the data and the uses to which the data are put. The design and implementation considerations, including usability and other implementation issues, are discussed in Chaps. 4 and 6.

1.1.2 Nonknowledge-Based Clinical Decision Support Systems

Unlike knowledge-based decision support systems, some of the nonknowledge-based CDSS use a form of artificial intelligence called machine learning, which allows the computer to learn from past experiences and/or to recognize patterns in the clinical data [26]. This type of approach is described briefly in Chap. 2 and in detail in Chap. 3. Artificial neural networks and genetic algorithms are two types of nonknowledge-based systems. These types of systems will become more important in the future as data analytics and other "big data" applications become more widely used in healthcare [9, 27].

Although, as Ozaydin et al. describe in Chap. 3, research has shown that CDSS based on pattern recognition and machine learning approaches may be more accurate than the average clinician in diagnosing the targeted diseases [28–30], many physicians are hesitant to use these CDSS in their practice because the reasoning behind them is not transparent [29]. Most of the systems that are available today involve knowledge-based systems with rules, guidelines, or other compiled knowledge derived from the medical literature. The research on the effectiveness of CDSS has come largely from a few institutions where these systems were developed, although in recent years as commercial systems have become more widespread, there is a growing literature on their effectiveness in a variety of settings [31, 32].

1.2 Effectiveness of Clinical Decision Support Systems

Clinical decision support systems have been shown to improve both patient outcomes, as well as the cost of care. Many of the published studies have come out of a limited number of institutions including LDS Hospital, Partners' Healthcare, Regenstrief Medical Institute and, Vanderbilt University [31]. Chapter 13 describes Partners' system, Chap. 14 describes the CDSS deployed in the HELP system at LDS Hospital and Intermountain Health Care, and Chap. 15 describes the system at Vanderbilt. It is interesting that all three of these pioneering institutions are now moving to commercial EHRs, but the lessons they have learned over the years will also be useful for using CDSS in commercial systems.

In addition, systematic reviews include an increasing number of studies from other places that have shown positive impact [32, 33]. Chapter 9 by Lobach provides a framework for evaluating CDSS and discusses the evaluation data on CDSS in more detail. CDSS can minimize errors by alerting the physician to potentially dangerous drug interactions, and the diagnostic programs have also been shown to improve physician diagnoses [34–37]. The reminder and alerting programs can potentially minimize problem severity and prevent complications. They can warn of early adverse drug events that have an impact on both cost and quality of care [4, 37–40]. These data have prompted the Leapfrog Group and others to advocate their use in promoting patient safety [3]. The Leapfrog Group also has developed an evaluation tool to help hospitals check the safety of their systems [41]. Many of the studies that have shown the strongest impact on reducing medication errors have been done at institutions with very sophisticated, internally developed systems, and where use of an EHR, CPOE, and CDSS are a routine and accepted part of the work environment [31]. As more places that do not have that cultural milieu, or a good understanding of the strengths and limitations of the systems, begin to adopt CDSS, integration of these systems may prove more difficult [42].

Several published reviews of CDSS have emphasized the dearth of evidence of similar effectiveness on a broader scale and have called for more research, especially qualitative research, that elucidates the factors which lead to success outside the development environment [43, 44]. More recent studies have examined some of these factors [45]. Studies of the Leeds University abdominal pain system, an early CDSS for diagnosis of the acute abdomen, showed success in the original environment and much more limited success when the system was implemented more broadly [46, 47]. As Chap. 9 shows, while the evidence is increasing, there are still limited systematic, broad-scale studies of the effectiveness of CDSS. In the future those data are likely to be more available. Not only is there a lack of studies on the impact of the diffusion of successful systems, but actual use of CDSS is variable [48]. However, use has clearly been increasing over the last decade. In 2003, for instance, there were few places utilizing CDSS [49, 50]. The KLAS research and consulting firm conducted an extensive survey of the sites that had implemented CPOE systems [50]. As KLAS defined these systems, CPOE systems usually included CDSS that were defined as, ". . . alerting, decision logic and knowledge tools to help eliminate errors during the ordering process"[50]. Although most of the CPOE systems provided for complex decision support, the results of the KLAS survey showed that most sites did not use more than ten alerts and that many sites did not use any of the alerting mechanisms at order entry [50]. By 2013, The Office of the National Coordinator for Health Information Technology (ONC) found that 74 % of physicians were using CDSS that provided warnings of drug interactions or contraindications and 57 % had implemented at least one clinical decision support rule that provided reminders for guideline-based interventions or screening tests [48].

Metzger and McDonald report anecdotal case studies of successful implementation of CDSS in ambulatory practices [13]. While such descriptions can motivate others to adopt CDSS, they are not a substitute for systematic evaluation of implementation in a wide range of settings. Unfortunately, when such evaluations are done, the results have sometimes been disappointing. A study incorporating guideline-based decision support systems in 31 general practice settings in England found that, although care was not optimal before implementing the computer-based guidelines, there was little change in health outcomes after the system was implemented. Further examination showed that, although the guideline was triggered appropriately, clinicians did not go past the first page and essentially did not use it [25]. Alert overrides are also a frequent occurrence [51] and there are suggestions that physician characteristics influence the overrides [52]. Another study found that clinicians did not follow the guideline advice because they did not agree with it

[53]. Configuring systems to avoid these problems is a challenge that ONC has tried to address [54]. In addition, Payne et al provided recommendations for improving the usability of CDSS for medication ordering [54].

There is a body of research that has shown that physicians have many unanswered questions during the typical clinical encounter [55, 56]. This situation should provide an optimal opportunity for the use of CDSS, yet a study tracking the use of a diagnostic system by medical residents indicated very little use [57]. This is unusual given that this group of physicians in training should have even more "unanswered questions" than more experienced practitioners, but this may be partially explained by the fact that the system was a stand-alone system not directly integrated into the workflow. Also, Teich et al. suggest that reminder systems and alerts usually work, but systems that challenge the physicians' judgment, or require them to change their care plans, are much more difficult to implement [58]. A case study of a CDSS for notification of adverse drug events supports this contention. The study showed that despite warnings of a dangerous drug level, the clinician in charge repeatedly ignored the advice. The article describes a mechanism of alerting a variety of clinicians, not just the patient's primary physician, to assure that the alerts receive proper attention [24]. Bria made analogies to making some alerts impossible to ignore. He used the example of the shaking stick in an airplane to alert the pilots to really serious problems [59]. In addition to the individual studies, Kawamoto et al. [45] examined factors associated with CDSS success across a variety of studies. They found that four factors were the main correlates of successful CDSS implementation. The factors were:

1. Providing alerts/reminders automatically as part of the workflow;
2. Providing the suggestions at a time and location where the decisions were being made;
3. Providing actionable recommendations; and
4. Computerizing the entire process.

Thus, although these systems can potentially influence the process of care, if they are not used, they obviously cannot have an impact. Integration into both the culture and the process of care is going to be necessary for these systems to be optimally used. Institutions that have developed such a culture provide a glimpse of what is potentially possible (see Chaps. 13, 14, and 15). However, Wong et al., in an article published in 2000, suggested that the incentives for use were not yet aligned to promote wide-scale adoption of CDSS [42]. With the availability of the incentives for meaningful use of Health IT from 2010 onward, there has been more adoption of EHRs in general, as well as CDSS, but there are also complaints about the usability of the systems. Chapter 4 explores the usability issues of CDSS and Chap. 6 describes strategies for optimal design and implementation of CDSS.

There are several reasons why implementation of CDSS is challenging. Some of the problems include issues of how the data are entered. Other issues include the development and maintenance of the knowledge base and issues around the vocabulary and user interface. Finally, since these systems may represent a change in the usual way patient care is conducted, there is a question of what will motivate their use, which also relates to how the systems are evaluated.

1.3 Implementation Challenges

The first issue concerns data entry, or how the data will actually get into the system. Some systems require the user to query the systems and/or enter some or all of the patient data manually. This is especially likely with the diagnostic decision support systems [34]. Not only is this "double data entry" disruptive to the patient care process, it is also time consuming, and, especially in the ambulatory setting, time is scarce. It is even more time consuming if the system is not mobile and/or requires a lengthy logon. Much of this disruption can be mitigated by integrating the CDSS with the EHR. As mentioned above, today most EHRs have integrated decision support capabilities. What that means is if the data are already entered into the medical record, the data are there for the decision support system to act upon, and, in fact, many systems are potentially capable of drawing from multiple ancillary systems as well. This is a strength, but not all clinical decision support systems are well-integrated, and without technical standards assuring integration of ancillary systems, such linkages may be difficult. There are also a number of stand-alone systems, including some of the diagnostic systems and some drug interaction systems, for example. This means that patient data have to be entered twice—once into the medical record system, and again, into the decision support system. For many physicians, this double data entry can limit the usefulness of such systems.

A related question is who should enter the data in a stand-alone system or even in the integrated hospital systems. Physicians are usually the key decision makers, but they are not always the people who interact with the EHR. In fact, in recent years, non-physician medical scribes are often the main people interacting with the EHR [60]. One of the reasons for linking CDSS with physician order entry is that it is much more efficient for the physician to receive the alerts and reminders from decision support systems. The issue concerns not just order entry, but also mechanisms of notification. The case study mentioned earlier described a situation where the physician who received the alert ignored it [24]. These systems can be useful, but their full benefits cannot be gained without collaboration between the information technology professionals and the clinicians.

Although it might not seem that vocabularies should be such a difficult issue, it is often only when clinicians actually try to use a system, either a decision support system or electronic health record or some other system with a controlled vocabulary, that they realize either the system cannot understand what they are trying to say or, worse yet, that it uses the same words for totally different concepts or different words for the same concept. The problem is there are no standards that are universally agreed upon for clinical vocabulary and, since most of the decision support systems have a controlled vocabulary, errors can have a major impact.

1.4 Future Uses of Clinical Decision Support Systems

Despite the challenges in integrating CDSS, when properly used they have the potential to make significant improvements in the quality of patient care. While more research still needs to be done evaluating the impact of CDSS outside the development settings and the factors that promote or impede integration, it is likely that increased commercialization will continue. CDSS for non-clinician users such as patients are likely to grow as well (see Chap. 10). There is increasing interest in clinical computing and, as mobile computing become more widely adopted, better integration into the process of care may be easier.

Similarly, trends in cloud computing and service oriented architecture are leading to new approaches for delivering CDSS to the user (see Chap. 5 for more details on service oriented architecture for CDSS) [61]. As discussed in Chap. 12, genomic data will become increasingly available for use in clinical care and CDSS that can be used with decisions around genomic medicine will also be needed. Finally, as the data for electronic health records become more standardized and shareable, the use of decision support in the public health arena is likely to increase.

In addition, the concerns over medical errors, patient safety, and meaningful use of health IT (see Chap. 7) have prompted a variety of initiatives that will lead to increased incorporation of CDSS. Physicians are legally obligated to practice in accordance with the standard of care, which at this time does not mandate the use of CDSS. However, that may be changing. The issue of the use of information technology in general, and clinical decision support systems in particular, to improve patient safety, has received a great deal of attention [1, 2]. Healthcare administrators, payers, and patients, are concerned, now more than ever before, that clinicians use the available technology to reduce medical errors. The Leapfrog Group [3] early on advocated physician order entry (with an implicit coupling of CDSS to provide alerts to reduce medication errors) as one of their main quality criteria, and CPOE, e-prescribing and clinical decision support are required for meaningful use (see Chap. 7).

Even if the standard of care does not yet require the use of such systems, there are some legal and ethical issues that have not yet been well addressed (see Chap. 8 for a fuller discussion of these issues). One interesting legal case that has been mentioned in relation to the use of technology in health care is the Hooper decision. This case involved two tugboats (the T.J. Hooper and its sister ship) that were pulling barges in the 1930s when radios (receiving sets) were available, but not widely used on tugboats. Because the boats did not have a radio, they missed storm warnings and their cargo sank. The barge owners sued the tugboat company, even though the tugboat captains were highly skilled and did the best they could under the circumstances to salvage their cargo. They were found liable for not having the radio, even though it was still not routinely used in boats. Parts of the following excerpt from the Hooper decision have been cited in other discussions of CDSS [62].

> . . . whole calling may have unduly lagged in the adoption of new and available devices. It never may set its own tests, however persuasive be its usages. Courts must in the end say

what is required; there are precautions so imperative that even their universal disregard will not excuse their omission. But here there was no custom at all as to receiving sets; some had them, some did not; the most that can be urged is that they had not yet become general. Certainly in such a case we need not pause; when some have thought a device necessary, at least we may say that they were right, and the others too slack. [63]

It has been suggested that as CDSS and other advanced computer systems become more available, the Hooper case may not only provide legal precedent for liability for failure to use available technology, but the legal standard of care may also change to include using available CDSS [64]. Since this area is still new, it is not clear what type of legal precedents will be invoked for hospitals or practices that choose to adopt, or avoid adopting, CDSS. It has been suggested that while the use of CDSS may lower a hospital's risk of medical errors, healthcare systems may incur new risks if the systems either cause harm or are not implemented properly [65, 66]. In any case, there are some guidelines that users can follow that may help ensure more appropriate use of CDSS.

1.5 Guidelines for Selecting and Implementing Clinical Decision Support Systems[1]

Osheroff et al. offer practical suggestions for steps to be taken in the implementation of CDSS [14]. The "five rights" of clinical decision support (right **information** to the right **person** in the right **intervention format** through the right **channel** at the right **time** in workflow) that Osheroff et al. advocate are a good summary of what needs to be done. The guidelines below address other issues such as those involved in selecting CDSS, interacting with vendors, and assuring that user expectations for CDSS are appropriate. They also touch on legal and ethical issues that are discussed in more detail in Chap. 8.

1.5.1 Assuring That Users Understand the Limitations

In 1986, Brannigan and Dayhoff highlighted the often different philosophies of physicians and software developers [67]. Brannigan and Dayhoff mention that physicians and software developers differ in regard to how "perfect" they expect their "product" to be when it is released to the public [67]. Physicians expect perfection from themselves and those around them. Physicians undergo rigorous training, have to pass multiple licensing examinations, and are held in high esteem by society for

[1] Significant parts of this section and smaller parts of other sections were reprinted with permission from Berner ES. Ethical and Legal Issues in the Use of Clinical Decision Support Systems. J. Healthcare Information Management, 2002;16(4):34–37.

their knowledge and skills. In contrast, software developers often assume that initial products will be "buggy" and that eventually most errors will be fixed, often as a result of user feedback and error reports. There is usually a version 1.01 of almost any system almost as soon as version 1.0 has reached most users. Because a CDSS is software that in some ways functions like a clinician consultant, these differing expectations can present problems, especially when the knowledge base and/or reasoning mechanism of the CDSS is not transparent to the user. The vendors of these systems have an obligation to inform the clinicians using the CDSS of its strengths and limitations.

1.5.2 Assuring That the Knowledge Is from Reputable Sources

Users of CDSS need to know the source of the knowledge if they purchase a knowledge-based system. What rules are actually included in the system and what is the evidence behind the rules? How was the system tested before implementation? This validation process should extend not just to testing whether the rules fire appropriately in the face of specific patient data (a programming issue), but also to whether the rules themselves are appropriate (a knowledge-engineering issue). Sim et al. advocate the use of CDSS to promote evidence-based medical practice, but this can only occur if the knowledge base contains high quality information [68].

1.5.3 Assuring That the System Is Appropriate for the Local Site

Vendors need to alert the client about idiosyncrasies that are either built into the system or that need to be added by the user. Does the clinical vocabulary in the system match that in the EHR? What are the normal values assumed by a system alerting to abnormal laboratory tests, and do they match those at the client site? In fact, does the client have to define the normal values as well as the thresholds for the alerts? The answers to the questions about what exactly the user is getting are not always easy to obtain.

When users ask questions about the sources of knowledge or its content, they may find that the decision support system provided is really just an expert system shell and that local clinicians need to provide the "knowledge" that determines the rules. For some systems, an effort has been made to use standards that can be shared among different sites, for example, the Arden syntax for medical logic modules [69], but local clinicians must still review the logic in shared rules to assure that they are appropriate for the local situation. Using in-house clinicians to determine the rules in the CDSS can assure its applicability to the local environment, but that means extensive development and testing must be done locally to assure the CDSS operates appropriately. Often a considerable amount of physician time is needed. Without adequate involvement by clinicians, there is a risk that the CDSS may include rules that are inappropriate for the local situation, or, if there are no built-in rules, that the CDSS may have only limited functionality. On the other hand, local development of the logic behind the rules may also mean that caution should be exercised if the rules are used at different sites. The important thing is for the user to learn at the outset what roles the vendor and the client will have to play in the development and maintenance of the systems. Although systems have decision support capabilities, the effort involved in customizing the CDSS for the local site may be considerable, and the result may be that CDSS capabilities are underutilized.

1.5.4 Assuring That Users Are Properly Trained

Just as the vendor should inform the client how much work is needed to get the CDSS operational, the vendor should also inform the client how much technical support and/or clinician training is needed for physicians to use the system appropriately and/or understand the systems' recommendations. As CDSS for genomic medicine (see Chap. 12) become available this new area may require even more training, since users may be unfamiliar with the medical content as well as the CDSS. It is not known whether the users of some CDSS need special clinical expertise to be able to use it properly, in addition to the mechanics of training on the use of the CDSS. For instance, systems that base their recommendations on what the user enters directly or on what was entered into the medical record by clinicians have been shown to reach faulty conclusions or make inappropriate recommendations if the data on which the CDSS bases its recommendations are incomplete or inaccurate [70]. Also, part of the reason for integrating CDSS with physician order entry is that it is assumed the physician has the expertise to understand, react to, and determine whether to override the CDSS recommendation. Diagnostic systems, for instance, may make an appropriate diagnostic suggestion that the user fails to recognize [36, 71, 72]. Thus, vendors of CDSS need to be clear about what expertise is assumed in using the system, and those who implement the systems need to assure that only the appropriate users are allowed to respond to the CDSS advice.

As these systems mature and are more regularly integrated into the healthcare environment, another possible concern about user expertise arises. Will users lose their ability to determine when it is appropriate to override the CDSS? This "deskilling" concern is similar to that reported when calculators became commonplace in elementary and secondary education, and children who made errors in using the calculator could not tell that the answers were obviously wrong. Galletta et al. report that when a computerized spell checker program provided incorrect advice, their research subjects made more errors than they did without the spell-checker [73]. Similar results were found in a study using the decision support programs that provide diagnostic interpretations for electrocardiograms [74]. The solution to the problem is not to remove the technology, but to remain alert to both the positive and negative potential impact on clinician decision making.

1.5.5 Monitoring Proper Utilization of the Installed Clinical Decision Support Systems

Simply having a CDSS installed and working does not guarantee that it will be used. Systems that are available for users if they need them, such as online guidelines or protocols, may not be used if the user has to choose to consult the system, and especially if the user has to enter additional data into the system. Automated alerting or reminder systems that prompt the user can address the issue of the user not recognizing the need for the system, but another set of problems arises with the more automated systems. They must be calibrated to alert the user often enough to prevent serious errors, but not so frequently that they will be ignored eventually. What this means is that testing the system with the users, and monitoring its use, is essential for the CDSS to operate effectively in practice as well as in theory.

1.5.6 Assuring the Knowledge Base Is Monitored and Maintained

Once the CDSS is operational at the client site, a very important issue involves the responsibility for updating the knowledge base in a timely manner. New diseases are discovered, new medications come on the market, and issues like the threat of bioterrorist actions prompt a need for new information to be added to the CDSS. Does the vendor have an obligation to provide regular knowledge updates? Such maintenance can be an expensive proposition given both rapidly changing knowledge and systems with complex rule sets. Who is at fault if the end user makes a decision based on outdated knowledge, or, conversely, if updating one set of rules inadvertently affects others, causing them to function improperly? Such questions were raised over 30 years ago [75], but because CDSS are still not in widespread use, the legal issues have not really been tested or clarified.

The Food and Drug Administration (FDA) is charged with device regulation and has recently begun to reevaluate its previous policy on software regulation. Up until recently, many CDSS have been exempt from FDA device regulation because they required "competent human intervention" between the CDSS' advice and anything being done to the patient [76]. In 2014, the FDA, ONC and the Federal Communications Commission (FCC), in the FDASIA Health IT Report, adopted a risk-based framework to clarify what types of software required more extensive oversight [77]. Even if the rules change and CDSS are required to pass a pre-market approval process, monitoring would need to be ongoing to ensure the knowledge does not get out of date, and that what functioned well in the development process still functions properly at the client site. For this reason, local software review committees, which would have the responsibility to monitor local software installations for problems, obsolete knowledge, and harm as a result of use, have been advocated [78].

1.6 Conclusion

There is now growing interest in the use of CDSS. More vendors of information systems are incorporating them. As skepticism about the usefulness of computers for clinical practice decreases, the wariness about accepting the CDSS' advice, that many clinicians currently exhibit, is likely to decrease. As research has shown, if CDSS are available and convenient, and if they provide what appears to be good information, they are likely to be heeded by clinicians. The remaining chapters in this book explore the issues raised here in more depth. Underlying all of them is the perspective that, as CDSS become widespread, we must continue to remember that the role of the computer should be to enhance and support the human who is ultimately responsible for the clinical decisions.

References

1. Kohn LT, Corrigan JM, Donaldson MS, editors. To err is human: building a safer health system. Washington, DC: National Academy Press; 2000.
2. Institute of Medicine. Crossing the quality chasm: a new health system for the 21st century. Washington, DC: National Academy Press; 2001.
3. The Leapfrog Group. www.leapfroggroup.org.
4. Bates DW, Leape LL, Cullen DJ, et al. Effect of computerized physician order entry and a team intervention on prevention of serious medical errors. JAMA. 1998;280:1311–6.
5. Blumenthal D, Tavenner M. The "meaningful use" regulation for electronic health records. N Engl J Med. 2010;363(6):501–4.
6. Bitton A, Flier LA, Jha AK. Health information technology in the era of care delivery reform: to what end? JAMA. 2012;307(24):2593–4
7. Oliveira J. A shotgun wedding: business decision support meets clinical decision support. J Healthc Inf Manage. 2002;16:28–33.
8. DeGruy KB. Healthcare applications of knowledge discovery in databases. J Healthc Inf Manage. 2000;14:59–69.
9. Simpao AF, Ahumada LM, Gálvez JA, Rehman MA. A review of analytics and clinical informatics in health care. J Med Syst. 2014;38(4):45.
10. Raghupathi W, Raghupathi V. Big data analytics in healthcare: promise and potential. Health Inf Sci Syst. 2014;2:3.
11. Sittig DF, Wright A, Meltzer S, Simonaitis L, Evans RS, Nichol WP, Ash JS, Middleton B. Comparison of clinical knowledge management capabilities of commercially-available and leading internally-developed electronic health records. BMC Med Inform Decis Mak. 2011;11:13.

12. Perreault LE, Metzger JB. A pragmatic framework for understanding clinical decision support. In: Middleton B, ed. Clinical decision support systems. J Healthc Inf Manage. 1999;13:5–21.
13. Metzger J, MacDonald K. Clinical decision support for the independent physician practice. Oakland: California Healthcare Foundation; 2002.
14. Osheroff JA, Teich JM, Levick D, Saldana L, Ferdinand T, Sitting DF, et al. Improving outcomes with clinical decision support, an implementer's guide. Chicago: HIMSS; 2012.
15. Shortliffe EH, Axline SG, Buchanan BG, Merigan TC, Cohen SN. An artificial intelligence program to advise physicians regarding antimicrobial therapy. Comput Biomed Res. 1973;6(6):544–60.
16. Miller RA, Pople Jr HE, Myers JD. Internist-I, an experimental computer-based diagnostic consultant for general internal medicine. N Engl J Med. 1982;307:468–76.
17. Barness LA, Tunnessen Jr WW, Worley WE, Simmons TL, Ringe Jr TB. Computer-assisted diagnosis in pediatrics. Am J Dis Child. 1974;127(6):852–8.
18. Miller RA, McNeil MA, Challinor S, Masarie Jr FE, Myers JD. Internist-I, quick medical reference project-status report. West J Med. 1986;145:816–22.
19. Miller RA, Masarie Jr FE. The demise of the "Greek Oracle" model for medical diagnostic systems. Methods Inf Med. 1990;29:1–2.
20. Tan JKH, Sheps S. Health decision support systems. Gaithersburg: Aspen Publishers; 1998.
21. Kuperman GJ, Teich JM, Bates DW, et al. Detecting alerts, notifying the physician, and offering action items: a comprehensive alerting system. Proc AMIA Annu Fall Symp. 1996:704–8.
22. Shabot MM, LoBue M, Chen J. Wireless clinical alerts for physiologic, laboratory and medication data. Proc AMIA Symp 2000:789–93.
23. Geissbuhler A, Miller RA. Clinical application of the UMLS in a computerized order entry and decision-support system. Proc AMIA Symp. 1998:320–4.
24. Galanter WL, DiDomenico RJ, Polikaitis A. Preventing exacerbation of an ADE with automated decision support. J Healthc Inf Manage. 2002;16(4):44–9.
25. Eccles M, McColl E, Steen N, et al. Effect of computerised evidence based guidelines on management of asthma and angina in adults in primary care: cluster randomised controlled trial. BMJ. 2002;325:941.
26. Marakas GM. Decision support systems in the 21st century. Upper Saddle River: Prentice Hall; 1999.
27. Murdoch TB, Detsky AS. The inevitable application of big data to health care. JAMA. 2013;309(13):1351–2.
28. Baxt WG. Application of artificial neural networks to clinical medicine. Lancet. 1995;346:1135–8.
29. Holst H, Astrom K, Jarund A, et al. Automated interpretation of ventilation- perfusion lung scintigrams for the diagnosis of pulmonary embolism using artificial neural networks. Eur J Nucl Med. 2000;27:400–6.
30. Olsson SE, Ohlsson M, Ohlin H, Edenbrandt L. Neural networks—a diagnostic tool in acute myocardial infarction with concomitant left bundle branch block. Clin Physiol Funct Imaging. 2002;22:295–9.
31. Chaudhry B, Wang J, Wu S, Maglione M, Mojica W, Roth E, Morton SC, Shekelle PG. Systematic review: impact of health information technology on quality, efficiency, and costs of medical care. Ann Intern Med. 2006;144(10):742–52.
32. Jones SS, Rudin RS, Perry T, Shekelle PG. Health information technology: an updated systematic review with a focus on meaningful use. Ann Intern Med. 2014;160(1):48–54.
33. Bright TJ, Wong A, Dhurjati R, Bristow E, Bastian L, Coeytaux RR, Samsa G, Hasselblad V, Williams JW, Musty MD, Wing L, Kendrick AS, Sanders GD, Lobach D. Effect of clinical decision-support systems: a systematic review. Ann Intern Med. 2012;157(1):29–43.
34. Ramnarayan P, Kapoor RR, Coren M, et al. Measuring the impact of diagnostic decision support on the quality of decision-making: development of a reliable and valid composite score. J Am Med Inform Assoc. 2003;10:563–57234.

35. Berner ES, Maisiak RS, Cobbs CG, Taunton OD. Effects of a decision support system on physicians' diagnostic performance. J Am Med Inform Assoc. 1999;6:420–7.
36. Friedman CP, Elstein AS, Wolf FM, et al. Enhancement of clinicians' diagnostic reasoning by computer-based consultation. A multisite study of 2 systems. JAMA. 1999;282:1851–6.
37. Berner ES. Clinical decision support systems: state of the art. AHRQ publication No.09-0069-EF. Rockville: Agency for Healthcare Research and Quality; 2009.
38. Evans RS, Pestotnik SL, Classen DC, et al. A computer-assisted management program for antibiotics and other antiinfective agents. N Engl J Med. 1998;338:232–8.
39. Doolan DF, Bates DW. Computerized physician order entry systems in hospitals: mandates and incentives. Health Aff. 2002;21:180–8.
40. Kucher N, Koo S, Quiroz R, et al. Electronic alerts to prevent venous thromboembolism among hospitalized patients. N Engl J Med. 2005;352:969–77.
41. Leung AA, Keohane C, Lipsitz S, Zimlichman E, Amato M, Simon SR, Coffey M, Kaufman N, Cadet B, Schiff G, Seger DL, Bates DW. Relationship between medication event rates and the Leapfrog computerized physician order entry evaluation tool. J Am Med Inform Assoc. 2013;20(e1):e85–90.
42. Wong HJ, Legnini MW, Whitmore HH. The diffusion of decision support systems in healthcare: are we there yet? J Healthc Manage. 2000;45:240–9. discussion 249–253.
43. Garg AX, Adhikari NK, McDonald H, et al. Effects of computerized clinical decision support systems on practitioner performance and patient outcomes: a systematic review. JAMA. 2005;293:1223–38.
44. Kaplan B. Evaluating informatics applications—clinical decision support systems literature review. Int J Med Inform. 2001;64:15–37.
45. Kawamoto K, Houlihan CA, Balas EA, Lobach DF. Improving clinical practice using clinical decision support systems: a systematic review of trials to identify features critical to success. BMJ. 2005;330(7494):765.
46. de Dombal FT. The diagnosis of acute abdominal pain with computer assistance: worldwide perspective. Ann Chir. 1991;45:273–7.
47. Adams ID, Chan M, Clifford PC, et al. Computer aided diagnosis of acute abdominal pain: a multicentre study. BMJ. 1986;293:800–4.
48. Office of the National Coordinator for Health Information Technology. 'Percent of Physicians with Selected Computerized Capabilities Related to Meaningful Use Objectives,' Health IT Quick-Stat#9.dashboard.healthit.gov/quickstats/pages/FIG-physicians-with-meaningful-use--functionalities-in-their-EHR.php. January 2014.
49. Burt CW, Hing E. Use of computerized clinical support systems in medical settings. United States, 2001–2003, Advance data from vital and health statistics, vol. 353. Hyattsville: National Center for Health Statistics; 2005.
50. KLAS Research and Consulting Firm. CPOE digest (computerized physician order entry; 2003.
51. Isaac T, Weissman JS, Davis RB, Massagli M, Cyrulik A, Sands DZ, Weingart SN. Overrides of medication alerts in ambulatory care. Arch Intern Med. 2009;169(3):305–11.
52. Cho I, Slight SP, Nanji KC, Seger DL, Maniam N, Fiskio JM, Dykes PC, Bates DW. The effect of provider characteristics on the responses to medication-related decision support alerts. Int J Med Inform. 2015;84(9):630–9.
53. Keefe B, Subramanian U, Tierney WM, et al. Provider response to computer- based care suggestions for chronic heart failure. Med Care. 2005;43:461–5.
54. Payne TH, Hines LE, Chan RC, Hartman S, Kapusnik-Uner J, Russ AL, Chaffee BW, Hartman C, Tamis V, Galbreth B, Glassman PA, Phansalkar S, Vander Sijs H, Gephart SM, Mann G, Strasberg HR, Grizzle AJ, Brown M, Kuperman GJ, Steiner C, Sullins A, Ryan H, Wittie MA, Malone DC. Recommendations to improve the usability of drug-drug interaction clinical decision support alerts. J Am Med Inform Assoc. 2015. [Epub ahead of print], pii: ocv011. doi: 10.1093/jamia/ocv011.
55. Covell DG, Uman GC, Manning PR. Information needs in office practice: are they being met? Ann Intern Med. 1985;103:596–69.

56. Gorman PN, Helfand M. Information seeking in primary care: how physicians choose which clinical questions to pursue and which to leave unanswered. Med Decis Making. 1995;15:113–9.
57. Berner ES, Maisiak RS, Phelan ST, Kennedy JI, Heudebert GR, Young KR. Use of a diagnostic decision support system by internal medicine residents. Unpublished study; 2002.
58. Teich JM, Merchia PR, Schmiz JL, Kuperman GJ, Spurr CD, Bates DW. Effects of computerized physician order entry on prescribing practices. Arch Intern Med. 2000;160:2741–7.
59. Bria WF. Clinical decision support and the parable of the stick shaker. J Healthc Info Manage. 2005;19:8–9.
60. Gellert GA, Ramirez R, Webster SL. The rise of the medical scribe industry: implications for the advancement of electronic health records. JAMA. 2015;313(13):1315–6.
61. Goldberg HS, Paterno MD, Rocha BH, Schaeffer M, Wright A, Erickson JL, Middleton B. A highly scalable, interoperable clinical decision support service. J Am Med Inform Assoc. 2014;21(e1):e55–62.
62. Weed LL, Weed L. Opening the black box of clinical judgment—an overview. BMJ. 1999;319:1279. Data Supplement–Complete Version. Available from: http://www.bmj.org/cgi/content/full/319/7220/1279/DC1.
63. The T.J. Hooper. 60 F.2d 737 (2d Cir. 1932).
64. Osler Harkins, Harcourt Law Firm. Ten commandments of computerization. Reprinted with permission by the Canadian Information Processing Society; 1992. Available from: http://www.cips.ca/it/resources/default.asp?load= practices.
65. Terry NP. When the machine that goes "ping" causes harm: default torts rules and technologically-mediated health care injuries. St Louis Univ Law J. 2002;45:37–59.
66. Coiera E1, Westbrook J, Wyatt J. The safety and quality of decision support systems. Yearb Med Inform. 2006:20–5.
67. Brannigan VM, Dayhoff RE. Medical informatics. The revolution in law, technology and medicine. J Leg Med. 1986;7:1–53.
68. Sim I, Gorman P, Greenes RA, Haynes RB, Kaplan B, Lehmann H, Tang PC. Clinical decision support for the practice of evidence-based medicine. J Am Med Inform Assoc. 2001;8:527–34.
69. Poikonen J. Arden syntax: the emerging standard language for representing medical knowledge in computer systems. Am J Health Syst Pharm. 1997;54:281–4.
70. Hsieh TC, Kuperman GJ, Jaggi T, et al. Characteristics and consequences of drug allergy alert overrides in a computerized physician order entry system. J Am Med Inform Assoc. 2004;11:482–91.
71. Berner ES, Maisiak RS, Heudebert GR, Young KR Jr. Clinician performance and prominence of diagnoses displayed by a clinical diagnostic decision support system. AMIA Annual Symp. Proc. 2003:76–80.
72. Friedman CP, Gatti GG, Franz TM, et al. Do physicians know when their diagnoses are correct? Implications for decision support and error reduction. J Gen Intern Med. 2005;20:334–9.
73. Galletta DF, Durcikova A, Everard A, Jones BM. Does spell-checking software need a warning label? Commun ACM. 2005;48(7):82–6.
74. Tsai TL, Fridsma DB, Gatti G. Computer decision support as a source of interpretation error: the case of electrocardiograms. J Am Med Inform Assoc. 2003;10(5):478–83.
75. Miller RA, Schaffner KF, Meisel A. Ethical and legal issues related to the use of computer programs in clinical medicine. Ann Intern Med. 1985;102:529–36.
76. Young FE. Validation of medical software: present policy of the Food and Drug Administration. Ann Intern Med. 1987;106(4):628–9.
77. U.S. Food and Drug Administration [Internet]. Silver Spring, MD: FDA; 2015. FDASIA Health IT Report. 2014. Available from: http://www.fda.gov/downloads/AboutFDA/CentersOffices/OfficeofMedicalProductsandTobacco/CDRH/CDRHReports/UCM391521.pdf.
78. Miller RA, Gardner RM. Recommendations for responsible monitoring and regulation of clinical software systems. J Am Med Inform Assoc. 1997;4:442–57.

Chapter 2
Mathematical Foundations of Decision Support Systems

S. Andrew Spooner

Abstract Health information technology can support decisions in a variety of ways, ranging from the passive display of information to intensive computation designed to model complex clinical reasoning. This chapter reviews the basics of the mathematics behind the methods that involve computation, including set theory, probability, Boolean logic, Bayesian reasoning, and nonknowledge-based systems.

Keywords Bayes theorem • Mathematics • Logic • Probability • Set theory • Electronic health records

Many computer applications may be considered to be clinical decision support systems. Programs that perform PubMed [1] searches do support decisions, but they are not "clinical decision support systems" in the usual sense. What we usually mean by a clinical decision support system (CDSS) is a program that supports a reasoning task carried out behind the scenes and based on clinical data. For example, a program that accepts thyroid panel results and generates a list of possible diagnoses is what we usually recognize as a *diagnostic* decision support system, a particular type of CDSS. General-purpose programs that accept clinical findings and generate diagnoses are typical diagnostic decision support systems. These programs employ numerical and logical techniques to convert clinical input into the kind of information that a physician might use in performing a diagnostic reasoning task. While one might suspect that such functionality might be useful within an electronic health record (EHR) system, this type of support is seldom found there; the usefulness of the EHR in decision support turns out to be less about sophisticated expert systems and more about access to needed information [2, 3].

Forms of decision support that are commonly found in EHR systems include alerts for medication prescribing [4], order sets that guide clinicians to use the correct antibiotic [5] to diagnostic decision support that converts findings into a list of diagnoses worth considering [6–8]. While the latter is not in widespread use; simpler methods like order sets, documentation templates, and drug alerts are practi-

S.A. Spooner, M.D., M.S. (✉)
Cincinnati Children's Hospital Medical Center,
3333 Burnet Avenue, MLC 9009, Cincinnati, OH 45229, USA
e-mail: andrew.spooner@cchmc.org

E.S. Berner (ed.), *Clinical Decision Support Systems*, Health Informatics,
DOI 10.1007/978-3-319-31913-1_2

cally universal in EHRs today. Nonetheless, the mathematics of diagnostic decision support is worth reviewing. Essential to the understanding of CDSS is familiarity with the basic principles of logic and probability. A brief review of these areas, followed by a description of a general model of CDSS, as well as exceptions to the model, will help in understanding how some CDSS perform reasoning tasks. We end with a discussion of the mathematical challenges in the evaluation of simple alerts as they are commonly deployed in EHRs today.

2.1 Review of Logic and Probability

2.1.1 Set Theory

A brief review of basic concepts in set theory is helpful in understanding logic, probability, and many other branches of mathematics. A *set* is a collection of unique objects. For example, the major Jones criteria [9] for patients at low risk for rheumatic fever is a set:

$$\text{JONES}-\text{CRITERIA}-\text{MAJOR} = \begin{Bmatrix} \text{carditis, migratory polyarthritis,} \\ \text{erythema marginatum, chorea,} \\ \text{subcutaneous nodules} \end{Bmatrix}$$

Likewise, the minor criteria make a set:

$$\text{JONES}-\text{CRITERIA}-\text{MINOR} = \begin{Bmatrix} \text{fever, arthralgia, elevated acute phase reactants,} \\ \text{prolonged P}-\text{R interval on electrocardiogram} \end{Bmatrix}$$

To complete our description of the Jones criteria, we need a third set:

$$\text{GROUP}-\text{A}-\text{STREP}-\text{EVIDENCE} = \begin{Bmatrix} \text{positive culture, positive rapid antigen,} \\ \text{antibody rise or elevation} \end{Bmatrix}$$

To apply the Jones criteria, one compares the patient's findings with the items in the various sets above. A patient is highly likely to have rheumatic fever if there is evidence of group A streptococcal infection *and* the patient has *either* two major criteria *or* one major and two minor criteria.

Each *element* or *member* of the set is distinguishable from the others. A *subset* is any collection of elements of a known set. Using the first of the criteria above, a patient must have a subset of clinical findings containing at least two of the elements of JONES-CRITERIA-MAJOR to meet the Jones criteria for rheumatic fever. If a patient has the clinical findings:

$$\text{FINDINGS} = \{\text{migratory polyarthritis, chorea, subcutaneous nodules}\}$$

then we say that FINDINGS is a subset of JONES-CRITERIA-MAJOR, or, in set terminology:

$$\text{FINDINGS} \subseteq \text{JONES} - \text{CRITERIA} - \text{MAJOR}$$

The *cardinality* or *size* of a set is simply the number of elements in the set. For our two examples, the cardinalities (written by placing a vertical bar before and after the symbol for the set) are:

$$|\text{FINDINGS}| = 3$$
$$|\text{JONES} - \text{CRITERIA} - \text{MAJOR}| = 5$$

The basic set operations are *intersection* and *union*. The intersection of two sets is the set of elements the two sets have in common. For example, if there is a patient with the following set of clinical findings:

$$\text{CLINICAL} - \text{FINDINGS} = \begin{Bmatrix} \text{heart murmur,} \\ \text{migratory polyarthritis,} \\ \text{chorea, subcutaneous nodules,} \\ \text{cough} \end{Bmatrix}$$

then the intersection of this set and JONES-CRITERIA-MAJOR is written:

$$\text{CLINICAL} - \text{FINDINGS} \cap \text{JONES} - \text{CRITERIA} - \text{MAJOR}$$

It is easy to see that the intersection of these two sets is simply the set FINDINGS. The union of two sets is the set of all elements that belong to either set. Since, by definition, a set's elements must be distinguishable from one another, the set resulting from the union of our patient's findings and the Jones major criteria is written:

$$\text{CLINICAL} - \text{FINDINGS} \cup \text{JONES} - \text{CRITERIA} - \text{MAJOR}$$
$$= \begin{Bmatrix} \text{heart murmur, migratory polyarthritis, chorea, subcutaneous} \\ \text{nodules, cough, carditis, erythema marginatum, chorea} \end{Bmatrix}$$

Anyone who has done a PubMed search in which two sets of literature citations are combined has performed these set operations; the AND function in PubMed is like set intersection, and the OR function is like set union.

Diagnostic criteria like the Jones criteria are good examples of how sets can be used to represent diagnostic rules. The full low-risk Jones criteria, represented in set theoretical terminology, might read like this (assuming we have sets JONES-

CRITERIA-MINOR and GROUP-A-STREP-EVIDENCE as described at the beginning of this section):

If CLINICAL-FINDINGS is the set of a given patient's symptoms, signs, and laboratory test results, then the patient is highly likely to have rheumatic fever if either of two conditions are met:

$$|\text{CLINICAL}-\text{FINDINGS} \cap \text{JONES}-\text{CRITERIA}-\text{MAJOR}| \geq 2 \quad (2.1)$$

and

$$|\text{CLINICAL}-\text{FINDINGS} \cap \text{GROUP}-\text{A}-\text{STREP}-\text{EVIDENCE}| \geq 1$$

$$|\text{CLINICAL}-\text{FINDINGS} \cap \text{JONES}-\text{CRITERIA}-\text{MAJOR}| = 1 \quad (2.2)$$

and

$$|\text{CLINICAL}-\text{FINDINGS} \cap \text{JONES}-\text{CRITERIA}-\text{MINOR}| \geq 2$$

and

$$|\text{CLINICAL}-\text{FINDINGS} \cap \text{GROUP}-\text{A}-\text{STREP}-\text{EVIDENCE}| \geq 1$$

There are other set operations besides union and intersection. For example, the phenomenon of *set covering* has applications in decision making [10]. A cover of a set is a set of subsets in which each element of the covered set appears at least once as a member of one of the sets in the cover set. An example makes this definition clearer. Suppose you were asked to recommend a list of antibiotics for your hospital's emergency department. Your objective is to stock the minimum number of antibiotics that will be effective for 95 % of the pathogenic organisms you've found in cultures at your hospital. For the sake of simplicity, suppose that there are six pathogens, each designated by a letter, which account for 95 % of the infections seen in your hospital.

You might represent this set of pathogens as:

$$\text{PATHOGENS} = \{\text{A, B, C, D, E, F}\}$$

You have the following set of antibiotics from which to choose:

$$\text{ANTIBIOTICS} = \{\text{A}-\text{Cillin}, \text{B}-\text{Cillin}, \text{C}-\text{Cillin}, \text{D}-\text{Cillin}, \text{E}-\text{Cillin}, \text{F}-\text{Cillin}\}$$

Each antibiotic is described by the set of pathogens for which that antibiotic is effective. Here is a list of your antibiotics, with their covered pathogen sets (each of which is a subset of PATHOGENS):

$$\begin{aligned}
\text{A}-\text{Cillin} &= \{\text{A,C}\} \\
\text{B}-\text{Cillin} &= \{\text{A,B,E}\} \\
\text{C}-\text{Cillin} &= \{\text{C,D,E}\} \\
\text{D}-\text{Cillin} &= \{\text{F}\} \\
\text{E}-\text{Cillin} &= \{\text{B,D,F}\} \\
\text{F}-\text{Cillin} &= \{\text{E}\}
\end{aligned}$$

What you seek is a set cover of the set PATHOGENS; in other words, you want to pick a set of antibiotics which contains at least one antibiotic that is effective for each pathogen. It's clear that all six antibiotics taken together make a set cover, but your job is to find the minimum number of antibiotics that will get the job done. Casual inspection shows that the set {A-Cillin, E-Cillin, F-Cillin} does the job as a set cover, in that at least one antibiotic in that set is effective for each one of the pathogens in PATHOGENS.

There are many other set operations which can be applied to real-world decision problems, but the brief introduction presented here should suffice to illuminate the concepts presented in this book. Generally speaking, sets are used to formalize logical operations in a way that a machine—usually a computer—can understand.

Before we leave the topic of sets, fuzzy sets are worth a brief mention. Under conventional principles of set theory, an element is either a member of a set or it isn't. Heart murmur, for example, is definitely not a member of the set JONES-CRITERIA-MAJOR. Under *fuzzy set theory*, membership in a set is not an all or nothing phenomenon. In a fuzzy set, an element is a member of the set with a certain probability; e.g., cough is a member of the set COLD-SYMPTOMS with a probability of 80 % (a four out of five chance). Fuzzy set theory has created new ways of looking at sets and new methods for applying set theory to solve decision-making problems: fuzzy logic [11–13]. Fuzzy logic has been used to tackle decision-making problems in which uncertainty plays a role.

2.1.2 Boolean Logic

Anyone who has performed a search of the medical literature using the PubMed system has used logic. When referring to common logical operations like combining two sets of literature citations using AND or OR, we often refer to these operations as "Boolean" logic, in honor of George Boole (1815–1864), a British mathematician who published seminal works on formal logic. Indeed, PubMed is not a bad way to learn about Boolean algebra, since its connection to set theory is made so clear by the sets of literature citations that we manipulate in that system.

Suppose we have performed two literature searches. The result of one search, set A, represents all the literature citations in the PubMed database that relate to rheumatoid arthritis. Set B consists of all the literature citations on immune globulin. By asking the PubMed program to give us a new set that is the result of combining A and B using the AND operator, we have a new set, C, that contains literature citations on the use of immune globulin in rheumatoid arthritis. When we combine two sets of citations using the AND function of our PubMed program, we are asking the computer to give us all citations that appear in both sets. This corresponds roughly to the English use of the word *and*.

The word OR in Boolean logic has a slightly different meaning than in English. In everyday usage, *or* usually has an exclusive meaning; the statement, "You may opt for chemotherapy or radiation therapy," usually means that one may have one or the other therapy, but not both. The Boolean OR is different. If one were to perform another pair of PubMed searches, this time for all articles that have asthma as a keyword (set A) and those that mention "reactive airway disease" in the text of the abstract (set B), one could combine sets A and B with the OR function to get a comprehensive set of citations on asthma. Because the OR function takes all citations that appear in one or both of sets A and B, the OR function is said to be *inclusive*.

There are other Boolean operators, like XOR (exclusive OR: "either A or B but not both") and NAND ("A and not B"), but AND and OR are the basic operators with which we are familiar.

How is Boolean logic used in CDSS? The mathematical subjects of statement logic and predicate logic give us formal definitions of how statements can be combined to produce new conclusions. For example, consider the following statements:

1. Urine cultures with colony counts of 10,000 or more are considered positive if they are obtained by bladder catheterization.
2. This patient's urine culture shows more than 10,000 colonies of E. coli.
3. All patients with positive urine cultures should be treated for urinary tract infections.

The statements can be combined intuitively, without the use of formal mathematics, into the conclusion:

This patient needs to be treated for a UTI.

The logic that gave us the conclusion so easily, comes from our medical intuition, but computers have no intuition. They must be programmed to generate even the most obvious conclusions. To understand logic as it is implemented on a computer, one must understand the basics of predicate logic and deductive reasoning.

The above example about UTIs is a sloppy instance of a syllogism. A syllogism is a form of deductive reasoning consisting of a major premise, a minor premise, and a conclusion. The premises are combined, using rules of predicate logic, into a conclusion. For example, a syllogism in a ventilator management decision support system might be:

Major Premise: All blood gas determinations that show carbon dioxide to be abnormally low indicate an over-ventilated patient.

Minor Premise: The current patient's carbon dioxide is abnormally low.

Conclusion: Therefore, the current patient is over-ventilated.

Again, this conclusion is obvious, but by representing the above syllogism using symbols, where the symbol Low-CO_2 represents the state of abnormally low carbon dioxide and the symbol OVERVENTILATED represents the state of an over-ventilated patient, the syllogism looks more computer friendly:

$$\begin{aligned}&\text{Major Premise}: \text{Low}-\text{CO2} \Rightarrow \text{OVERVENTILATED}\\&\text{Minor Premise}: \text{Low}-\text{CO2}\\&\text{Conclusion}: \text{OVERVENTILATED}\end{aligned}$$

Extending this example, suppose we have another statement in our CDSS that over-ventilation should cause a High Rate alarm to sound (we can represent this by the symbol HIGH-RATE-ALARM), then we can construct the syllogism:

$$\begin{aligned}&\text{Major Premise}: \text{Low}-\text{CO2} \Rightarrow \text{OVERVENTILATED}\\&\text{Minor Premise}: \text{OVERVENTILATED} \Rightarrow \text{HIGH}-\text{RATE}-\text{ALARM}\\&\text{Conclusion}: \text{Low}-\text{CO2} \Rightarrow \text{HIGH}-\text{RATE}-\text{ALARM}\end{aligned}$$

Thus, we have generated a new rule for the system, where the intermediate state of overventilation is bypassed. This simplification of two rules into a new one may or may not help our understanding of the system, but the results the system gives are the same: a low carbon dioxide value sets off the High Rate alarm. One can imagine how large sets of rules can be combined with each other to reduce complex reasoning tasks to simple ones.

The syllogism above is an example of rule chaining, where two rules are chained together to form a new conclusion. Specifically, the simple system outlined above is a *forward-chaining deduction system*, because the system starts with *if* statements and moves to a *then* statement. In real life, though, we often start with the "then" portion of a logical rule. For instance, consider the clinical rule:

If your patient has asthma, then give an influenza immunization each fall.

There are many other rules in real clinical practice with the same "then" portion ("give a flu vaccine"). The question a clinician might ask is not "Does this patient have asthma? If so, I should give a flu shot," but more likely the question would be simply "Does this patient need a flu shot?" We start with the "then" portion of this set of flu shot rules. A *backward-chaining deduction system* does this—it starts with the "then" end of a set of rules and works backwards to answer questions based on its rule set. In the flu shot example, a backward-chaining system would start with the "Does this patient need a flu shot" question and immediately learn that the diagnosis of asthma would cause this rule to be satisfied. The system might then ask the user or query a clinical database about the presence of this diagnosis.

An example of a backward-chaining deduction system in medicine was the MYCIN system developed at Stanford [14], MYCIN's domain was the selection of antibiotics for the treatment of bacterial infections based on clinical and microbiological information. An example of a forward-chaining system in medicine was

GermWatcher, developed at Barnes Hospital in St. Louis, [15, 16] GermWatcher used as its rules the Centers for Disease Control and Prevention's National Nosocomial Infections Surveillance System [17]. Using a forward-chaining reasoning system called CLIPS (C Language Integrated Production System, Software Technology Branch, National Aeronautics and Space Administration, Johnson Space Center, Houston, TX), expert system shell GermWatcher worked in a large hospital microbiology laboratory to identify hospital-acquired infections early from culture data.

CDSS that use logic like the simple management system above have limited application, since the range of truth encompassed by this logical system includes only true (e.g., the High Rate alarm needs to be sounded) or false (e.g., the High Rate alarm does not need to be sounded). Not many applications in medicine can be reduced to such simple truths. There may be situations where the High Rate alarm might not always have to be sounded for a low carbon dioxide reading (e.g., for a head injury patient who needs low carbon dioxide to preserve cerebral blood flow). To accommodate these situations, it would be helpful if the response from the system were something like "the high rate alarm should probably be sounded." Such a system would then need to be able to handle probabilities, as well as certainties, which most CDSS do. MYCIN, for example, reported its conclusions in terms of their likelihood. The next section covers basic concepts of probability.

2.1.3 Probability

Everyday medical practice contains many examples of probability. We often use words such as *probably*, *unlikely*, *certainly*, or *almost certainly* in all conversations with patients. We only rarely attach numbers to these terms, but computerized systems must use some numerical representation of likelihood in order to combine statements into conclusions.

Probability is represented numerically by a number between 0 and 1. Statements with a probability of 0 are false. Statements with a probability of 1 are true. Most statements from real life fall somewhere in the middle. A probability of 0.5 or 50 % is just as likely to be true as false. A round, opacified area seen in the lungs on a chest radiograph is probably pneumonia; one might assign a probability of 0.8, or 80 %, (a four in five chance) to this statement. Based on the high probability of pneumonia, one might elect to treat this condition without performing further testing—a lung biopsy, perhaps—that would increase the probability of pneumonia to greater than 80 %. We are accustomed to accepting the fact that our diagnoses have a certain probability of being wrong, so we counsel patients about what to do in the event (we might use the term "unlikely event") that things don't work out in the expected way.

Probabilities can be combined to yield new probabilities. For example, the two statements:

$$\Pr(\text{diabetes}) = 0.6$$
$$\Pr(\text{hypertension}) = 0.3$$

mean that the probability of diabetes is 0.6, or 60 %, (three in five chance), and the probability of hypertension is 0.3, or 30 %, (three in ten chance). We have not specified the clinical context of these statements, but suppose these probabilities applied to a particular population. Suppose further that the two conditions are independent; that is, the likelihood of patients having one disease is unaffected by whether they have the other (not always a safe assumption!). If we then want to know what the probability is of finding a patient in our specified population with both diseases, we simply multiply the two probabilities (0.6 and 0.3) to get 0.18, or 18 %. If the two clinical conditions are not independent, (e.g., pulmonary emphysema and lung cancer) then we cannot combine the probabilities in such a simple, multiplicative manner. This is much like the AND function in PubMed or the interaction function as applied to sets.

The familiar "OR" function from our PubMed program also has a mathematical meaning in combining probabilities. If we wanted to know how many patients in the above example had diabetes *or* hypertension (remember: this would also include those with both diseases in the usual mathematical sense of *or*), we would compute:

$$\Pr(\text{diabetes OR hypertension}) = \Pr(\text{diabetes}) + \Pr(\text{hypertension}) - \Pr(\text{diabetes AND hypertension})$$

The last term in the above equation we already know to be $0.6 \times 0.3 = 0.18$, so:

$$\Pr(\text{diabetes OR hypertension}) = 0.6 + 0.3 - 0.18 = 0.72.$$

Conditional probability is another type of probability often used in medicine. A conditional probability is the probability of an event (or the probability of the truth of a statement) *given the occurrence of another event* (or the truth of another statement). The most familiar case of conditional probability in medicine arises in the interpretation of diagnostic tests. For example, the probability of pneumonia given a round density on a chest radiograph is what we need to know in interpreting that diagnostic test if it is positive. In mathematical notation, this conditional probability is written this way:

$$\Pr(\text{Pneumonia} \mid \text{Round Density on CXR}).$$

One reads this notation, "The probability of pneumonia given a round density on chest radiograph." This notation is convenient in the explanation of Bayes' rule, which is the cornerstone of the logic in many decision support systems.

2.1.4 Bayes' Rule

If we have a patient with jaundice, how likely is it that he has hepatitis? Written another way, we seek to learn:

$$\Pr(\text{hepatitis} \mid \text{jaundice}),$$

which is read as "the probability of hepatitis given the presence of jaundice." We may not have this probability at our fingertips, but we might be able to find a slightly different probability more easily:

$$\Pr(\text{jaundice} \mid \text{hepatitis}),$$

which is, simply, the probability of jaundice given the presence of hepatitis. The latter probability could be found by studying a series of patients with proven hepatitis (it would be easy to get this data by looking up diagnosis codes in the medical records department) and computing the percentage of these patients who present with jaundice. However, this does not directly answer our original question. Bayes' rule allows us to compute the probability we *really* want—Pr(hepatitis | jaundice)—with the help of the more readily available number Pr(jaundice | hepatitis). Bayes' rule [18] is simply this:

$$\Pr(\text{hepatitis} \mid \text{jaundice}) = \frac{\Pr(\text{hepatitis}) \times \Pr(\text{jaundice} \mid \text{hepatitis})}{\Pr(\text{jaundice})}$$

Notice that to solve this equation, we need not only Pr(jaundice | hepatitis), but Pr(hepatitis)—the probability of hepatitis independent of any given symptom—and Pr(jaundice)—the probability of jaundice independent of any particular disease. These two independent probabilities are called *prior probabilities*, since they are the probabilities prior to the consideration of other factors.

The derivation of Bayes' rule is very simple. We already know that the probability of any two events occurring simultaneously is simply the product of their individual probabilities. For example, the joint probability we already computed of diabetes and hypertension in a hypothetical population was:

$$\Pr(\text{diabetes AND hypertension}) = \Pr(\text{diabetes}) \times \Pr(\text{hypertension})$$
$$= 0.6 \times 0.3 = 0.18.$$

We were free to multiply these together, because in our hypothetical population, the likelihood of one disease occurring in an individual was independent of the other. In other words:

$$\text{Pr(hypertension)} = \text{Pr(hypertension} \mid \text{diabetes) and}$$
$$\text{Pr(diabetes)} = \text{Pr(diabetes} \mid \text{hypertension).}$$

In this population, one's chance of having one disease is unaffected by the presence of the other disease.

In medicine, we are often faced with the question of the likelihood of two interrelated events occurring simultaneously in a patient. The case of a diagnostic test and the disease it is supposed to test for is a good example: what is the probability of an abnormal chest radiograph and pneumonia occurring in the same patient simultaneously? The question asks for this probability:

$$\text{Pr(pneumonia AND abnormal CXR).}$$

Can't we simply find out what the incidence of pneumonia in the population is, and multiply it by the incidence of abnormal chest radiographs in the population? A moment's reflection should show that this simple calculation is not sufficient. For example, if the incidence of pneumonia is 1 in 1,000, and the incidence of abnormal chest radiograph is 1 in 100, then the erroneous probability would be computed:

$$\text{WRONG: Pr(pneumonia AND abnormal CXR)} = 1/1000 \times 1/100 = 0.00001 = 0.001\%$$

This does not fit with our clinical intuition very well, since we know that people with pneumonia tend to have abnormal chest films. Our intuition says that the probability of the two events occurring together should be pretty close to the probability of having pneumonia alone, since a majority of those patients will have abnormal chest films. What we *really* need to compute is this:

$$\text{Pr(pneumonia AND abnormal CXR)} = \text{Pr(pneumonia)} \times \text{Pr}\begin{pmatrix}\text{abnormal CXR} \mid \\ \text{pneumonia}\end{pmatrix}.$$

This is the probability of pneumonia multiplied by the probability of an abnormal chest radiograph given that pneumonia exists. If we take Pr(abnormal CXR | pneumonia) to be 90 %, then the computation matches our intuition much better.

In general, for any two events A and B:

$$\text{Pr(A AND B)} = \text{Pr(A)} \times \text{Pr(B} \mid \text{A)and}$$
$$\text{Pr(B AND A)} = \text{Pr(B)} \times \text{Pr(A} \mid \text{B).}$$

But since Pr(A AND B) must surely equal Pr(B AND A), we can say that the right-hand sides of the equations above are equal to each other:

$$\text{Pr(A)} \times \text{Pr(B} \mid \text{A)} = \text{Pr(B)} \times \text{Pr(A} \mid \text{B)}$$

Rearranging this equation, we have Bayes' rule:

$$\Pr(A \mid B) = \frac{\Pr(A) \times \Pr(B \mid A)}{\Pr(B)}$$

At an intuitive level, we use Bayes' rule when making seat-of-the-pants estimates of disease probability in patients. For example, if we designate hepatitis by A and jaundice by B, and there were an ongoing epidemic of hepatitis (i.e., Pr(A) was high), then our index of suspicion for hepatitis in a jaundiced person would be increased. Likewise, if the likelihood of jaundice due to other causes was high (i.e., Pr(B) was high), then our estimation of the probability of hepatitis as a specific diagnosis would be lowered. Similarly, if jaundice were pathognomonic of hepatitis (i.e., Pr(A | B) was 1 or near to it), then our hepatitis diagnosis would be greatly increased. By using numerical estimates of the probability of diseases, findings, and conditional probabilities, Bayes' rule can help make medical decisions.

One might imagine a simple CDSS in which one enters a single symptom and receives the probability of the presence of a disease given that symptom. A problem arises when one wishes to get disease probabilities given multiple symptoms. The number of data points needed to do Bayesian calculations on multiple simultaneous symptoms is huge. For example, in a system which handles only single symptoms, if one had a database of 1,000 symptoms and 200 diseases, one would need to create $1{,}000 \times 200 = 200{,}000$ conditional probabilities, 1,000 symptom probabilities, and 200 disease probabilities, for a total of about 200,000 numbers. Since most of these numbers are 0 (many symptoms are unrelated to many diseases), this may be a reasonable amount of numbers to collect into a knowledge base. When one starts considering the probabilities needed to do computations on two simultaneous symptoms, this number climbs from 200,000 to about 200,000,000! If one wanted to design a system that could handle the very realistic situation of five or six simultaneous symptoms, estimating the number of numbers needed to support the calculation would be intractable. Modifying the system to handle multiple simultaneous "diseases" adds even more to the complexity. Only after making the simplifying assumption that most disease findings are independent of one another [19] do many diagnostic CDSS use Bayesian approaches. One such system, Iliad [20], successfully employed this assumption.

2.1.5 *Informal Logic*

Even if we create a reasoning system that follows all the rules of logic and probability, it would be difficult to come up with all the numbers that must be assigned to each event in even a small clinical database. Many successful CDSS have circumvented this difficulty by employing informal rules of logic to accomplish the reasoning task, without creating an intractable data gathering task. In the early development of one of the most famous CDSS, MYCIN [14, 21, 22], the creators of the system developed their own logic system (heuristic) that made intuitive sense. This system employed "certainty factors" which ranged from −1 (false) to +1 (true). A certainty factor of 0 indicated no belief in either direction in the statement's veracity. In combining several statements with the AND function into a single combined statement in MYCIN, one simply takes the minimum certainty factor of all the statements as the certainty factor of the combined statement. This makes a certain intuitive sense: we cannot be any more certain of an AND statement than we are of the least certain part. Later development of the MYCIN project showed a sound probabilistic basis for the certainty factor rules, but the point here is that sometimes cutting mathematical corners can still yield a useful system. In other early CDSS (QMR [23] and DXplain, [8, 24]), there is a knowledge base of diseases and findings (a finding is an item from the history, physical examination, laboratory data, or radiographic data). Each disease is defined by a particular set of findings. Each disease-finding relationship is assigned a frequency (of the finding among people with the disease) and an evoking strength (of how strongly a finding would evoke the possibility of a disease) on an ordinal scale (1–5 for frequency; 0–5 for evoking strength). These two factors make intuitive sense, and the system works, but the manipulation of these factors within these systems is very different from the formal algebra of logic and probability.

2.2 The General Model of Knowledge-Based Decision Support Systems

There are similarities between physician and CDSS reasoning, although a CDSS might arrive at a similar conclusion to a physician without employing the same model of reasoning. Physicians do use some probabilistic information when they make decisions. For instance, a physician might make a diagnosis of influenza more often during the winter when influenza is more prevalent (probable) than in the summer. However, physicians use this information in informal ways; in other words, they do not use precise numbers in formulas to make diagnostic decisions [25, 26]. Another feature of real-life clinical decision making is that physicians do not require complete information to make a decision. Most doctors are comfortable making decisions based on incomplete or contradictory information [27]. In contrast, CDSS rely on well defined numerical techniques to do their reasoning, and they do require sufficient information to complete their formulae. While physicians can fall back on their knowledge of pathophysiology, CDSS are not well suited to situations in which hard data are unknown. To understand how these systems operate, and under what conditions they are best used, it is important to appreciate a general model of CDSS.

Figure 2.1 shows a general model of a CDSS. There is input to the system and output from it. The CDSS has a reasoning (inference) engine and a knowledge base. Understanding these basic components provides a useful framework for under-

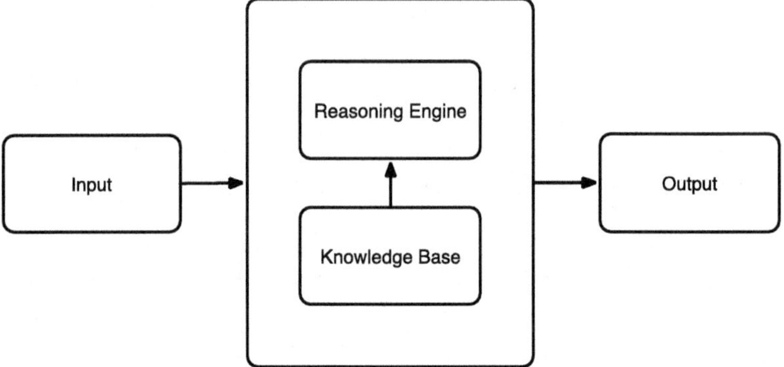

Fig. 2.1 A general model of a clinical diagnostic decision support system

standing most CDSS and their limitations. There are systems which do not follow this model which will be discussed briefly later in this chapter and in Chap. 3 in more detail.

The user supplies input appropriate to the system (i.e., terms from the system's controlled vocabulary to represent clinical data), and the system supplies output (e.g., a differential diagnosis or a therapy suggestion). The reasoning engine applies formal or informal rules of logic to the input and often relies on additional facts encoded in the system's knowledge base. The knowledge base is the compilation of the relationships between all of the diseases in the system and their associated manifestations (e.g., signs, symptoms, laboratory and radiographic tests). Maintaining the knowledge base is the most significant bottleneck in the maintenance of such systems, since the knowledge base needs to be expanded and updated as medical knowledge grows.

2.2.1 Input

The manner in which clinical information is entered into the CDSS (user interface) varies from system to system, but most diagnostic systems require the user to select terms from their specialized, controlled vocabulary. Comprehension of natural language has been an elusive goal in the development of CDSS. While it would be highly desirable to be able to speak or type the query "What are the diagnostic possibilities for a 4-year-old child with joint swelling and fever for a month," most who have used such systems are accustomed to the task of reformatting this question in terms the particular CDSS can understand. We might, for example, break the above query into components:

- Age: 4 years
- Gender: unspecified
- Symptom: joint swelling

- Duration: 1 month
- Time course: unknown

This breakdown of the original query might work on one system, but another system might demand that we break it down another way:

- Age: less than 12 years
- Finding: arthritis

Notice that the second description describes the age in vague terms, and it forces us to eschew joint swelling for the more specific term arthritis (usually defined as joint pain, redness, warmth, and swelling). In the vocabulary of the program, the age of 4 years (as opposed to 10 years) is unimportant, and joint swelling, without other signs of inflammation, is undefined.

Any physician who has assigned diagnostic and procedural codes in billing systems understands the limitations of controlled vocabularies. In a CDSS, it is common for the user's input to be restricted to a finite set of terms and modifiers. How well the system works in a given clinical situation may depend on how well the system's vocabulary matches the terms the clinician uses. CDSS take a variety of terms, called findings, which encompass items from the medical history, physical examination, laboratory results, and other pieces of clinical information. What constitutes a valid finding in a given program is entirely up to the program; there is no "standard" set of findings for all CDSS. For general purpose CDSS, items from the history and physical examination are going to be the findings. In specialized domains, e.g., an arterial–blood–gas expert system, the input vocabulary will be entirely different and much more restrictive.

Entering "chest pain" as a finding in a CDSS may be insufficient to capture the essence of the symptom. "Chest pain radiating to the left arm" may be sufficient, but usually there are pertinent temporal factors related to symptoms that are difficult to express in a controlled vocabulary. For example, "sudden onset, 20 min ago, of chest pain radiating to the left arm" has a very different meaning from "five-year history of continuous chest pain radiating to the left arm." While CDSS often include a vocabulary of severity and location modifiers, temporal modifiers are more difficult to build into a system, since minute changes in the timing of onset and duration can make a big difference in the conclusion the system reaches. Some CDSS make simplifying assumptions about broad categories of timing (acute, subacute, chronic) to aid in the temporal description of findings. Although users may experience frustration in being unable to enter temporal information, the research is equivocal in its impact.

One solution to the problem of temporal modeling in CDSS is to use an explicit model of time, in which the user is asked to specify intervals and points in time, along with temporal relationships between events (e.g., event A occurred before event B), in order to drive a temporal reasoning process within the CDSS. Clearly, this complicates the matter of entering data (to say nothing of programming the system). A simpler approach is to model time implicitly. In implicit time [28], temporal information is built into the data input elements of the CDSS; no special temporal reasoning procedures are required. For example, one input item could be "history of recent exposure to strep." By joining the concept "history of" with the concept of a particular bacterial pathogen, one successfully abstracts the temporal nature of this finding, which would be pertinent in the diagnosis of rheumatic fever or post-streptococcal glomerulonephritis. Note that no explicit definition of "recent" is part of this representation; if for some reason one needed to distinguish infection 2 weeks ago from infection 3 months ago, this abstraction would not suffice. Thus, there is a disadvantage to this simplification. Nonetheless, CDSS which use implicit temporal abstractions seem to perform well for time-sensitive clinical cases.

2.2.2 Inference Engine

There are many ways of programming an inference engine. The inference engine is the portion of the CDSS that combines the input and other data according to some logical scheme for output. Users of the system do not usually know—or need to know—how the engine works to achieve the results.

One such scheme for an inference engine is the Bayesian network. Recall that Bayes' rule helps us express conditional probabilities—the likelihood of one event given that another has occurred. A Bayesian network is a way to put Bayes' rule to work by laying out graphically which events influence the likelihood of occurrence of other events. Figure 2.2 shows a Bayesian network for the diagnosis of pneumonia.

The arrows in the diagram indicate all of the conditional relationships between findings and diagnoses. Note that the symptoms listed are not necessarily independent; since febrile patients are often tachypneic, even in the absence of lung disease, one cannot say the two are as independent as Bayesian reasoning requires. Conceptually, this network simply states that the diagnosis of pneumonia is supported by the presence of three symptoms. The strength of association—that is, how strongly pneumonia is suggested by each of the three symptoms—varies with each symptom–disease pairing. By "activating" all three nodes (cough, fever, and tachypnea) the probability of pneumonia is maximized. Of course, each of these three nodes might be tied to other disease states in the knowledge base (like lung cancer or upper respiratory infection).

Bayesian networks can be complex, but their usefulness comes from their ability to represent knowledge in an intuitively appealing way. Inference engines that operate on the basis of a network simply adjust probabilities based on simple mathematical relationships between nodes in the network. Iliad [20, 29], an early CDSS, was one such program that was built on Bayesian reasoning, and whose reasoning engine can be described as a Bayesian network. Bayesian network systems have been designed and validated for a variety of clinical situations, including tumor classification, cancer prognosis, and ectopic pregnancy detection [30–33]. Inputs to these systems include data ordinarily found in the EHR, although none of these have found their way into commercial use.

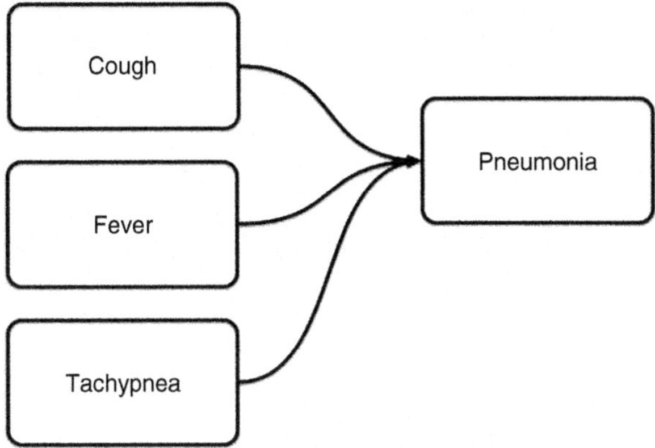

Fig. 2.2 A Bayesian network for the diagnosis of pneumonia

Production rule systems are another method of programming an inference engine. The rules of predicate logic dictate the functioning of such an engine as it combines statements to form new conclusions. MYCIN, described earlier, uses a production rule system. Production rules are an intuitively attractive way to start thinking about CDSS, since so much of the care physicians give in daily practice follows certain well known rules (e.g., giving patients with asthma an influenza vaccine each year). Other CDSS using production rules include Care Assistant, a general purpose, rule-based tool developed at the Childrens Hospital of Philadelphia that accepts input from an EHR via Web services and delivers decision support to the EHR user for immunizations and other treatment guidelines [34–37]. Chapter 5 describes this type of CDS via Web services in more detail. While this system was a customized add-on to the EHR, today some of this functionality is available in commercial EHR products, especially on the domain of immunizations.

An appealing solution to the problem of constructing inference engines in a clinical setting is to develop a cognitive model of actual clinical reasoning. In other words, one could study the reasoning that a physician uses and attempt to create a computerized version of that cognitive task. Workers in the field of artificial intelligence, in modeling human cognition, have developed the notion of "frames" or schemes, as a reasonable cognitive model. A frame consists of a set of "slots" into which fit details of a particular kind of information. For example, a disease frame may have a slot for etiologic agent and time course. Frames can be used to construct a semantic network model of the world, which may then be searched for answers to questions based on a particular situation. One such application of frames in medicine is the criterion-table method of diagnosing diseases like rheumatoid arthritis or Kawasaki disease. By applying a list of criteria, physicians can classify patients by diagnosis. The AI/Rheum system [38, 39] employed this familiar device in an inference engine that could have been used outside its original domain of rheumatologic diseases.

2.2.3 *Knowledge Base*

For CDSS to work, they must possess some form of medical knowledge. Obviously, the method of encoding this knowledge must match the inference engine design. For example, a CDSS based on a Bayesian network must contain probabilities—prior, conditional, and posterior—of diseases and findings. A big obstacle to building such a knowledge base is that many relevant probabilities are not known. While the medical literature can surely help with this task, and CDSS developers use the literature to varying degrees in building their knowledge bases, knowledge base developers must resort to estimates of probabilities, based on the clinical judgment of experts, to fill in the needed numbers. Unfortunately, physicians can exhibit markedly variable behavior in supplying such numbers, and probabilities can vary from situation to situation, even with the same disease entities (e.g., variations in disease prevalence with different populations).

Once one creates a knowledge base and populates it with some amount of data, the next task is to create a way to maintain it. Since many CDSS begin as funded academic research projects, it is no wonder that development of their knowledge bases often halts after the grant funds cease. Since knowledge base maintenance takes a tremendous amount of time, and since the market for some CDSS is rather small, many CDSS become too expensive to maintain. The knowledge-acquisition bottleneck [40] has been recognized as a problem in CDSS research.

2.2.4 *Output*

The output of CDSS is usually in the form of a list of possibilities, ranked in some order of probability. Sometimes probability is not the only criterion on which results are evaluated; for example, in the DXplain output, diseases which are not necessarily very likely, but whose misdiagnosis would be catastrophic, are flagged with a special disease-importance tag to call attention to the possibility [24]. Very often, physicians are not interested in the most likely diagnosis from a CDSS; for experienced physicians, the most likely diagnosis is obvious. It is the less likely diagnosis that one might fail to consider that interests physicians in CDSS, yet clearly it is difficult to draw the line between the rare and the ultra-rare.

2.3 Nonknowledge-Based Systems

The systems discussed so far have been knowledge-based in the sense that an expert must expressly encode medical knowledge into numerical form for the systems to work. The knowledge-based systems cannot simply "learn" how to do the reasoning task from modeling human experts; the human expert must put the knowledge into the system explicitly and directly.

2.3.1 Neural Networks

There are systems that can learn from examples. Neural networks are the most widely recognized of these types of systems, and there are regular reports in the medical literature on their use in diverse fields [41–47].

Artificial neural networks are constructed in a fashion similar to biological neural networks. Neuron bodies ("nodes") are connected to one another by axons and dendrites ("links"). Nodes may be turned on or off, just as a biological neuron can be in an activated or inactivated state. Activation of a node causes activation of a signal on a link. The effect of that signal depends on the weight assigned to that link. In most learning neural networks, some nodes are input nodes and some are output nodes. In the CDSS context, the input nodes would be findings and the output nodes would be possible diseases. To understand how a neural network might work, consider the problem of determining whether a person with a sore throat has streptococcal infection (as opposed to a harmless viral infection). There are many input nodes to this decision, and perhaps two output nodes, strep infection and viral infection. By presenting to a neural network many thousands of cases of sore throat (where the outcome is known), the neural network would "learn," for example, that the presence of cough decreases the likelihood of strep, and the height of fever increases this likelihood.

The appealing feature of neural networks—and what separates this technique from other methods of discovering relationships among data, like logistic regression—is the ability of the system to learn over time. A neural network changes its behavior based on previous patterns. In a domain where the relationship between findings and diseases might change, like infectious disease surveillance, this changing behavior can be desirable. Another desirable feature of neural networks is the lack of necessity to understand complex relationships between input variables; the network learns these relationships as it changes the links between its nodes. This is the principal difference between neural networks and Bayesian networks. In the latter, one explicitly constructs the network based on one's knowledge of pathophysiology and known probabilities. With neural networks, the links are established as the network is developed, often on the basis of a learning process, without regard to pathophysiologic facts. A disadvantage of neural networks, however, is that unlike the other systems discussed, the "rules" that the network uses do not follow a particular logic and are not explicitly understandable.

2.3.2 Genetic Algorithms

Genetic algorithms represent another nonknowledge-based method for constructing CDSS. Genetic algorithms take their name from an analogy to the molecular rearrangements that take place in chromosomes. Genes rearrange themselves randomly; such rearrangements give rise to variations in an individual, which can affect the individual's ability to pass on genetic material. Over time, the species as a whole incorporates the most adaptive features of the "fittest" individuals. Genetic algorithms take a similar approach. To use a genetic algorithm, the problem to be solved must have many components (e.g., a complex cancer treatment protocol with multiple drugs, radiation therapy, and so on). By selecting components randomly, a population of possible solutions is created. The fittest of these solutions (the one with the best outcome) is selected, and this subpopulation undergoes rearrangement, producing another generation of solutions. By iteratively extracting the best solutions, an optimal solution can be reached. The main challenge in using genetic algorithms is in creating the criteria by which fitness is defined. Since the computing power required to use both genetic algorithms and neural networks is considerable, these techniques have had only limited use in medicine.

2.4 Model for Evaluating the Appropriateness of CDSS

In a technology environment dominated by electronic health record (EHR) systems [48–51] most of the decision support that clinicians today face comes in the form of alerts presented during the normal use of the EHR [52]. The mathematics behind these alerts is usually a straightforward application of conditional logic, e.g.:

If current order's medication is in Nephrotoxic-Drug-Group,
And Creatinine-Clearance > Age-Specific-Threshold,
Then Display warning "Use caution when prescribing nephrotoxic drugs in this patient."

Studies of this kind of decision support suggest that clinicians ignore such alerts at high rates [53, 54]. The usual explanation is "alert fatigue" [55] but more complex sociotechnical factors affect the impact alerts have on quality of care [56, 57]. In any case, simple alerting as a form of decision support in EHRs has been shown to be of limited effectiveness, in contrast to other sources of information that clinicians use to make decisions. The ways laboratory tests are evaluated may help us formulate a way to develop metrics for quantifying the physician response to alerts. For example, in the case of laboratory test results, the classic method of evaluation of this kind of clinical data is the 2 × 2 table, shown in Fig. 2.3.

In this case, one can calculate several metrics that can inform the clinical user about the performance of the test:

Fig. 2.3 Typical 2×2 table for a common laboratory test, indicating the four possible outcomes of applying the test in a population of patients, some of whom have the disease in question. The letters serve as a convenient way to refer to each cell of the table (see text)

	Strep throat present	Strep throat absent
Rapid strep test positive	*a* True positive	*b* False positive
Rapid strep test negative	*c* False negative	*d* True negative

Fig. 2.4 Possible 2×2 table for an alert embedded in an electronic health record. The alert would fire under the circumstances for which it was programmed, but typically the programming would not detect the condition perfectly. Again, the letters serve as a convenient way to refer to cells of this table

	Condition present	Condition absent
Alert fires	*a* True positive	*b* False positive
Alert does not fire	*c* False negative	*d* True negative

- Sensitivity (true positive rate among those with disease) = $a / (a + c)$
- Specificity (true negative rate among those without disease) = $d / (b + d)$
- Positive predictive value (PPV; true positive rate among positive tests) = $a / (a + b)$
- Negative predictive value (NPV; true negative rate among negative tests) = $d / (c + d)$

A highly sensitive test picks up a high proportion of those who have the disease. A highly specific test means there will be very few false positives. Using these metrics, one can judge the usefulness of a laboratory test as a decision support aid. For example, one could design guideline recommendations based on whether a test was highly sensitive (useful for ruling *out* disease) or highly specific (more useful for ruling *in* disease). There are other methods of using these metrics in the interpretation of laboratory test results that are beyond the scope of this chapter.

For EHR-based alerts, one might like to have a similar 2×2 table in order to make judgments about the usefulness of the alert (Fig. 2.4).

If one could gather data from one's EHR to fill in this table, one could gain an appreciation for the performance of an alert, and be able to make decisions about whether an alert was valuable. For example, one could deploy a highly sensitive alert to screen for a condition (in a manner similar to a lab test), but a more specific alert in a part of the workflow where condition confirmation is more important. In theory, it is possible to gather data to fill in this table, but given that the manual chart review and data collection is expensive, one usually uses data from a report in which the EHR system displays when the alert fired (boxes *a* and *b* in 2.4). The EHR cannot report on box *c* (condition present but alert did not fire) since, had the EHR been able to detect the condition, those data would have gone to boxes *a* or *b*. In other words, it is a logical impossibility for a computer system to present a report on something it is not programmed to know. As a result, we are left with the ability to calculate only the true positive rate, and cannot obtain the other metrics without an infeasible amount of manual data collection. Reliance on true positive rate only—what one might call the "tyranny of box *a*" generates false contentment that a given alert is effective. The question of "how good is this alert?" often remains unanswered among the numerous safety-driven requests to add more alerts that must be accommodated in a typical EHR implementation.

2.5 Summary

Understanding clinical decision support systems requires a basic understanding of probability and logic. Set theory, familiar to most practitioners who have manipulated collections of literature citations in PubMed, provides the basis for understanding probability and other computational methods for reasoning. Probability—in particular, conditional probability—is the principle behind most modern CDSS, but non-probabilistic heuristic techniques have been used to good effect in the past.

Understanding CDSS can be facilitated by considering four basic components of the CDSS process: input, reasoning engine, knowledge base, and output. Input is often constrained by controlled vocabularies or limitations in temporal expression of clinical features. Reasoning engines take on different designs, but their operation is usually transparent to the user of a CDSS. Knowledge bases contain data from which the reasoning engine takes rules, probabilities, and other constructs required to convert the input into output. Output can take many forms, including a differential diagnosis list or simply a probability of a particular diagnosis. Nonknowledge-based systems use techniques of machine learning to generate methods of turning input into meaningful output, regardless of an explicit representation of expert knowledge. While very important to do, it is a challenge to develop appropriate metrics to judge the appropriateness of CDSS performance.

References

1. NCBI. PubMed: National Center for Biotechnology Information. 2015 [cited 2015 7/4/2015]. Available from: http://www.ncbi.nlm.nih.gov/pubmed/.
2. Schiff GD, Bates DW. Can electronic clinical documentation help prevent diagnostic errors? N Engl J Med. 2010;362(12):1066–9. doi:10.1056/NEJMp0911734.

3. Richardson JE, Ash JS. A clinical decision support needs assessment of community-based physicians. J Am Med Inform Assoc. 2011;18 Suppl 1:i28–35. doi:10.1136/amiajnl-2011-000119. PubMed PMID: 21890874, PubMed Central PMCID: PMC3241161.
4. Kuperman GJ, Bobb A, Payne TH, Avery AJ, Gandhi TK, Burns G, et al. Medication-related clinical decision support in computerized provider order entry systems: a review. J Am Med Inform Assoc. 2007;14(1):29–40. doi:10.1197/jamia.M2170. PubMed PMID: 17068355, PubMed Central PMCID: PMC2215064.
5. Brokel J. Evidence-based clinical decision support improves the appropriate use of antibiotics and rapid strep testing. Evid Based Med. 2014;19(3):118. doi:10.1136/eb-2013-101625.
6. Henderson EJ, Rubin GP. The utility of an online diagnostic decision support system (Isabel) in general practice: a process evaluation. JRSM Short Rep. 2013;4(5):31. doi:10.1177/2042533313476691. PubMed PMID: 23772310; PubMed Central PMCID: PMCPMC3681231.
7. Bond WF, Schwartz LM, Weaver KR, Levick D, Giuliano M, Graber ML. Differential diagnosis generators: an evaluation of currently available computer programs. J Gen Intern Med. 2012;27(2):213–9. doi:10.1007/s11606-011-1804-8. PubMed PMID: 21789717; PubMed Central PMCID: PMCPMC3270234.
8. Hoffer EP, Feldman MJ, Kim RJ, Famiglietti KT, Barnett GO. DXplain: patterns of use of a mature expert system. AMIA Annu Symp Proc. 2005:321–5. PubMed PMID: 16779054; PubMed Central PMCID: PMC1560464.
9. Gibofsky A. Clinical manifestations and diagnosis of acute rheumatic fever. In: Post TW, editor. UpToDate. Waltham: Wolters Kluwer Health; 2013.
10. Reggia JA, Nau DS, Wang PY. Diagnostic expert systems based on a set covering model. Int J Man Mach Stud. 1983;19(5):437–60.
11. Hsieh YZ, Su MC, Wang PC. A PSO-based rule extractor for medical diagnosis. J Biomed Inform. 2014;49:53–60. doi:10.1016/j.jbi.2014.05.001.
12. Leite CR, Sizilio GR, Neto AD, Valentim RA, Guerreiro AM. A fuzzy model for processing and monitoring vital signs in ICU patients. Biomed Eng Online. 2011;10:68. doi:10.1186/1475-925X-10-68. PubMed PMID: 21810277, PubMed Central PMCID: PMC3162941.
13. Miranda GH, Felipe JC. Computer-aided diagnosis system based on fuzzy logic for breast cancer categorization. Comput Biol Med. 2014. doi:10.1016/j.compbiomed.2014.10.006.
14. Yu VL, Buchanan BG, Shortliffe EH, Wraith SM, Davis R, Scott AC, et al. Evaluating the performance of a computer-based consultant. Comput Programs Biomed. 1979;9(1):95–102.
15. Doherty J, Noirot LA, Mayfield J, Ramiah S, Huang C, Dunagan WC, et al. Implementing GermWatcher, an enterprise infection control application. AMIA Annu Symp Proc. 2006:209–13. PubMed PMID: 17238333; PubMed Central PMCID: PMC1839697.
16. Kahn MG, Steib SA, Dunagan WC, Fraser VJ. Monitoring expert system performance using continuous user feedback. J Am Med Inform Assoc. 1996;3(3):216–23. PubMed PMID: 8723612, PubMed Central PMCID: PMC116303.
17. Martone WJ, Gaynes RP, Horan TC, Danzig L, Emori TG, Monnet D, et al. National Nosocomial Infections Surveillance (NNIS) semiannual report, May 1995. A report from the National Nosocomial Infections Surveillance (NNIS) System. Am J Infect Control. 1995;23(6):377–85.
18. Bayes T. An essay towards solving a problem in the doctrine of chances. 1763. MD Comput. 1991;8(3):157–71.
19. Warner HR, Toronto AF, Veasey LG, Stephenson R. A mathematical approach to medical diagnosis: application to congenital heart disease. 1961. MD Comput. 1992;9(1):43–50.
20. Warner Jr HR, Bouhaddou O. Innovation review: Iliad – a medical diagnostic support program. Top Health Inf Manag. 1994;14(4):51–8.
21. Shortliffe EH, Davis R, Axline SG, Buchanan BG, Green CC, Cohen SN. Computer-based consultations in clinical therapeutics: explanation and rule acquisition capabilities of the MYCIN system. Comput Biomed Res. 1975;8(4):303–20.

22. Vincent WR, Martin CA, Winstead PS, Smith KM, Gatz J, Lewis DA. Effects of a pharmacist-to-dose computerized request on promptness of antimicrobial therapy. J Am Med Inform Assoc. 2009;16(1):47–53. doi:10.1197/jamia.M2559. Epub 2008/10/28doi: M2559 [pii].
23. Miller RA. A history of the INTERNIST-1 and Quick Medical Reference (QMR) computer-assisted diagnosis projects, with lessons learned. Yearb Med Inform. 2010:121–36.
24. Elkin PL, Liebow M, Bauer BA, Chaliki S, Wahner-Roedler D, Bundrick J, et al. The introduction of a diagnostic decision support system (DXplain) into the workflow of a teaching hospital service can decrease the cost of service for diagnostically challenging Diagnostic Related Groups (DRGs). Int J Med Inform. 2010;79(11):772–7. doi:10.1016/j.ijmedinf.2010.09.004. PubMed PMID: 20951080, PubMed Central PMCID: PMC2977948.
25. Norman GR, Eva KW. Diagnostic error and clinical reasoning. Med Educ. 2010;44(1):94–100. doi:10.1111/j.1365-2923.2009.03507.x.
26. Poses RM, Anthony M. Availability, wishful thinking, and physicians' diagnostic judgments for patients with suspected bacteremia. Med Decis Mak. 1991;11(3):159–68.
27. Groopman J. How doctors think. Boston: Houghton Mifflin Publishing Co.; 2008.
28. Aliferis CF, Cooper GF, Miller RA, Buchanan BG, Bankowitz R, Giuse N. A temporal analysis of QMR. J Am Med Inform Assoc. 1996;3(1):79–91.
29. Lau LM, Warner HR. Performance of a diagnostic system (Iliad) as a tool for quality assurance. Comput Biomed Res. 1992;25(4):314–23.
30. Chen R, Wang S, Poptani H, Melhem ER, Herskovits EH. A Bayesian diagnostic system to differentiate glioblastomas from solitary brain metastases. Neuroradiol J. 2013;26(2):175–83.
31. Gevaert O, De Smet F, Kirk E, Van Calster B, Bourne T, Van Huffel S, et al. Predicting the outcome of pregnancies of unknown location: Bayesian networks with expert prior information compared to logistic regression. Hum Reprod. 2006;21(7):1824–31. doi:10.1093/humrep/del083.
32. Gevaert O, De Smet F, Timmerman D, Moreau Y, De Moor B. Predicting the prognosis of breast cancer by integrating clinical and microarray data with Bayesian networks. Bioinformatics. 2006;22(14):e184–90. doi:10.1093/bioinformatics/btl230.
33. Sesen MB, Peake MD, Banares-Alcantara R, Tse D, Kadir T, Stanley R, et al. Lung cancer assistant: a hybrid clinical decision support application for lung cancer care. J R Soc Interface. 2014;11(98):20140534. doi:10.1098/rsif.2014.0534. PubMed PMID: 24990290, PubMed Central PMCID: PMC4233704.
34. Bell LM, Grundmeier R, Localio R, Zorc J, Fiks AG, Zhang X, et al. Electronic health record-based decision support to improve asthma care: a cluster-randomized trial. Pediatrics. 2010;125(4):e770–7. doi:10.1542/peds.2009-1385.
35. Fiks AG, Grundmeier RW, Biggs LM, Localio AR, Alessandrini EA. Impact of clinical alerts within an electronic health record on routine childhood immunization in an urban pediatric population. Pediatrics. 2007;120(4):707–14. doi:10.1542/peds.2007-0257.
36. Fiks AG, Hunter KF, Localio AR, Grundmeier RW, Bryant-Stephens T, Luberti AA, et al. Impact of electronic health record-based alerts on influenza vaccination for children with asthma. Pediatrics. 2009;124(1):159–69. doi:10.1542/peds.2008-2823.
37. Forrest CB, Fiks AG, Bailey LC, Localio R, Grundmeier RW, Richards T, et al. Improving adherence to otitis media guidelines with clinical decision support and physician feedback. Pediatrics. 2013;131(4):e1071–81. doi:10.1542/peds.2012-1988.
38. Athreya BH, Cheh ML, Kingsland 3rd LC. Computer-assisted diagnosis of pediatric rheumatic diseases. Pediatrics. 1998;102(4), E48.
39. Bernelot Moens HJ. Validation of the AI/RHEUM knowledge base with data from consecutive rheumatological outpatients. Methods Inf Med. 1992;31(3):175–81.
40. Musen MA, van der Lei J. Knowledge engineering for clinical consultation programs: modeling the application area. Methods Inf Med. 1989;28(1):28–35.
41. Azimi P, Mohammadi HR, Benzel EC, Shahzadi S, Azhari S, Montazeri A. Artificial neural networks in neurosurgery. J Neurol Neurosurg Psychiatry. 2015;86(3):251–6. doi:10.1136/jnnp-2014-307807.

42. Zhang F, Feng M, Pan SJ, Loy LY, Guo W, Zhang Z, et al. Artificial neural network based intracranial pressure mean forecast algorithm for medical decision support. Conf Proc IEEE Eng Med Biol Soc. 2011;2011:7111–4. doi:10.1109/IEMBS.2011.6091797.
43. Santhiyakumari N, Rajendran P, Madheswaran M. Medical decision-making system of ultrasound carotid artery intima-media thickness using neural networks. J Digit Imaging. 2011;24(6):1112–25. doi:10.1007/s10278-010-9356-8. PubMed PMID: 21181487, PubMed Central PMCID: PMC3222553.
44. Xie X, Wang L, Wang A. Artificial neural network modeling for deciding if extractions are necessary prior to orthodontic treatment. Angle Orthod. 2010;80(2):262–6. doi:10.2319/111608-588.1.
45. Larder B, Wang D, Revell A. Application of artificial neural networks for decision support in medicine. Methods Mol Biol. 2008;458:123–36.
46. Shimada T, Shiina T, Saito Y. Detection of characteristic waves of sleep EEG by neural network analysis. IEEE Trans Biomed Eng. 2000;47(3):369–79. doi:10.1109/10.827301.
47. Somoza E, Somoza JR. A neural-network approach to predicting admission decisions in a psychiatric emergency room. Med Decis Making. 1993;13(4):273–80.
48. Grinspan ZM, Banerjee S, Kaushal R, Kern LM. Physician specialty and variations in adoption of electronic health records. Appl Clin Inf. 2013;4(2):225–40. doi:10.4338/ACI-2013-02-RA-0015. PubMed PMID: 23874360; PubMed Central PMCID: PMCPMC3716415.
49. Hsiao CJ, Hing E, Socey TC, Cai B. Electronic medical record/electronic health record Systems of office-based physicians: United States, 2009 and preliminary 2010 state estimates. In: Statistics NCfH, editor. Washington, DC: Centers for Disease Control; 2010.
50. Jha AK, DesRoches CM, Kralovec PD, Joshi MS. A progress report on electronic health records in U.S. hospitals. Health Aff (Millwood). 2010;29(10):1951–7. doi:10.1377/hlthaff.2010.0502. hlthaff.2010.0502 [pii].
51. Leu MG, O'Connor KG, Marshall R, Price DT, Klein JD. Pediatricians' use of health information technology: a national survey. Pediatrics. 2012;130(6):e1441–6. doi:10.1542/peds.2012-0396.
52. Mann D, Knaus M, McCullagh L, Sofianou A, Rosen L, McGinn T, et al. Measures of user experience in a streptococcal pharyngitis and pneumonia clinical decision support tools. Appl Clin Inf. 2014;5(3):824–35. doi:10.4338/ACI-2014-04-RA-0043. PubMed PMID: 25298820, PubMed Central PMCID: PMC4187097.
53. Nanji KC, Slight SP, Seger DL, Cho I, Fiskio JM, Redden LM, et al. Overrides of medication-related clinical decision support alerts in outpatients. J Am Med Inform Assoc. 2014;21(3):487–91. doi:10.1136/amiajnl-2013-001813.
54. Slight SP, Nanji KC, Seger DL, Cho I, Volk LA, Bates DW. Overrides of clinical decision support alerts in primary care clinics. Stud Health Technol Inf. 2013;192:923.
55. Lo HG, Matheny ME, Seger DL, Bates DW, Gandhi TK. Impact of non-interruptive medication laboratory monitoring alerts in ambulatory care. J Am Med Inform Assoc. 2009;16(1):66–71. doi:10.1197/jamia.M2687. Epub 2008/10/28M2687 [pii].
56. Ash J, Sittig D, Campbell E, Guappone K, Dykstra R. Some unintended consequences of clinical decision support systems. AMIA Annu Symp Proc. 2007:26–30.
57. Ash J, Sittig D, Dykstra R, Campbell E, Guappone K. The unintended consequences of computerized provider order entry: findings from a mixed methods exploration. Int J Med Inform. 2009;78 Suppl 1:S69–76.

Chapter 3
Data Mining and Clinical Decision Support Systems

Bunyamin Ozaydin, J. Michael Hardin, and David C. Chhieng

Abstract Data mining is a process of pattern and relationship discovery within large sets of data. Because of the large volume of data generated in healthcare settings, it is not surprising that healthcare organizations have been interested in data mining to enhance physician practices, disease management, and resource utilization. This chapter discusses a variety of data mining techniques that have been used to develop clinical decision support systems, including decision trees, neural networks, logistic regression, nearest neighbor classifiers. In addition, genetic algorithms, biologic and quantum computing, and big data analytics as well as methods of evaluating and comparing the different approaches are also discussed.

Keywords Statistical pattern recognition • Data mining • Neural networks • Decision trees • Genetic algorithms • Big data analytics • Quantum computing

3.1 Introduction

Data miningis a process of pattern and relationship discovery within large sets of data. The context encompasses several fields, including pattern recognition, statistics, computer science, and database management. Thus, the definition of data mining largely depends on the point of view of the writer giving the definitions. For example, from the perspective of pattern recognition, data mining is defined as the process of identifying valid, novel, and easily understood patterns within the data set [1].

B. Ozaydin, Ph.D. (✉)
School of Health Professions, Department of Health Services Administration,
University of Alabama at Birmingham, SHPB 590H, 1720 2nd Ave S,
Birmingham, AL 35294-1212, USA
e-mail: bozaydin@uab.edu

J.M. Hardin, Ph.D.
Academic Affairs, Samford University, 800 Lakeshore Drive, Birmingham, AL 35229, USA
e-mail: mhardin@samford.edu

D.C. Chhieng, M.D., M.B.A., M.S.H.I., M.S.E.M.
Pathology, Mount Sinai Health System, 1 Gustave L. Levy Place, New York, NY 10029, USA
e-mail: david.chhieng@mountsinai.org

E.S. Berner (ed.), *Clinical Decision Support Systems*, Health Informatics,
DOI 10.1007/978-3-319-31913-1_3

In still broader terms, the main goal of data mining is to convert data into meaningful information. More specifically, one major primary goal of data mining is to discover new patterns for the users. The discovery of new patterns can serve two purposes: description and prediction. The former focuses on finding patterns and presenting them to users in an interpretable and understandable form. Prediction involves identifying variables or fields in the database and using them to predict future values or behavior of some entities.

Data mining is well suited to provide decision support in healthcare settings. Healthcare organizations face increasing pressures to improve the quality of care while reducing costs. Because of the large volume of data generated in healthcare settings, it is not surprising that healthcare organizations have been interested in data mining to enhance physician practices, disease management, and resource utilization.

Example 3.1 One early application of data mining to health care was done in the early 1990s by United HealthCare Corporation. United HealthCare Corporation was a managed-care company, and developed its first data mining system, Quality Screening and Management (QSM), to analyze treatment records from its members [2]. QSM examined 15 measures for studying patients with chronic illness and compared the care received by its members to that recommended by national standards and guidelines. Results of the analyses were then used to identify appropriate quality management improvement strategies, and to monitor the effectiveness of such actions. Although not providing direct support for decision making at the point of care, these data could be used to improve the way clinical guidelines are used.

3.2 Data Mining and Clinical Decision Support Systems

With the advent of computing power and medical technology, large data sets as well as diverse and elaborate methods for data classification have been developed and studied. As a result, data mining has attracted considerable attention during the past several decades, and has found its way into a large number of applications that have included both data mining and clinical decision support systems. Decision support systems refer to a class of computer-based systems that aids the process of decision making [3]. Table 3.1 lists some examples of decision support systems that utilize data mining tools in healthcare settings.

A typical decision support system consists of five components: the data management, the model management, the knowledge engine, the user interface, and the user(s) [29]. One of the major differences between decision support systems employing data mining tools and those that employ rule-based expert systems rests in the knowledge engine. In the decision support systems that utilize rule-based expert systems, the inference engine must be supplied with the facts and the rules associated with them that, as described in Chap. 2, are often expressed in sets of "if–then" rules. In this sense, the decision support system requires a vast amount of

Table 3.1 Examples of clinical decision support systems and data mining tools

System (reference)	Description
Medical imaging recognition and interpretation system	
Monitoring tumor response to chemotherapy [4]	Computer-assisted texture analysis of ultrasound images aids monitoring of tumor response to chemotherapy
Diagnosis of neuromuscular disorder [5]	Classification of electromyographic (EMG) signals, based on the shapes and firing rates of motor unit
Detection of neonatal epileptic seizures [6]	Quantum neural networks are evaluated in detecting epileptic seizures in the neonatal electroencephalogram (EEG)
Gene and protein expression analysis	
Screening for prostate cancer [7]	Early detection of prostate cancer based on serum protein patterns detected by surface enhanced laser description ionization time-of-flight mass spectometry (SELDI-TOF MS)
Educational system	
Mining biomedical literature [8]	Automated system to mine MEDLINE for references to genes and proteins and to assess the relevance of each reference assignment
Laboratory system	
ISPAHAN [9]	Classification of immature and mature white blood cells (neutrophils series) using morphometrical parameters
Histologic diagnosis of Alzheimer's disease [10]	Analysis of digital images of tissue sections to identify and quantify senile plagues for diagnosing and evaluating the severity of Alzheimer's disease
Diagnosis of inherited metabolic diseases in newborns [11]	Identification of novel patterns in high-dimensional metabolic data for the construction of classification system to aid the diagnosis of inherited metabolic diseases
Acute care system	
Identification of potential quality problems [12]	Using logistic regression models to compare hospitals based on risk-adjusted death within 30 days of non-cardiac surgery
Evaluation of fetal well-being [13]	Using support vector machines and genetic algorithms to classify normal vs pathological cardiotocograms (CTGs)
Pneumonia and readmission prediction [14]	Multiple machine learning techniques used to construct intelligible models to predict inpatient pneumonia risk and 30-day readmission
Expert selection for diagnosis [15]	Context-adaptive algorithms used to discover the best clinic and expert to use to give a diagnosis based on patient's contexts using breast cancer data
Extensive pathology ordering [16]	CDSS combining data mining techniques with case-based reasoning to help general practitioners make more evidential informed decision in pathology ordering
Disease prediction, diagnosis, or progression system	
Prevailing diseases [17]	Decision support system to predict prevailing diseases to improve survivability using multiple data mining techniques
Disease progression [18]	Unsupervised learning algorithm is used to model progression of slowly progressing chronic diseases

(continued)

Table 3.1 (continued)

System (reference)	Description
Heart diseases [19–21]	Various studies using data mining techniques and big data to predict heart disease risk levels and heart attack and provide personalized diagnosis and treatment
Glaucoma [22–24]	Various studies using neural networks and comparing their performance to other methods in classifying glaucomatous and normal eyes using visual field analyzer and confocal scanning laser ophthalmoscopy and determining the effects of input data in neural network performance
Other diseases [25–28]	Various studies using data mining and machine learning techniques to predict early childhood obesity, cerebrovascular disease, and type 2 diabetes risk factors and provide a decision support system to diagnose chronic renal failure

a priori knowledge on the part of the decision maker in order to provide the right answers to well-formed questions. On the contrary, the decision support systems employing data mining tools do not require a priori knowledge on the part of the decision maker. Instead, the system is designed to find new and unsuspected patterns and relationships in a given set of data; the system then applies this newly discovered knowledge to a new set of data. This technique is most useful when a priori knowledge is limited or nonexistent.

Many successful clinical decision support systems using rule-based expert systems have been developed for very specialized areas in health care [30–36]. One early example of a rule-based expert system is MYCIN, which used its rules to identify micro-organisms that caused bacteremia and meningitis [36]. However, such systems can be challenging to maintain due to the fact that they often contain several thousand rules or more. In addition, these "if–then" rule systems have difficulty dealing with uncertainty. Bayesian systems (see Chap. 2) are one way of addressing uncertainty. Statistical pattern recognition approaches are another.

3.3 Data Mining and Statistical Pattern Recognition

Pattern recognition is a field within the area of data mining. It is the science that seeks analytical models with the ability to describe or classify data/measurements. The objective is to infer from a collection of data/measurements mechanisms to facilitate decision-making processes [37, 38]. With time, pattern recognition methodologies have evolved into an interdisciplinary field that covers multiple areas, including statistics, engineering, computer science, and artificial intelligence. Because of cross-disciplinary interest and participation, it is not surprising that pattern recognition is comprised of a variety of approaches. One approach to pattern recognition is called statistical pattern recognition.

Statistical pattern recognition implies the use of a statistical approach to the modeling of measurements or data [39]. Briefly, each pattern is represented by a set of features or variables related to an object. The goal is to select features that enable the objects to be classified into one or more groups or classes.

3.4 Supervised Versus Unsupervised Learning

Data mining and predictive modeling can be understood as learning from data. In this context, data mining comes in two categories: supervised learning and unsupervised learning.

3.4.1 Supervised Learning

Supervised learning, also called directed data mining, assumes that the user knows ahead of time what the classes are and that there are examples of each class available (Fig. 3.1a). This knowledge is transferred to the system through a process called training. The data set used in this process is called the training sample. The training sample is composed of dependent or target variables, and independent variables or input. The system is adjusted based on the training sample and the error signal (the difference between the desired response and the actual response of the system). In other words, a supervised learning system can be viewed as an operation that attempts to reduce the discrepancy between the expected and observed values as the training process progresses. With enough examples in the training data, the discrepancy will be minimized and the pattern recognition will be more accurate.

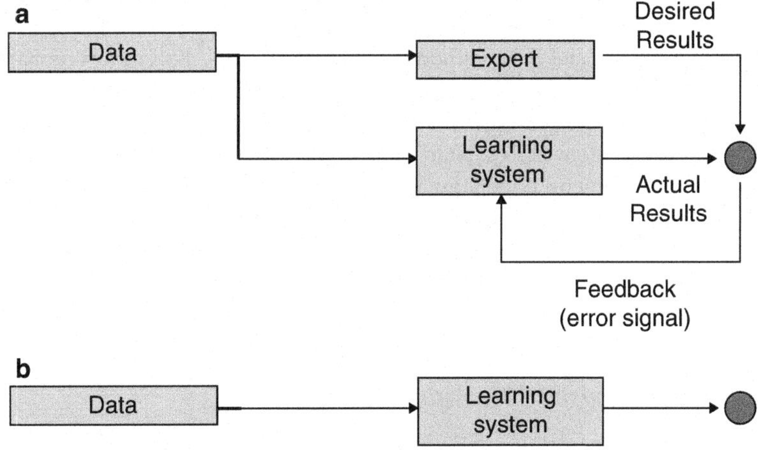

Fig. 3.1 (**a**) Supervised learning; (**b**) unsupervised learning

The goal of this approach is to establish a relationship or predictive model between the dependent and independent variables. Predictive modeling falls into the category of supervised learning because one variable is designated as the target that will be explained as a function of other variables. Predictive models are often built to predict the future values or behavior of an object or entity. The nature of the target/dependent variable determines the type of model: a model is called a classification model if the target variable is discrete; and a regression model if the target variable is continuous.

Example 3.2 Goldman et al. described the construction of a clinical decision support system to predict the presence of myocardial infraction in a cohort of 4,770 patients presenting with acute chest pain at two university hospitals and four community hospitals [40]. Based on the patient's symptoms and signs, the clinical decision support system had similar sensitivity (88.0 % versus 87.8 %) but a significantly higher specificity (74 % versus 71 %) in predicting the absence of myocardial infarction when compared to physicians' decisions if the patients were required to be admitted to the coronary care unit. If the decision to admit was based solely on the decision support system, the admission of patients without infarction to the coronary care unit would have been reduced by 11.5 % without adversely affecting patient outcomes or quality of care. The system was referred to as the Goldman algorithm and its performance was tested again by other researchers a decade later, confirming its success [41].

3.4.2 A Priori Probability

In supervised learning, the frequency distribution, or a priori probability, of the classes of a certain training set (or a sample taken from the general population) may be quite different from that of the general population to which the classifier is intended to be applied. In other words, the training set/sample may not represent the general population. For example, a particular training set may consist of 50 % of the subjects with disease and 50 % without the disease. In this case, a priori probabilities of the two classes in the training set are 0.5 for each class. However, the actual a priori probability or the actual prevalence of disease may be very different (less than or greater than 0.5) from that of the training set. In some instances, the actual a priori probability of the general population may be unknown to the researchers. This may have a negative effect on the performance of the classifier when applied to a real world data set. Therefore, it is necessary to adjust the output of a classifier with respect to the new condition to ensure the optimal performance of the classifier [42].

3.4.3 Unsupervised Learning

In unsupervised or undirected learning, the system is presented with a set of data but no information is available as to how to group the data into more meaningful classes (Fig. 3.1b). Based on perceived similarities that the learning system detects within the data set, the system develops classes or clusters until a set of definable patterns begins to emerge. There are no target variables; all variables are treated the same way without the distinction between dependent and independent variables.

Example 3.3 Avanzolini et al. analyzed 13 commonly monitored physiological variables in a group of 200 patients in the six-hour period immediately following cardiac surgery in an attempt to identify patients who were at risk for developing postoperative complications [43]. Using an unsupervised learning (clustering) method, the investigators showed the existence of two well defined categories of patients: those with low risk of developing postoperative complications and those with high risk.

Example 3.4 In a more recent study, Mullins et al. investigated the potential value of searching a large cohort of 667,000 inpatient and outpatient electronic records from an academic medical system, using three unsupervised methods: CliniMiner®, Predictive Analysis, and Pattern Discovery from IBM's HealthMiner®. The dataset included biological, clinical, and administrative data and they concluded that these approaches have the potential to expand research capabilities through identification of potentially novel clinical disease associations [44].

3.4.4 Classifiers for Supervised Learning

In supervised learning, classification refers to the mapping of data items into one of the predefined classes. In the development of data mining tools and clinical decision support systems that use statistical approaches like those described here, one of the critical tasks is to create a classification model, known as a classifier, which will predict the class of some entities or patterns based on the values of the input attributes. Choosing the right classifier is a critical step in the pattern recognition process. A variety of techniques have been used to obtain good classifiers. Some of the more widely used and well known techniques that are used in data mining include decision trees, logistic regression, neural networks, and nearest neighbor approach.

3.4.5 Decision Trees

The use of decision trees is perhaps the easiest to understand and the most widely used method that falls into the category of supervised learning. Figure 3.2 is the graphical representation of a simple decision tree using two attributes.

A typical decision tree system adopts a top-down strategy in searching for a solution. It consists of nodes where predictor attributes are tested. At each node, the algorithm examines all attributes and all values of each attribute with respect to determining the attribute and a value of the attribute that will "best" separate the data into more homogeneous subgroups with respect to the target variable. In other words, each node is a classification question and the branches of the tree are

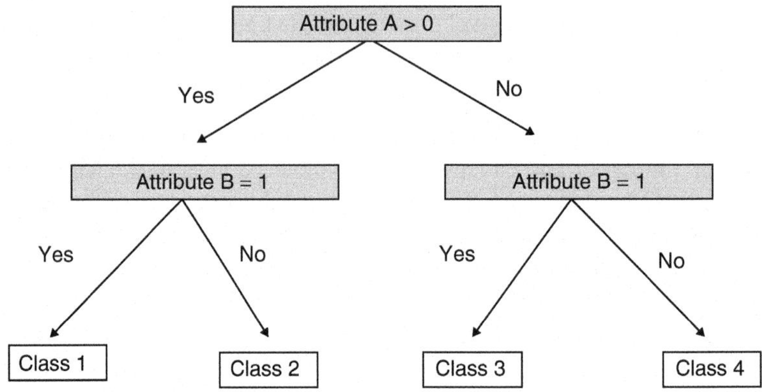

Fig. 3.2 A simple decision tree with the tests on attributes A and B

partitions of the data set into different classes. This process repeats itself in a recursive, iterative manner until no further separation of the data is feasible or a single classification can be applied to each member of the derived subgroups. Therefore, the terminal nodes at the end of the branches of the decision tree represent the different classes.

Example 3.5 An example of a clinical decision support system using decision trees can be found in a study by Gerald et al. [45]. The authors developed a decision tree that assisted health workers in predicting which contacts of tuberculosis patients were most likely to have positive tuberculin skin tests. The model was developed based on 292 consecutive cases and close to 3,000 contacts and subsequently tested prospectively on 366 new cases and 3,162 contacts. Testing showed that the decision tree model had a sensitivity of 94 %, a specificity of 28 %, and a false negative rate of 7 %. The authors concluded that the use of decision trees would decrease the number of contacts investigated by 25 % while maintaining a false negative rate that was close to that of the presumed background rate of latent tuberculosis infection in the region.

3.4.6 Logistic Regression

Logistic regression is used to model data in which the target or dependent variable is binary, i.e., the dependent variable can take the value 1 with a probability of success p, or the value 0 with the probability of failure $1 - p$. The main objective is to develop a regression type model relating the binary variable to the independent variables. As such it is a form of supervised learning. It can also be used to examine the variation in the dependent variable that can be explained by the independent variables, to rank the independent variables based on their relative importance in predicting the target variable, and to determine the interaction effects among independent variables. Rather than predicting the values of the dependent variable, logistic regression estimates the probability that a dependent variable will have a given value. For example, instead of predicting whether a patient is suffering from a certain disease, logistic regression tries to estimate the probability of the patient having the disease. If the estimated probability is greater than 0.5, then there is a higher probability of the patient having the disease than not having the disease. The function relating the probabilities to the independent variables is not a linear function and is represented by the following equation:

$$p(y) = 1/\left\{1 + e^{(-a-bx)}\right\}$$

where $p(y)$ is the probability that y, the dependent variable, occurs based on x, the value of an attribute/independent variable, a is the constant, and b is the coefficient of the independent variable. Figure 3.3 shows a graphical representation of the logistic regression model which fits the relationship between the value of the independent variable, x and the probability of dependent variable, y occurring with a special S-shaped curve that is mathematically constrained to remain within the range of 0.0–1.0 on the Y axis. Logistic regression is a well-established and powerful statistical method and it is often recommended that more recent data mining techniques, like the ones mentioned in the remainder of this chapter be compared to logistic regression to measure their relative performance [46].

Example 3.6 The following is an example that applies logistic regression to decision making. In the earliest stage of the epidemic of severe acute respiratory syndrome (SARS) when reliable rapid confirmatory tests were lacking, a group of researchers from Taiwan attempted to establish a scoring system to improve accuracy in diagnosing SARS [47]. The scoring system was developed based on the clinical and laboratory findings of 175 suspected cases using a multivariate, stepwise logistic regression model. The authors then applied the scoring system to 232 patients and were able to achieve a sensitivity and specificity of 100 % and 93 %, respectively, in diagnosing SARS.

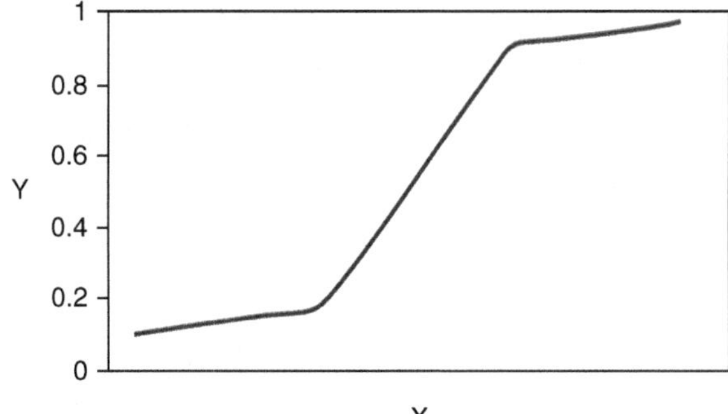

Fig. 3.3 Logistic regression model

Example 3.7 In another study, the authors applied texture analysis to images of breast tissue generated by magnetic resonance imaging (MRI) for differentiating between benign and malignant lesions [48]. Using logistic regression analysis, a diagnostic accuracy of 0.8 ± 0.07 was obtained with a model requiring only three parameters.

3.4.7 Neural Networks

The original development of the neural network programs was inspired by the way the brain recognizes patterns. A neural network is composed of a large number of processors known as neurons (after the brain cells that perform a similar function) that have a small amount of local memory and are connected unidirectionally (Fig. 3.4).

Each neuron can have more than one input and operates only on the inputs it receives via the connections. Like some of the data mining tools, neural networks can be supervised or unsupervised. In supervised neural networks, examples in the form of the training data are provided to the network one at a time. For each example, the network generates an output that is compared with the actual value as a form of feedback.

Once the output of the neural network is the same as the actual value, no further training is required. If the output differs from the actual value, the network adjusts those parameters that contributed to the incorrect output. Once adjustment is made, another example is presented to the network and the whole process is repeated. The process terminates when all parameters are stabilized. The size and representativeness of the training data are obviously very important, since a neural network could work fine on the training set, but not generalize to a broader sample.

This generalization problem led to the development of Support Vector Machines (SVMs). While neural networks try to minimize the error between the actual value

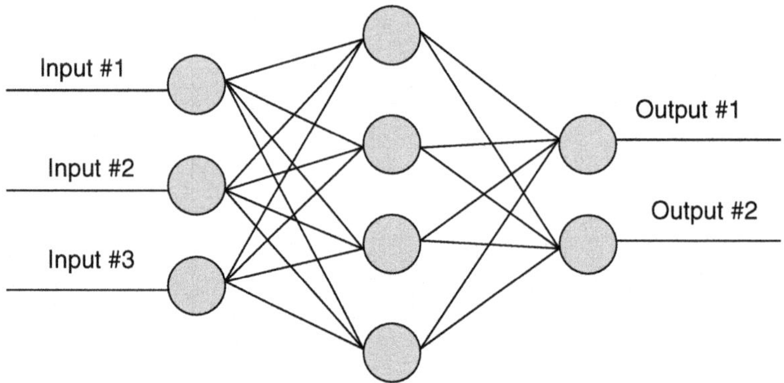

Fig. 3.4 Neural network

and their output for the training data, SVMs use the Structural Risk Minimization (SRM) principle to minimize an upper bound on the expected error risk [49]. SVMs have been gaining popularity over traditional neural networks due to their empirical performance.

Example 3.8 One example of a neural network is the computer-aided diagnosis of solid breast nodules. In one study, ultrasonographic features were extracted from 300 benign and 284 malignant biopsy-confirmed breast nodules [50]. The neural network was trained with a randomly selected data set consisting of half of the breast nodule ultrasonographic images. Using the trained neural network, surgery could be avoided in over half of the patients with benign nodules with a sensitivity of 99 %.

Example 3.9 In another example, a neural network was used to detect the disposition in children presenting to the emergency room with bronchiolitis (inflammation of small airways) [51]. The neural network correctly predicted the disposition in 81 % of test cases.

Example 3.10 The performance of a support vector machine method was compared to neural network, decision tree, and naïve Bayes methods in a study to develop a clinical decision support system for diagnosing patients with chronic renal failure. The data set included 102 patient records with 15 attributes. SVM was shown to be the most accurate with 93.1 %, compared to the other methods [25].

3.4.8 Nearest Neighbor Classifier

When a system uses the nearest neighbor (NN) classification, each attribute is assigned a dimension to form a multidimensional space. A training set of objects, whose classes are known, are analyzed for each attribute; each object is then plotted within the multidimensional space based on the values of all attributes. New objects, whose classes are yet to be determined, are then classified according to a simple rule; each new object is analyzed for the same set of attributes and is then plotted within the multidimensional space based on the value of each attribute. The new object is assigned to the same class of its closest neighbor based on appropriate metrics/measurements. In other words, the NN rule assumes that observations which are the closest together (based on some form of measurement) belong to the same category (Fig. 3.5). The NN rule is often used in situations where the user has no knowledge of the distribution of the categories.

One extension of this approach is the k-nearest neighbor approach (k- NN). Instead of comparing to a single nearest prototype, one can take into account k-neighboring points when classifying a data point, if the number of preclassified points is large. For each new pattern, the class is assigned by finding the most prominent class among the k-nearest data points in the training set (Fig. 3.5). This

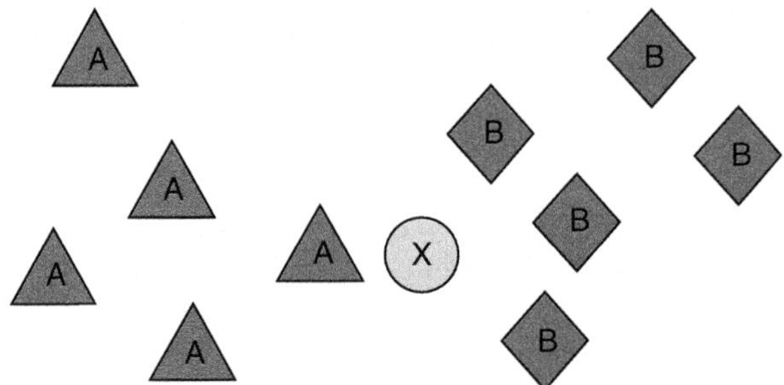

Fig. 3.5 Nearest neighbor (*NN*) classifier. There are two classes, A (*triangles*) and B (*diamonds*). The *circle* represents the unknown sample, X. For the NN rule the nearest neighbor of X comes from class A, so it would be labeled class A. Using the k-NN rule with k=4, three of the nearest neighbors of sample X come from class B, so it would be labeled as B

approach works very well in cases where a class does not form a single coherent group but is a collection of more than one separate group.

Example 3.11 By applying the k-NN classifier, Burroni et al. developed a decision support system to assist clinicians with distinguishing early melanoma from benign skin lesions, based on the analysis of digitized images obtained by epiluminescence microscopy [52]. Digital images of 201 melanomas and 449 benign nevi were included in the study and were separated into two groups, a learning set and a test set. A k-NN pattern recognition classifier was constructed using all available image features and trained for a sensitivity of 98 % with the learning set. Using an independent test set of images, a mean specificity of 79 % was achieved with a sensitivity of 98 %. The authors concluded that this approach might improve early diagnosis of melanoma and reduce unnecessary surgery.

3.5 Evaluation of Classifiers

3.5.1 ROC Graphs

In statistical pattern recognition, the goal is to map entities to classes. Therefore, the ultimate question is: which classifiers are more accurate in performing this classification task? Suppose one wanted to identify which classifiers would be best to determine whether a patient has cancer or not based on the results of certain laboratory tests. Given a classifier and an instance, there are four possible outcomes. If the patient has cancer and is diagnosed with cancer, based on the classifier, it is considered a true positive; if the patient is declared healthy by the classifier, but really has cancer, it is considered a false negative. If the patient has no cancer and is declared healthy, it is considered a true negative; if he is diagnosed as having cancer when he is really healthy, it is considered a false positive.

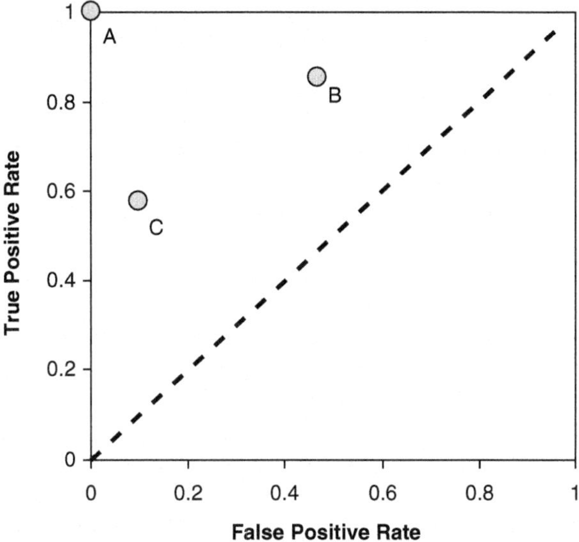

Fig. 3.6 ROC curve. Point *A* represents perfect performance. The performance of *C* is more conservative than *B*

We can plot the true positive rate on the Y axis and the false positive rate on the X axis; a receiver operating characteristic (ROC) graph results (Fig. 3.6).

The true positive rate (also known as sensitivity) is obtained by dividing the number of true positives by the sum of true positives and false negatives. The false positive rate is obtained by dividing the number of false positives by the sum of true negatives and false positives; the false positive rate can also be expressed as "1 minus specificity," where specificity is equal to true negatives divided by the sum of true negatives and false positives. The ROC graph is a two-dimensional graph that depicts the tradeoffs between benefits (detecting cancer correctly, or true positive) and costs (false alarm or false positive). Each classifier generates a pair of true positive and false positive rates, which corresponds to a point on the ROC graph. The point (0, 1) represents perfect classification, i.e., 100 % true positive rate and 0 % false positive rate. One classifier is considered superior to another if it has a higher true positive rate and a lower false positive rate, corresponding to a more "northwest" location relative to the other on the ROC graph. In general, the false alarm rates go up as one attempts to increase the true positive rate. Classifiers with points on the southwest corner of an ROC graph are more "conservative" since they make positive predictions only with strong evidence; therefore there is a low true positive rate, but also few false positive errors. On the other hand, classifiers on the northeast corner of an ROC graph are more "liberal" since they make positive prediction with weak evidence; therefore they have high true positive rates, but also high false positive rates.

Some classifiers, such as neural networks, yield a numeric value which can be in the form of a numeric score or probability that represents the likelihood an object belongs to a certain class. These classifiers can be converted into discrete, binary (yes versus no) classifiers by setting a threshold, i.e., if the output score is above the threshold, the classifier produces a “Yes", else a "No”. By choosing a different threshold, a different point in the ROC graph is produced. As a result, varying the thresholds will produce a curve in the ROC graph for a particular classifier. Given an ROC curve, one can select the threshold corresponding to a particular point on the ROC that produces the desired binary classifier with the best true positive rate (correctly diagnosed cancer) within the constraints of an acceptable false positive rate (false alarm). This is chosen based on the relative costs of the two types of errors: missing a diagnosis of cancer (type I error) versus creating a false alarm (type II error).

The area under the ROC curve (AUC) provides a single statistic (the C- Statistic) for comparing classifiers. It measures the accuracy of the classifiers. Consider the situation in which a classifier attempts to separate patients into two groups; those with disease and those without. One can randomly pick a patient from the disease group and one from the non-disease group and apply the classifier on both. The area under the curve represents the percentage of randomly drawn pairs where the classifier correctly classifies the two patients in the random pair. The value of AUC ranges from 0.5 to 1. A classifier with an AUC of 0.5 would be a poor classifier, roughly equivalent to flipping a coin to decide the class membership. A classifier with an AUC close to 1 results in better classification of entities to classes. For example, in Example 3.8, the resulting trained neural network model yielded a normalized area under the ROC curve of 0.95.

Computing the AUC is complex and beyond the scope of this chapter. Briefly, there are two commonly used methods. One method is based on the construction of trapezoids under the curve as an approximation of the area. The other method employs a maximum likelihood estimator to fit a smooth curve to the data points. Both methods are available as computer programs and give an estimate of area and standard error that can be used to compare different classifiers.

3.5.2 Kolmogorov-Smirnov Test

While the AUC provides a way of distinguishing groups overall, there are other statistical tests used to provide a more refined comparison of groups or subgroups. The Kolmogorov-Smirnov test, or KS test, is used to determine whether the distributions of two samples differ from each other or whether the distribution of a sample differs from that of the general population. The KS test provides what is called the D-statistic for comparison of classifiers [53].

3.6 Unsupervised Learning

3.6.1 Cluster Analysis

Unsupervised classification refers to situations where the goal is to classify a diverse collection of unlabeled data into different groups based on different features in a data set. Unsupervised classification, also known as cluster analysis or clustering, is a general term to describe methodologies that are designed to find natural groupings or clusters based on measured or perceived similarities among the items in the clusters using a multidimensional data set (Fig. 3.7). There is no need to identify the groupings desired or the features that should be used to classify the data set. In addition, clustering offers a generalized description of each cluster, resulting in better understanding of the data set's characteristics and providing a starting point for exploring further relationships.

Clustering techniques are very useful in data mining because of the speed, reliability, and consistency with which they can organize a large amount of data into distinct groupings. Despite the availability of a vast collection of clustering algorithms in the literature, they are based on two popular approaches: hierarchical clustering and nonhierarchical clustering. The former, which is the most frequently used technique, organizes data in a nested sequence of groups that can be displayed in a tree-like structure, or dendrogram.

There are several problems that are associated with clustering. One problem is that data can be grouped into clusters with different shapes and sizes. Another problem is the resolution or granularity, i.e., fine versus coarse, with which the data are viewed. This problem is most obvious when one tries to delineate a region containing a high density of patterns compared to the background. Therefore, some authors define a cluster as one that consists of a relatively high density of points separated from other clusters by a relatively low density of points, whereas some define clusters containing samples that share more similarities to each other than to samples of different clusters. As a result, the selection of an appropriate measure of similarity to define clusters is a major challenge in cluster analysis.

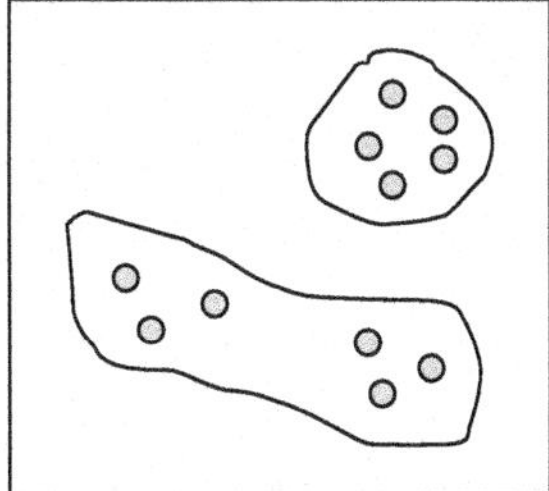

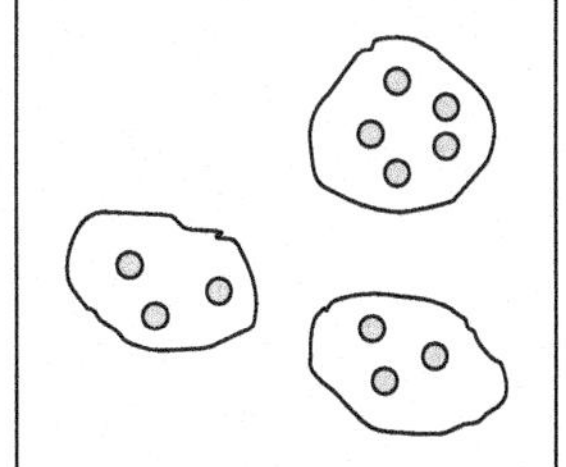

Fig. 3.7 Cluster analysis. Two clusters of data (*left*); three clusters (*right*) using the same set of data

3.6.2 Gene Expression Data Analysis

One of the applications of cluster analysis in medicine is the analysis of gene expression. With the completion of the human genome project, which identified more than 30,000 gene sequences, researchers have been able to examine the expression of several thousand genes from blood, body fluids, and tissue samples at the same time, in an attempt to identify gene subsets that are associated with various disease characteristics. The pace of gene expression data analysis has been further accelerated by the "Precision Medicine" initiative that takes into account individual variability in genes, when approaching disease treatment and prevention [54]. Since information is obtained from hundreds and thousands of gene sequences, an astronomical body of data is generated. Common research questions often fall under the following categories: class discovery, class prediction, and gene identification. Class prediction refers to the classification of samples based on certain behaviors or properties such as response to therapy, whereas gene identification involves the discovery of genes that are differentially expressed among different disease groups.

Class discovery refers to the discovery of previously unknown categories or subtypes based on some similarity measure calculated from the gene expression data. Cluster analysis is often the method of choice in accomplishing this task, because samples are clustered into groups based on the similarity of their gene expressions without utilizing any knowledge of any predefined classification schemes such as known histological tumor classification.

Example 3.12 Genomic data is already being incorporated into clinical decision support systems to refine both diagnosis and therapy. The following is an example that used clustering to explore breast cancer classification using genomic data. In this study, Perou et al. evaluated the pattern of gene expression of 8,102 human genes in 65 breast cancers obtained from 42 patients [55]. Using hierarchical cluster analysis, the authors were able to classify 65 breast cancer samples into three distinct subtypes. One subtype was cancers that overexpressed the oncogene *erbB-2*. The remaining two subtypes were unknown prior to this study; they were estrogen receptor-positive luminal-like cancers and basaloid cancers. Subsequent survival analyses on a group of patients with locally advanced breast cancer showed significantly different outcomes for the patients belonging to different subtypes; patients with basaloid cancers had a poor survival rate [56]. In the same study by Perou et al., the samples contained 20 primary tumors that were biopsied twice, before and after the completion of chemotherapy. Using clustering, the authors demonstrated that gene expression patterns were similar among samples from the same patients taken at different time points but not between samples taken from different patients.

Example 3.13 A more comprehensive study of the use of genomic data for predicting clinical outcomes compares several naïve Bayes methods, logistic regression, a version of linear regression, a faster version of a neural network, and a support vector machine. The researchers used a hundred 1,000-single nucleotide polymorphism (SNP) simulated datasets, ten 10,000-SNP datasets, six semi-synthetic sets, and two real genome-wide association studies (GWAS) datasets and concluded that the support vector machine performed best on the 1,000-SNP dataset, while the Bayesian network-based methods performed best on the other datasets, with the efficient Bayesian multivariate classifier (EBMC) method showing the best overall performance [57].

3.7 Other Techniques

The goal of any tool that is used for pattern recognition is to arrive at an optimal solution within a given set of complex constraints. The development of sophisticated computer-based computation techniques has enabled analysts to attain better solutions than previous techniques. As improved techniques are developed to handle increasingly complex problems, there is a corresponding need for more innovative methods for arriving at optimal solutions. Genetic algorithms, biologic and quantum computing, Big Data analytics, and hybrid methods are examples of innovative techniques that have gained increasing acceptance and application in the field of pattern recognition and data mining.

3.7.1 Genetic Algorithms

The fundamental concept of genetic algorithms has its roots in Darwin's evolutionary theories of natural selection and adaptation. According to Darwin, organisms that come up with successful solutions to best support them and protect themselves from harm survive, whereas those organisms that fail to adapt to their environment become extinct. Based on the same idea of "survival of the fittest," a genetic algorithm initially tries to solve a given problem with random solutions. These solutions are often referred to as the genomes, or a collection of genes. The gene represents the smallest unit of information for the construction of possible solutions. The next step is to evaluate or quantify the fitness of all the available genomes or solutions based on a fitness function. The latter returns a value of goodness or fitness so that a particular genome or solution may be ranked against all other genomes or solutions. Those solutions with better fit are ranked higher among others and are allowed to "breed." Once the initial evaluation is completed, the genetic algorithms examine new solutions by letting all the current solutions "evolve" through mutual exchange of "genetic materials" among solutions to improve the genomes and/or mutation (i.e., randomly changing the genetic materials) to "create" new solutions. The new solutions are then evaluated using the same fitness functions to determine which solutions are good and which are not and need to be eliminated. Thus the process repeats itself until an "optimal" solution is attained.

There are many benefits of genetic algorithms. One major advantage is that a genetic algorithm almost always guarantees finding some reasonable solution to problems, particularly those that we have no idea how to solve. Further, the final solution is often superior to the initial collection of possible solutions. Another benefit is that genetic algorithms tend to arrive at a solution much faster than other optimization techniques. Also, the strength of the genetic algorithm does not depend upon complex algorithms but rather on relatively simple concepts. Despite the power of genetic algorithms, however, some parameters, such as the size of the solution population, the rate of mutation and crossover, and the selection methods and criteria, can significantly affect their performance. For example, if the solution population size is too small, the genetic algorithm may have exhausted all the available solutions before the process can identify an optimal solution. If the rate of genetic mutation is too high, the process may be changing too fast for the selection to ever bring about convergence, resulting in the failure of generating an optimal solution.

Example 3.14 Genetic algorithms have been used to construct clinical decision support systems. In a study by Zellner et al., the authors evaluated the performance of a logistic regression model in diagnosing brain tumors with magnetic resonance spectroscopy using the genetic algorithms approach [58]. The genetic algorithm approach was superior to the conventional approach in 14 out of 18 trials, and the genetic algorithm had fewer false negatives and false positives. In addition, the authors also pointed out that the genetic algorithm approach was less costly.

Example 3.15 Genetic algorithms have also been used as a data mining technique in healthcare operations. One study investigated whether genetic algorithms could be used to predict the risk of in-hospital mortality of cancer patients [59]. A total of 201 cancer patients, over a 2-year period of time, was retrospectively evaluated. Compared to other methods, such as multivariate logistic regression, neural networks, and recursive partitioning analysis, genetic algorithms selected the least number of explanatory variables with a comparable proportion of the cases explained (79 %). The authors concluded that genetic algorithms reliably predicted in-hospital mortality of cancer patients and were as efficient as the other data mining techniques examined.

Example 3.16 In a more recent study, an improved adaptive genetic algorithm method was used to create a decision support system to assess fetal well-being based on cardiotocogram (CTG) data. The classification resulted in a satisfactory accuracy rate of 94% [60].

3.7.2 Biological Computing

Biological computing is another discipline that has found its way into data mining applications. It cuts across two well established fields: computer science and biology. While the genetic algorithm approach uses the analogy of natural selection to develop computer algorithms, the idea of biological computing actually involves the use of living organisms or their components, e.g., DNA strands, to perform computing operations. The benefits include the ability to hold enormous amounts of information, the capability of massive parallel processing, self-assembly, self-healing, self- adaptation, and energy efficiency. Scientists have already created genetic logic gates that prove the existence of what is called the transcriptor, which is a biological version of transistors used in computer processors [61]. For now, a biological computer can only perform rudimentary functions, but its potential continues to emerge. For example, some scientists have been working on the development of tiny DNA computers that circulate in a person's body to monitor his/her well-being and release the right drugs to repair damaged tissue or fight off infections and cancers [62].

3.7.3 Quantum Computing

Quantum computing is also a relatively new and exciting discipline that promises similar benefits listed for biological computing. It is a vast discipline that studies subjects beyond computing, such as coding, cryptography, communication channels and error correction, and data mining, under the umbrella of quantum information science. All these subjects are studies from the perspective of ideas and tools introduced by the quantum mechanics. Entanglement and superposition are the two crucial concepts of quantum mechanics that make the quantum perspective so powerful, compared to the traditional/classical perspective. Quantum computing research has been conducted at very cold temperatures closer to absolute zero (−460 °F), because it has not been possible for the subatomic particles to be captured at a certain quantum state at higher temperatures. Because of this challenge, today's quantum computing capacity is very limited. However, experimental research has been promising: an international group of researchers have already been able to store data at room temperature for 39 min [63]. Most of the data mining methods inspired by techniques of quantum information science do not require quantum computers; they are simply quantum inspired algorithms of the data mining techniques discussed in this chapter. For example, Lu et al. developed a quantum-based evolving artificial neural network with few connections and high classification performance by optimizing the network structure and connection weights simultaneously. They tested the model using problematic and normal sample data for breast cancer, iris and heart related diseases, and diabetes and concluded that the quantum-based model performed better than traditional models included in the comparison [64].

3.7.4 Incorporating Fuzzy Logic and Other Hybrid Methods

The idea of fuzzy logic originated from the fuzzy set theory developed to deal with problems in control systems [65]. In essence, fuzzy logic deals with the cognitive uncertainty expressed in human language [66]. For example, when humans say "hot", there is a range of temperature measurements that would qualify as hot, depending on the context. On the other hand, computers are deterministic and unable to handle uncertainty. Fuzzy logic methods help data mining systems to incorporate cognitive uncertainty by allowing quantified partial membership of categories. For example, 30 °F could be considered only 2 % hot, where 95 °F is considered 90 % hot. Fuzzy logic supervised data mining systems allow degrees of membership to be determined during training. Although there is a lot of emphasis on codifying data in the era of electronic health records, there will always be situations where cognitive uncertainty cannot be avoided. Fuzzy logic methods are especially useful when mining such datasets. The fuzzy logic approach has been used with many of the data mining methods described in this chapter. For example, Nguyen et al. used a genetic fuzzy logic system and wavelets to classify breast cancer and heart disease datasets and found the proposed method to be superior to other classification methods [67].

The data mining methods described here are often used together to utilize particular strengths of each to address particular challenges a given project poses. In one such study, Seera and Lim compared the performance of a hybrid intelligent system (consisting of a fuzzy min-max neural network, a classification and regression tree, and a random forest model) in classifying breast cancer, diabetes, and liver disorder datasets. They found the hybrid system performed better than other systems reported in the literature [68].

3.7.5 Big Data Analytics

Although the unique challenges of health care led it to be slow in adopting Big Data analytics compared to other industries, the healthcare industry is now investing a lot of effort into large-scale integration and analysis of its challenging big data. This is especially apparent with the National Institutes of Health's (NIH) Big Data to Knowledge (BD2K) initiative for biomedical big data [69]. The data science community at NIH describes biomedical big data as a very large amount of data from a large number of data sources that is complex and diverse with many challenges and opportunities. The BD2K initiative that approaches the biomedical big data strategically, basically includes all of the data mining methods for clinical decision support systems that are discussed in this chapter and much more. Together with the "Precision Medicine" initiative mentioned above in the gene expression data analysis section, the BD2K initiative is likely to determine the path for data mining research for clinical decision support systems in the near future. Jensen et al. present a nice review of current resources and initiatives, challenges, and the outlook for mining electronic health records[70].

3.8 Conclusions

Data mining refers to the process of pattern and relationship discovery within large data sets. It holds promise in many areas of health care and medical research, with applications ranging from medical diagnosis to quality assurance. The power of data mining lies in its ability to allow users to consider data from a variety of perspectives in order to discover apparent or hidden patterns. There are two main divisions of classification: supervised learning or training and unsupervised learning. Supervised training requires training samples to be labeled with a known category or outcome to be applied to the classifier. There are many classifiers available and their performance can be assessed using an ROC curve. Unsupervised learning, also known as clustering, refers to methodologies that are designed to find natural groupings or clusters without the benefit of a training set. The goal is to discover hidden or new relationships within the data set. One application of clustering is the analysis of gene expression data. Genetic algorithms and biological and quantum computing, as well as Big Data analytics are newer disciplines that have found their way into data mining applications and clinical decision support systems.

References

1. Fayyad UM, Piatetsky-Shapiro G, Smyth P. Knowledge discovery and data mining: towards a unifying framework. Proceedings of the 2nd International Conference on Knowledge Discovery and Data Mining. Portland. pp. 82–88. August 1996. AAAI Press. Available from: http://ww-aig.jpl.nasa.gov.kdd96. Accessed 17 July 2006.
2. Leatherman S, Peterson E, Heinen L, Quam L. Quality screening and management using claims data in a managed care setting. QRB Qual Rev Bull. 1991;17:349–59.
3. Finlay PN. Introducing decision support systems. Cambridge, MA: Blackwell Publishers; 1994.
4. Huber S, Medl M, Vesely M, Czembirek H, Zuna I, Delorme S. Ultrasonographic tissue characterization in monitoring tumor response to neoadjuvant chemotherapy in locally advanced breast cancer (work in progress). J Ultrasound Med. 2000;19:677–86.
5. Christodoulou CI, Pattichis CS. Unsupervided pattern recognition for the classification of EMG signals. IEEE Trans Biomed Eng. 1999;46:169–78.
6. Karayiannis NB, Mukherjee A, Glover JR, Frost J, Hrachovy JR, Mizrahi EM. An evaluation of quantum neural networks in the detection of epileptic seizures in the neonatal electroencephalogram. Soft Comput. 2006;10:382–96.
7. Banez LL, Prasanna P, Sun L, et al. Diagnostic potential of serum proteomic patterns in prostate cancer. J Urol. 2003;170(2 Pt 1):442–26.
8. Leonard JE, Colombe JB, Levy JL. Finding relevant references to genes and proteins in Medline using a Bayesian approach. Bioinformatics. 2002;18:1515–22.

9. Bins M, van Montfort LH, Timmers T, Landeweerd GH, Gelsema ES, Halie MR. Classification of immature and mature cells of the neutrophil series using morphometrical parameters. Cytometry. 1983;3:435–8.
10. Hibbard LS, McKeel Jr DW. Automated identification and quantitative morphometry of the senile plaques of Alzheimer's disease. Anal Quant Cytol Histol. 1997;19:123–38.
11. Baumgartner C, Bohm C, Baumgartner D, et al. Supervised machine learning techniques for the classification of metabolic disorders in newborns. Bioinformatics. 2004;20:2985–96.
12. Gordon HS, Johnson ML, Wray NP, et al. Mortality after noncardiac surgery: prediction from administrative versus clinical data. Med Care. 2005;43:159–67.
13. Ocak H. A medical decision support system based on support vector machines and the genetic algorithm for the evaluation of fetal well-being. J Med Syst. 2013;37:1–9.
14. Caruana R, Lou Y, Gehrke J, Koch P, Sturm M, Elhadad N. Intelligible models for healthcare: predicting pneumonia risk and hospital 30-day readmission. Proceedings of the 21th ACM SIGKDD International Conference on Knowledge Discovery and Data Mining. 2015. pp. 1721–30.
15. Tekin C, Atan O, van der Schaar M. Discover the expert: context-adaptive expert selection for medical diagnosis. IEEE Trans Emerg Topics Comput. 2015;3:220–34. IEEE.
16. Zhuang ZY, Churilov L, Burstein F, Sikaris K. Combining data mining and case-based reasoning for intelligent decision support for pathology ordering by general practitioners. Eur J Oper Res. 2009;195:662–75.
17. Rane AL. Clinical decision support model for prevailing diseases to improve human life survivability. 2015 International Conference on Pervasive Computing (ICPC), 2015. pp. 1–5.
18. Wang X, Sontag D, Wang F. Unsupervised learning of disease progression models. Proceedings of the 20th ACM SIGKDD international conference on knowledge discovery and data mining. 2014. pp. 85–94.
19. Dilsizian SE, Siegel EL. Artificial intelligence in medicine and cardiac imaging: harnessing big data and advanced computing to provide personalized medical diagnosis and treatment. Curr Cardiol Rep. 2014;16:1–8.
20. Anooj P. Clinical decision support system: risk level prediction of heart disease using weighted fuzzy rules. J King Saud Univ-Comput Inf Sci. 2012;24:27–40.
21. Srinivas K, Rani BK, Govrdhan A. Applications of data mining techniques in healthcare and prediction of heart attacks. Int J Comput Sci Eng (IJCSE). 2010;2:250–5.
22. Bowd C, Chan K, Zangwill LM, Goldbaum MH, Lee T-W, Sejnowski TJ, et al. Comparing neural networks and linear discriminant functions for glaucoma detection using confocal scanning laser ophthalmoscopy of the optic disc. Investig Ophthalmol Vis Sci. 2002;43:3444–54.
23. Lin A, Hoffman D, Gaasterland DE, Caprioli J. Neural networks to identify glaucomatous visual field progression. Am J Ophthalmol. 2003;135:49–54.
24. Bengtsson B, Bizios D, Heijl A. Effects of input data on the performance of a neural network in distinguishing normal and glaucomatous visual fields. Invest Ophthalmol Vis Sci. 2005;46:3730–6.
25. Al-Hyari AY, Al-Taee AM, Al-Taee MA. Diagnosis and classification of chronic renal failure utilising intelligent data mining classifiers. Int J Inf Technol Web Eng (IJITWE). 2014;9:1–12.
26. Yeh D-Y, Cheng C-H, Chen Y-W. A predictive model for cerebrovascular disease using data mining. Expert Syst Applic. 2011;38:8970–7.
27. Lee BJ, Kim JY. Identification of type 2 diabetes risk factors using phenotypes consisting of anthropometry and triglycerides based on machine learning. IEEE J Biomed Health Inform. 2016;20(1):39–46. doi:10.1109/JBHI.2015.2396520.
28. Dugan T, Mukhopadhyay S, Carroll A, Downs S, et al. Machine learning techniques for prediction of early childhood obesity. Appl Clin Inform. 2015;6:506–20.
29. Marakas GM. Decision support systems. 2nd ed. Princeton: Prentice Hall; 2002.
30. Ambrosiadou BV, Goulis DG, Pappas C. Clinical evaluation of the DIABETES expert system for decision support by multiple regimen insulin dose adjustment. Comp Methods Programs Biomed. 1996;49:105–15.

31. Marchevsky AM, Coons G. Expert systems as an aid for the pathologist's role of clinical consultant: CANCER-STAGE. Mod Pathol. 1993;6:265–9.
32. Nguyen AN, Hartwell EA, Milam JD. A rule-based expert system for laboratory diagnosis of hemoglobin disorders. Arch Pathol Lab Med. 1996;120:817–27.
33. Papaloukas C, Fotiadis DI, Likas A, Stroumbis CS, Michalis LK. Use of a novel rule-based expert system in the detection of changes in the ST segment and the T wave in long duration ECGs. J Electrocardiol. 2002;35:27–34.
34. Riss PA, Koelbl H, Reinthaller A, Deutinger J. Development and application of simple expert systems in obstetrics and gynecology. J Perinat Med. 1988;16:283–7.
35. Sailors RM, East TD. A model-based simulator for testing rule-based decision support systems for mechanical ventilation of ARDS patients. Proc Ann Symp Comp Appl Med Care. 1994:1007. http://www.ncbi.nlm.nih.gov/pmc/articles/PMC2247879/.
36. Shortliffe EH, Davis R, Axline SG, Buchanan BG, Green CC, Cohen SN. Computer-based consultations in clinical therapeutics: explanation and rule acquisition capabilities of the MYCIN system. Comput Biomed Res. 1975;8:303–20.
37. Duda RO, Hart PE, Stork DG. Pattern classification and scene analysis. 2nd ed. New York: Wiley; 2000.
38. Fukunaga K. Introduction to statistical pattern recognition. 2nd ed. New York: Academic; 1990.
39. Schalkoff RJ. Pattern recognition: statistical, structural and neural approaches. New York: Wiley; 1991.
40. Goldman L, Cook EF, Brand DA, et al. A computer protocol to predict myocardial infarction in emergency department patients with chest pain. N Engl J Med. 1988;318:797–803.
41. Qamar A, McPherson C, Babb J, Bernstein L, Werdmann M, Yasick D, et al. The Goldman algorithm revisited: prospective evaluation of a computer-derived algorithm versus unaided physician judgment in suspected acute myocardial infarction. Am Heart J. 1999;138:705–9.
42. Scott AJ, Wild CJ. Fitting logistic models under case-control or choice based sampling. J Roy Stat Soc B. 1986;48:170–82.
43. Avanzolini G, Barbini P, Gnudi G. Unsupervised learning and discriminant analysis applied to identification of high risk postoperative cardiac patients. Int J Biomed Comp. 1990;25:207–21.
44. Mullins IM, Siadaty MS, Lyman J, Scully K, Garrett CT, Miller WG, et al. Data mining and clinical data repositories: insights from a 667,000 patient data set. Comput Biol Med. 2006;36:1351–77.
45. Gerald LB, Tang S, Bruce F, et al. A decision tree for tuberculosis contact investigation [see comment]. Am J Respir Crit Care Med. 2002;166:1122–7.
46. Bellazzi R, Zupan B. Predictive data mining in clinical medicine: current issues and guidelines. Int J Med Inform. 2008;77:81–97.
47. Wang TL, Jang TN, Huang CH, et al. Establishing a clinical decision rule of severe acute respiratory syndrome at the emergency department. Ann Emerg Med. 2004;43:17–22.
48. Gibbs P, Turnbull LW. Textural analysis of contrast-enhanced MR images of the breast. Magn Reson Med. 2003;50:92–8.
49. Haykin S. Neural networks and learning machines. New York: Prentice Hall/Pearson; 2009.
50. Joo S, Yang YS, Moon WK, Kim HC. Computer-aided diagnosis of solid breast nodules: use of an artificial neural network based on multiple sonographic features. IEEE Transact Med Imaging. 2004;23:1292–300.
51. Walsh P, Cunningham P, Rothenberg SJ, O'Doherty S, Hoey H, Healy R. An artificial neural network ensemble to predict disposition and length of stay in children presenting with bronchiolitis. Eur J Emerg Med. 2004;11:259–564.
52. Burroni M, Corona R, Dell'Eva G, et al. Melanoma computer-aided diagnosis: reliability and feasibility study. Clin Cancer Res. 2004;10:1881–6.
53. Press WH, Flannery BP, Teukolsky SA, Vetterling WT. Numerical recipes in FORTRAN example book: the art of scientific computing. 2nd ed. New York: Cambridge University Press; 1992.

54. Collins FS, Varmus H. A new initiative on precision medicine. New Engl J Med Mass Med Soc. 2015;372:793–5.
55. Perou CM, Sorlie T, Eisen MB, et al. Molecular portraits of human breast tumours. Nature. 2000;406:747–52.
56. Sorlie T, Perou CM, Tibshirani R, et al. Gene expression patterns of breast carcinomas distinguish tumor subclasses with clinical implications. Proc Natl Acad Sci U S A. 2001;98:10869–74.
57. Jiang X, Cai B, Xue D, Lu X, Cooper GF, Neapolitan RE. A comparative analysis of methods for predicting clinical outcomes using high-dimensional genomic datasets. J Am Med Inform Assoc. 2014;21:e312–9.
58. Zellner BB, Rand SD, Prost R, Krouwer H, Chetty VK. A cost-minimizing diagnostic methodology for discrimination between neoplastic and non-neoplastic brain lesions: utilizing a genetic algorithm. Acad Radiol. 2004;11:169–77.
59. Bozcuk H, Bilge U, Koyuncu E, Gulkesen H. An application of a genetic algorithm in conjunction with other data mining methods for estimating outcome after hospitalization in cancer patients. Med Sci Monit. 2004;10:CR246–51.
60. Ravindran S, Jambek AB, Muthusamy H, Neoh S-C. A novel clinical decision support system using improved adaptive genetic algorithm for the assessment of fetal well-being. Comput Math Methods Med. 2015;2015:283532. doi:10.1155/2015/283532.
61. Bonnet J, Yin P, Ortiz ME, Subsoontorn P, Endy D. Amplifying genetic logic gates. Science. 2013;340:599–603.
62. Benenson Y, Gil B, Ben-Dor U, Adar R, Shapiro E. An autonomous molecular computer for logical control of gene expression. Nature. 2004;429:423–9.
63. Saeedi K, Simmons S, Salvail JZ, Dluhy P, Riemann H, Abrosimov NV, et al. Room-temperature quantum bit storage exceeding 39 minutes using ionized donors in silicon-28. Science. 2013;342:830–3.
64. Lu T-C, Yu G-R, Juang J-C. Quantum-based algorithm for optimizing artificial neural networks. IEEE Trans Neural Netw Learn Syst. 2013;24:1266–78.
65. Zadeh LA. Fuzzy sets. Information and control. World Sci. 1965;8:338–53.
66. Rokach L. Using fuzzy logic in data mining. In: Maimon O, Rokach L, editors. Data mining and knowledge discovery handbook. New York: Springer; 2010. p. 505–20.
67. Nguyen T, Khosravi A, Creighton D, Nahavandi S. Classification of healthcare data using genetic fuzzy logic system and wavelets. Expert Syst Applic. 2015;42:2184–97.
68. Seera M, Lim CP. A hybrid intelligent system for medical data classification. Expert Syste Applic. 2014;41:2239–49.
69. Margolis R, Derr L, Dunn M, Huerta M, Larkin J, Sheehan J, et al. The National Institutes of health's big data to knowledge (BD2K) initiative: capitalizing on biomedical big data. JAMIA. 2014;21:957–8.
70. Jensen PB, Jensen LJ, Brunak S. Mining electronic health records: towards better research applications and clinical care. Nat Rev Genet. 2012;13:395–405.

Chapter 4
Usability and Clinical Decision Support

Yang Gong and Hong Kang

Abstract Clinical decision support systems (CDSS) link clinical observations with health knowledge to assist clinical decisions. The systems influence clinicians' decisions and consequently enhance healthcare quality. Unfortunately, widespread adoption and user acceptance have not been achieved in most clinical settings since CDSS are not immune to common usability problems of health information technology. This chapter describes clinical and technical issues related to the usability of CDSS.

The clinical issues that affect usability are mainly associated with workflow integration and the growing body of knowledge that needs to be incorporated in clinical decision making. Technical issues include those related to knowledge representation, knowledge base construction and maintenance, and system implementation. The chapter also includes discussions on reducing alert fatigue and improving human-computer interaction in CDSS. It is expected that integrating CDSS with electronic health records will improve healthcare quality and patient safety and improve the timeliness of the adoption of research into practice.

Keywords Usability • Ontology • Workflow integration • Alert fatigue • Knowledge base • Human-computer interaction • Knowledge representation

4.1 CDSS Usability and Functionality

"Clinical decision support systems (CDSS) are computer systems designed to assist clinicians in making decisions regarding individual patients at a specific point in time" [1]. By linking clinical observations with health knowledge, CDSS influence

Y. Gong, M.D., Ph.D. (✉)
School of Biomedical Informatics, University of Texas Health Science Center at Houston, 7000 Fannin St., Suite 165, Houston, TX 77030, USA
e-mail: Yang.Gong@uth.tmc.edu; gongyang@gmail.com

H. Kang, Ph.D.
Postdoctoral Fellow of UTHealth Innovation in Cancer Prevention Research Training Program, University of Texas Health Science Center at Houston, 7000 Fannin St., Suite 165, Houston, TX 77030, USA
e-mail: Hong.Kang@uth.tmc.edu

E.S. Berner (ed.), *Clinical Decision Support Systems*, Health Informatics, DOI 10.1007/978-3-319-31913-1_4

clinical decisions and consequently enhance healthcare quality. Researchers have been striving to produce viable CDSS to support all aspects of clinical tasks. However, except for minor successes in the pharmacy and billing sectors [2], most CDSS suffer from common problems in usability, which have received significant attention in the patient safety community [3–8].

Usability is widely accepted as a crucial feature in industrial product design in industries such as aviation, nuclear power, automobile, consumer software, consumer electronics, etc. In contrast, the use of usability principles in the design of Electronic Health Records (EHR) and CDSS has been sporadic and unsystematic, partly due to the lack of attention and effective design and assessment frameworks [9].

"Usability refers to how useful, usable and satisfying a system is for the intended users to accomplish goals in the work domain by performing certain sequences of tasks [10]." "Useful" is described by Zhang and Walji as "how well a system supports the work domain where users accomplish goals for their work independent of how the system is implemented"; how "usable" a system is can be measured by learnability, efficiency and error tolerance; "satisfaction" refers to the subjective impression of how useful, usable and likable a system is to a user [10].

Usability is an emergent quality that reflects the grasp and the reach of human-computer interaction (HCI). HCI is defined as "the study of how humans interact with computers, and how to design computer systems that are easy, quick and productive for humans to use" [11]. It is crucial that CDSS incorporate a greatly improved HCI paradigm for the presentation of both solicited and unsolicited recommendations. Sittig et al., in discussing what they refer to as "grand challenges" of CDSS, emphasize that one of the usability challenges for CDSS is to make them operate unobtrusively, in the background, yet still be effective and specific in reminding the users of things that they may have forgotten, misinterpreted, or overlooked or present new data prior to the decision, rather than correcting users after the fact [12]. Currently, a major concern has been the massive number of alerts presented to the user. When exposed to frequent and overwhelming alerts in daily practice, clinicians may become insensitive to the alerts and consequently may pay less attention, or even override them without offering meaningful reasons. This phenomenon is called "alert fatigue" and it reflects how busy clinicians become desensitized to safety alerts [13]. Alert fatigue can be extremely dangerous because the critical alerts that warn of impending or serious harm to the patient may be unheeded along with the bothersome or clinically meaningless alerts. Ironically, computer generated alerts intended to improve safety may result in increasing the chance of harm to the patient. Since EHR systems are being widely used in today's healthcare environment, alert fatigue has been recognized as a major, unintended consequence as well as a significant patient safety concern [14].

Usability problems of CDSS involve both clinical and technical challenges. The challenges are summarized below with the hope that further discussion and research endeavors will be directed toward this important area. By solving these critical challenges, the full benefits of CDSS are more likely to be achieved.

4.1.1 *Clinical Challenges*

Disseminating Existing Knowledge About CDSS

Although studies consistently demonstrate successful CDSS, there has not been an easy way to organize the lessons learned in these implementations and disseminate them widely, so that others can learn from them [12]. Sittig et al. argue say that there is a need to build on initial efforts in developing more robust methods to identify, describe, evaluate, collect, catalog, synthesize and disseminate best practices for clinical decision support (CDS) design, development, implementation, maintenance, and evaluation [12].

Clinical Workflow Integration

In the past, many CDSS were not well integrated with computer-based physician order entry (CPOE), and physicians chose to ignore CDSS just because of the "double data entry" requirement which is interruptive to the patient care process [1]. As more and more CDSS have been integrated into EHR systems, the double data entry issue is no longer a major problem for clinicians, although several diagnostic decision support systems remain standalone, not integrated into EHR systems.

A key success factor that is strongly supported by empirical studies and expert recommendations is that CDSS should be integrated into the clinical workflow [15, 16]. CDSS could be more effective when the support of workflow is integrated. For instance, if clinicians do not do their documentation while the patient is present, CDSS are unlikely to influence the clinician-patient interaction. Without feedback from users or observation of the care process, CDSS developers may not realize why their products are not being used effectively. Karsh describes a study where the researchers utilized rapid prototyping with iterative feedback in order to design a CDSS that would efficiently integrate into the workflow of the users. However, Karsh also indicates that care processes themselves are not standardized, making it difficult to develop a set of universally applicable guidelines for CDSS integration. There is no single "workflow"; rather each clinician often has a unique way to approach the care process [16]. More efforts for collaboration are needed between health information technology (HIT) professionals who integrate CDSS into the care process and clinicians who use CDSS in practice to better understand and effectively integrate clinical workflow with CDSS.

Keeping Abreast of New Clinical Research Developments

New clinical evidence is being published on an ongoing basis. Each year, tens of thousands of clinical trials are published [17], which means a large amount of new knowledge must be incorporated into the existing knowledge bases. Accordingly, reasoning modules in CDSS need to be re-evaluated or updated to reflect the advances in science. In some situations, the updates may trigger unexpected conflicts of rules between new knowledge and previous knowledge. Although computational power has been used to assist the updating and maintenance, labor-intensive manual work is still needed [18]. Most research groups cannot afford such an expense in the long run. As a result, CDSS projects that are initially grant funded may stop as soon as the funding ends. The vendors of commercial systems also suffer from similar financial challenges in providing the necessary, but costly, maintenance teams for a long period to support their products. Financial issues may lead to less frequent updates of the knowledge base, which can seriously impact the usability of the systems.

4.1.2 Technical Issues

Variety in Types of Data

A CDSS usually uses a wide range of relevant data, which may potentially increase the difficulty of selecting algorithms for data integration. For example, a CDSS might use data from an EHR such as a patient's symptoms, medical history, family history and it would not be a surprise in the near future if the EHR included genetic information as well. These data might be used in conjunction with the historical and geographical trends of disease occurrence. Such a large database may consist of many types of data including, but not limited to, discrete, continuous, binary, matrix, or even natural language represented in a free text format. Therefore, it may be technically challenging to handle the variety of types of data.

The integration of these data could generate patient summaries, which would be a great help to clinicians since it is not easy for them to recall the important facts and conclusions based on such complicated patient data [12]. Moreover, it has been a challenge to automate the filtering and summarizing of all of the clinical data in EHR systems [12]. The primary difficulty is that the data may be represented in both free text and coded formats, which are difficult to integrate. Furthermore, because of the different requirements of clinicians and their workflows, multiple versions of summaries may be needed to optimize the data output for better decision-making [19, 20].

In order to model or organize the challenging textual data, researchers have applied ontologies to describe the data. However, the lack of a universally accepted standard for clinical vocabulary limits the development of ontologies for CDSS. For example, CDSS may use different words for the same concepts or an identical word for totally different concepts. Although the Unified Medical Language System (UMLS) makes connections among prevailing controlled vocabularies such as International Classification of Diseases (ICD), Current Procedural Terminology (CPT), Logical Observation Identifiers Names and Codes (LOINC) and SNOMED Clinical Terms (SNOMED CT), etc., the problems of ambiguity and redundancy in vocabulary still exist.

Synthesizing Clinical Knowledge

Another challenge is that a large amount of clinical knowledge is waiting to be fully synthesized, developed, and put into use in CDSS. To reflect the clinical knowledge in a timely manner, there is a need for the creation, testing, and execution of the algorithms to make use of the data in EHR systems and other clinical repositories [12]. If clinical knowledge could be more easily synthesized and deployed in CDSS, the new clinical guidelines and CDS interventions would undoubtedly be helpful in promoting improved outcomes.

4.2 Strategies to Improve the Usability of CDSS

The implementations of CDSS often suffer from usability issues, which have a direct impact on the adoption and effectiveness of CDSS [21]. Imagine that a physician is trying to prescribe a medication to his patient, and the physician keeps suffering from all kinds of alerts in the process with the "help" of a CDSS. After carefully reading the first several alerts which are meaningless, the physician may start to override the rest of the alerts in order to speed up the process. Unfortunately, he may have missed an important drug-drug interaction. The prescription is then sent to the pharmacy with unfortunate results. Therefore, in real-world clinical settings, usability design and validation are some of the most important perspectives of successful CDSS implementation.

The most typical result due to poor usability is alert fatigue. This phenomenon has been regarded as a significant factor in several high-profile errors. For example, an article described an investigation where failure to attend to alarms in a patient monitoring system led to more than 200 deaths over 5 years [22]. Most alert fatigue events occur while using CPOE and CDSS, where a major class of alerts are those for drug-drug interactions or incorrect dosage of medications. Patient Safety Network (PSNet), an online journal and forum on patient safety and healthcare quality sponsored by the Agency for Healthcare Research and Quality (AHRQ) provides several suggestions on how to minimize alert fatigue in CDSS [23] as shown in Table 4.1.

The proposed solutions for alert fatigue issues, once being fully implemented, may significantly advance patient safety and healthcare quality. In addition, the patient safety community will also need to learn from other industries. For example,

Table 4.1 Solutions of alert fatigue in CDSS

	Potential solutions
1	Increase alert specificity. Examples of ways to increase specificity include classifying medications as individual agents (rather than by classes of medication) and specifying the route of administration.
2	Tier alerts according to severity. Presenting each alert level in a different way to users (e.g., different colors, different signal words) allows prescribers to identify important alerts quickly and may result in fewer important alerts being missed or overridden. This approach, although intuitive, is problematic due to the lack of widespread agreement regarding what constitutes a high-level or low-level alert.
3	Apply human factors principles when designing alerts (e.g., format, content, legibility, and color of alerts), and include only high-level (severe) alerts in an alert set. Low priority alerts have been shown to cause user frustration and slow down the medication ordering process. Low priority information could be presented in a non-interruptive way (e.g., as a hyperlink on the prescribing screen).
4	Tailor alerts to patient characteristics. As an example, integrate laboratory results into the alert system to ensure alerts are more patient-relevant. Other strategies include presenting pregnancy alerts only for patients who are pregnant, not all female patients in the hospital, and only presenting allergy alerts for patients in whom a complete list of allergies has been documented.
5	Customize alerts for physicians. Presenting specific alert types to specific specialties or skill levels would ensure that specialists with a high level of knowledge in an area do not receive alerts related to that area (e.g., nephrologists may not need to receive alerts about nephrotoxic drugs). This approach is sometimes viewed as problematic because computerized alerts are meant to serve as a safety net in times of forgetfulness or time pressure, even for experts.

From Baysari [23]. Available at: https://psnet.ahrq.gov/webmm/case/310/

in the aviation industry, the alerts in the cockpit are minimized so that only the most important ones are displayed to the pilots, thus allowing them to avoid the distractions of less important alerts. This approach can provide a useful model for CDSS design [13]. Tiered alerts are recommended, where only the most significant alerts require a hard stop [24].

The effectiveness of CDSS highly depends on the implementation of workflow integration and usability in complex healthcare settings [25]. Most CDSS were generally designed for healthcare providers, but might not fully consider the diversity of providers and their requirements, as well as their expertise levels. When using CDSS, physician experts may expect to make decisions more precisely and quickly, while nurses may hope to take care of their patients in a better way [26]. Sometimes, even patients are encouraged to get engaged in CDSS in retirement living communities, such as TigerPlace in Columbia, Missouri. In TigerPlace, smart home technologies are installed within the private apartments of the residents. The technologies may include devices for emergency communication, falls detection, gait and movement monitoring, cognitive reminder systems, and medication management. The devices are monitors, sensors, and even personal PDAs which need the residents to engage in the information collection [27, 28].

The increasing amount of knowledge represented by diverse types of data and purposes of potential users have an effect on the usability, even though the algorithms or reasoning approaches of CDSS may be well-designed and solid. For example, a multi-site study indicated that nurses routinely override CDSS recommendations that do not fit their local practice, leading to a potential increase in errors [29]. User-centered design can improve HCI by providing personalized and targeted support [30]. Improved HCI design may include individualized interfaces according to the user group and purpose, increased sensitivity to the needs of the current clinical scenario, or may even provide patient interfaces for some special CDSS such as those used for aging-in-place, in order to enhance the patients' self-efficacy and awareness to reduce patient safety events. Chapter 10 discusses patient-focused CDSS in more detail.

4.2.1 Perform User-Centered Design

Norman proposed the term user-centered design (UCD) in his co-authored book published in 1986 [31]. The term has become widely used since then. Norman and Draper presented seven principles of design which are essential for facilitating the designer's task [31]. Below we list and explain these principles (Norman and Draper's principles are italicized):

1. "*Use both knowledge in the world and knowledge in the head.*" To assist the user in building conceptual models about how a system works, one should write easy-to-understand manuals prior to the design to assist the user in understanding the system and which can also be a good reference tool. Writing the manual prior to designing the system may also aid in the design of the system itself.
2. "*Simplify the structure of tasks.*" Designers should not overload either the short-term memory, or the long term memory of the system user. The user's task should be consistent with mental aids, so that the user can easily retrieve information from long-term memory. Users should have control over the task.
3. "*Make things visible.*" The visibility should help users to figure out the use of an object, for example, by seeing the right buttons or devices for executing an operation.
4. "*Get the mappings right.*" The user needs to understand the relationship between what the user wants to do and how the system works. One way to improve this understanding is to use effective graphics.
5. "*Exploit the power of constraints, both natural and artificial.*" Design the system so the correct way to use it is obvious and make any incorrect ways of using the system impossible or difficult, so that the user is automatically guided to the correct way.
6. "*Design forerror.*" Assume that user will make errors and build in strategies to help recover from errors.

7. "*When all else fails, standardize.*" Standards are challenging to develop, but once the standards are agreed to, their use can make things much easier for the user.

Parallel design is an effective method in the UCD process. The design requires several people to create an initial design based on the same requirements. Before they complete their plans and share with the group, each designer should have worked independently. Then all the solutions will be considered by the design team, after which each designer will be allowed to further improve the ideas. The main tasks of designers include: (1) define layouts, (2) clarify the expectations on design fidelity, (3) if using a team approach, make sure team members have equivalent skills, (4) set up the evaluation criteria [32].

Prototyping is a widely used method, based on "a draft version of a product, allowing researchers to explore ideas and demonstrate the intention of a feature prior to the investment of time and money into real design" [33]. There is no limit for the prototype format which can be a paper draft or even a functional website. Using the prototyping method can significantly reduce the cost when changes need to be made before the final product is finished. Usability issues are already addressed since the feedback from users is gathered while researchers or companies are still planning and designing the product.

An individual interview is a direct way to gather information from users. This method allows researchers to probe the users' attitudes, beliefs, desires, and experiences to get a more comprehensive understanding about the requirements of potential users. Such an interview can be a face-to-face meeting, a phone call, or a video conference, or even a chat via instant messaging systems [34]. Surveys such as rating or ranking choices for the product content can also be processed during the interviews. During an individual talk, the interviewer can give the interviewee his full attention and adjust the interviewing style according to the interviewee's needs without being worried about the group dynamics. Individual interviews typically involve five to ten participants. Since the interviewers only talk to one person at a time, too many interviewees could extend the overall time, which may influence the quality of the discussion.

4.2.2 Create Approaches for Sharing CDS Knowledge, Modules and Services

To improve CDS research and development, there is an urgent need to establish approaches for sharing the practices and experiences. The primary task is to standardize the taxonomy of CDS interventions and outcomes which allows different systems and organizations to display and compare their practices and outcomes. With a goal of providing a platform for such sharing purposes, Sittig et al. suggest that "a set of standards-based interfaces to externally maintained clinical decision support services that any EHR could "subscribe to", in such a way that healthcare organizations and practices can implement new state of the art clinical decision support interventions with little or no extra effort on their part." [12]. Imagine a system where CDS knowledge modules can be executed everywhere because the modules are designed to be compatible with the local clinical system based on the standardized interface. In the near future, all novel CDS applications could be proposed collectively with standards-based, sharable CDS modules. It is also necessary to create Internet-accessible CDS repositories which could be easily shared by all the products using the standards-based interface [12]. Such a repository would provide an accurate source of knowledge and would allow individual healthcare facilities to avoid the arduous task of creating their own rules.

4.2.3 Enhance Quality of Knowledge Base to Support Multimorbidity Decisions

The multimorbidity issue is becoming a great challenge in healthcare [12]. Multimorbidity is defined as "any combination of chronic disease with at least one other acute or chronic disease, bio-psychosocial factor or somatic risk factor" [35]. Elderly patients almost always have multiple co-morbidities and a wide spectrum of medication prescriptions [36]. Studies have found that the following disease groups are likely to co-occur: cardiovascular diseases, diabetes mellitus, chronic kidney disease, chronic musculoskeletal disorders, chronic lung disorders, and mental health problems [37–39]. It is estimated that 84 % of total health expenditures involve patients with more than one condition in the United States [40]. The impact on public health and the economy of multimorbidity is significantly increasing [41].

To identify a technological approach for managing multimorbidity, evidence-based practice and involvement from both health professionals and patients are essential. As Sittig et al. argued, "the challenge is to create mechanisms to identify and eliminate redundant, contraindicated, potentially discordant, or mutually exclusive guideline-based recommendations for patients presenting with co-morbid conditions" [12]. Reviews on multimorbidity from the perspective of informatics indicate that CDSS can potentially improve patient safety for patients with multimorbidity [42, 43]. However, clinical guidelines are still far away from being fully utilized since they do not sufficiently address the multimorbidity issue, which may lead to the requirement of developing new strategies using computer science methods, such as logical and semantic approaches. To date, the most effective solution for the combination of clinical practice guidelines is to create ontologies including the criteria provided by experts [44].

As defined by Carter, "Knowledge bases are collections of facts about the real world, encoded in a manner that allows them to be used computationally" [45]. In fact, more sophisticated CDSS require a knowledge base for accessing facts and key concepts that underlie the domain. An ontology can provide structure to that knowledge. Communication, computational inference and reuse, and knowledge management are the three basic purposes when using ontologies [45]. In regard to communication, the information extracted and aggregated from different sources can be used to answer user queries or be regarded as input data to other applications, if all the terms are shared and published using the same underlying ontology [46]. The hierarchical structure of ontologies is helpful for functional and computational inference and data reuse in the investigated domains [47], which may consequently enhance the application value of the system. Ontologies are widely accepted in the next generation knowledge management systems focusing on conceptual models because they are an essential technology for activating semantic knowledge [48]. Thus, the use of ontologies can significantly enhance the quality of CDSSknowledge bases, especially in supporting multimorbidity decisions.

4.2.4 Integrate CDSS with the EHR

In a review of the effectiveness of CDSS, Moja et al. cite studies that show that CDSS "increase the use of preventive care in hospitalized patients, facilitate communication between providers and patients, enable faster and more accurate access to medical record data, improve the quality and safety of medication prescribing, and decrease the rate of prescription errors" [49]. CDSS should be integrated with the EHR so as to further improve the effectiveness.

Although EHR adoption is gaining momentum in healthcare systems, issues related to usability, workflow, and cognitive support are barriers to EHR meaningful use. Some of these barriers can be addressed by integrating the CDSS with the hospital information systems including but not limited to EHRs [1]. There are a number of commercial CDSS that are successful in narrowly defined domains, for instance, diagnostic decision support systems built into electrocardiograms (EKGs). However, they are still far from being well-integrated with the EHR. Similar to the process of knowledge standardization, EHRs also need uniform definitions prior to integrating CDSS. In addition, standardization is considered a priority to optimization. The Armed Forces Health Longitudinal Technology Application (AHLTA), the only EHR system used by healthcare providers of the U.S. Department of Defense (DoD) since 2004, allows central storage of standardized EHR data and shares patient information worldwide. Although this system is not immune to common issues shared with other EHR systems, AHLTA has been proven to be effective because of its standardization. Despite its strengths, the system is not as interoperable as it needs to be. In July 2015, the DoD announced that AHLTA will be replaced by a commercial system that is able to interact more effectively with civilian EHR systems [50]. This change reflects the inexorable trend of EHR standardization. The impact and benefit of CDSS linked to EHR will not be fully realized until the standardization of EHRs is further developed.

4.2.5 Reduce Errors by Learning from Previous Experience

Each year in the United States, 650,000 cancer outpatients receiving chemotherapy are at high-risk of developing infections [51]. The infections may lead to hospitalization, disruptions in chemotherapy schedules, or even death. This is just a fraction of preventable patient safety events which are highly repetitive and could be reduced. To learn from the recurring events, an event reporting system is regarded as an effective way to analyze accumulated events and similarities at a collective level. An ideal reporting system would generate actionable knowledge based upon patient safety event repository, and even suggest common solutions for similar events under investigation. Unfortunately, current reporting systems still remain in the primary stage transitioning from paper forms, lacking a logic-based organizational knowledge structure for comparison and analysis, and suffering from poor usability—all of which impede the development of the systems towards the ideal. Therefore, there is an urgent need for learning from patient safety event reporting systems. Based on structural knowledge, the learning mechanism can dynamically measure the similarities of patient safety events and thus promote a learning effect. By integrating semantic searching algorithms into a patient safety event reporting system, the system should have the ability to learn from previous events and provide hints or common solutions for current events. With this innovative idea, reporting systems will have more useful functions and potentially trigger a revolution for data management and analysis in the field of patient safety, and then become an important approach to enhance the usability of CDSS [52].

4.3 Safety-Enhanced Design and Usability Assessment

CDSS have the potential to dramatically improve healthcare quality and safety. To reach this goal, systems must be designed, developed, and implemented with a focus on usability and safe use [53]. In the last decade, considerable attention from both researchers and vendors has been directed towards usability and integration into the clinical setting. Usability assessment aims to measure the satisfaction of users when they learn or use a product to achieve their goals. The degree of satisfaction is based on user feedback which reflects a combination of various factors including intuitive design, ease of learning, efficiency of use, memorability, error frequency and severity, subjective satisfaction, etc. In order to collect and assess such feedback, there are plenty of competent methods such as safety-enhanced design (SED), rapid usability assessment (RUA), usability testing, heuristic evaluation, card sorting, first click testing, individual interviews, online surveys, and system usability scales (SUS), etc. Some of these methods can be used for both design and assessment. This section provides an overview of usability evaluation and presents several of these commonly used approaches.

4.3.1 Safety-Enhanced Design (SED)

Aiming at accommodating users rather than forcing users to adapt, there are six key principles of user-centered design (UCD) according to Usability.gov [54].

1. Design is based upon an explicit understanding of users, tasks and environments.
2. Users are involved throughout design and development.
3. Design is driven and refined by user-centered evaluation.
4. The process is iterative.
5. The design addresses the whole user experience.
6. The design team includes multidisciplinary skills and perspectives.

Safety-enhanced design (SED) is a design process to reduce design-based errors within EHR interfaces, thereby improving the quality and safety of EHR systems [55]. As part of the certification criteria for meaningful use [26] vendors are required to use a formal, user-centered design (UCD) process during EHR system development and perform summative usability testing for portions of their EHR products. The testing includes CPOE, drug-drug, drug-allergy interaction check, medication list, medication allergy list, CDS, electronic medication administration record, electronic prescribing, and clinical information reconciliation. To fulfill certification requirements, vendors must submit documentation specifying the UCD processes used, which allows for significant flexibility in achieving SED. However, few summative tests or UCD experience reports are available at the current stage. Growing the literature on UCD implementation is considered necessary [56].

4.3.2 Rapid Usability Assessment (RUA)

Rapid Usability Assessment (RUA) is a laboratory-based, analytical usability process which was proposed to identify usability challenges and estimate the efficiency in performing routine meaningful use related tasks [57]. As described by Walji et al., there are three main stages in RUA [57]:

1. Selection of meaningful use objectives. The National Institute of Standards and Technology (NIST) developed meaningful use test procedures which contain specific instructions and sample data to determine if a system has met a meaningful use objective. The test specified data must be recorded in a structured format using either ICD-10-CM or SNOMED-CT.
2. Use of a modeling tool to predict task completion times as an indicator of productivity. Specifically, predict an expert's routine task completion times using a modeling tool, then use these results as performance benchmarks for laboratory evaluations [58]. There are several cognitively grounded approaches that can be used to predict task completion times, such as Goals, Operators, Methods and Selection (GOMS) technique [59].

3. Identifying usability challenges through expert review. Expert review can be conducted rapidly, and has been found to be effective in identifying gross usability problems [60]. A typical type of expert review is Heuristic Evaluation which was initially proposed by Nielsen and modified for use in clinical settings, and has been successfully applied to health IT, including practice management, computerized provider order entry (CPOE), telemedicine, and medical devices [61–65]. It has also been successfully used for predicting usability issues that impact end user involvement [66–68].

4.3.3 *Usability Testing*

"Usability testing refers to evaluating a product or service by testing it with representative users" [69]. In the context of CDSS, usability testing refers to evaluating CDSS and the associated heath information system with clinicians or other types of users. During a typical usability test, participants will be asked to complete typical tasks (e.g. prescribe an order) while observers watch, listen with minimum interruption, and take notes or record the entire test session. The purpose of usability testing is to make sure the usability issues of products are identified and fixed before they go into production. The process of usability testing typically includes three main steps: develop a plan, recruit participants, choose a moderating technique and proceed to the testing. In order to make the whole schema more tangible, below is an example to further demonstrate the implementation of usability testing. The examples come from a description of the design of a voluntary patient safety reporting system [70].

1. Develop a plan. The plan should be made according to the purpose of the testing, such as what type of data you are going to collect. In the example, the researchers wanted to assess the usability of their user-centered voluntary patient safety reporting system. The problem of patient falls, a major patient safety event, was selected as the research target. The data to be captured from testing was execution times on five subtasks (answer initial questions, rate a harm score, enter patient related information, answer case-dependent multiple-choice questions, and document further comments). Further, the testing plan was designed to ask participants to report three patient fall events using the system and then complete the five subtasks.
2. Recruit participants. The participants should be a representative sample of the potential users of the product. The number of participants depends on the testing purpose. Although normally five participants will be able to generate the majority of the usability problems in most usability tests, ten subjects were recruited for the test in the example case because the tasks they needed to do were fairly complex.

3. Choose a moderating technique and proceed to the testing. A moderating technique should be chosen according to the goals once the plan and participants of the test are determined. Retrospective think aloud (RTA) was used in the study. This technique involved gathering the user's verbalizations of attitudes when the reporting session was completed instead of during the session. The obtrusive disturbances to users' cognition, which would happen when the thinking aloud were done concurrently with task performance, can be significantly reduced or even completely eliminated when using RTA. There are also several other methods that could have been used, such as concurrent think aloud (CTA), concurrent probing (CP), and retrospective probing (RP).

Card Sorting

Card sorting is applied to help design or assess the information architecture of a product [71]. Topics are organized in the form of cards and provided to participants who may help researchers label the groups according to whether the topics make sense to them. Rather than the actual cards, researchers can also choose other forms such as pieces of paper or even online card-sorting tools. Open card sort and closed card sort are two widely used sorting strategies based on different requirements. The only difference is whether the categories of topics are pre-defined prior to sorting. The open and closed card sort can also be used in a combination way that initially implements an open card sort to identify content categories and then applies a closed card sort to see how well the category labels work.

Online Surveys

Online surveys provide researchers a more flexible and low-cost way to learn from users' feedback, such as the potential user group, the purpose of users when using the product, and what kind of information users expect to gain [72]. Online surveys can be used at any stage of the development process according to the goal. A study on identifying the user requirements of UCD demonstrated a successful example of using online surveys to screen interview candidates and train the follow-up interview [34]. Aiming at figuring out both benefits and barriers of a voluntary patient safety event reporting system toward UCD, the investigators organized an online survey in the form of a questionnaire including questions about participant's role, assessment, and preference of the proposed UCD features in e-reporting. A Likert scale was used to measure the level of agreement for the questions. The online survey form and the easy-to-use scale made the survey more understandable and easy to complete [34].

4.4 Summary

While it is becoming increasingly clear that CDSS are effective in improving clinical processes when integrated with the clinical workflow, it may take some time to fully realize CDSS' potential in improving healthcare quality and outcomes. As Osheroff and colleagues state in the preface to their book, *Improving OutcomeswithClinical Decision Support*, "The challenge of improving healthcare has never been primarily due to a lack of innovations, but in failure to implement, evaluate, and disseminate the myriad promising innovations awaiting our attention" [73]. Fortunately, more researchers have been involved in this field over the past decade, especially those from other disciplines. As the researchers bring more innovative ideas, we hope to witness the revolution of CDSS with enhanced usability in the near future.

References

1. Berner ES, La Lande TJ. Overview of clinical decision support systems. In: Berner ES, editor. Clinical decision support systems. Theory and practice. 2nd ed. New York: Springer; 2007. p. 3–22.
2. Curtain C, Peterson GM. Review of computerized clinical decision support in community pharmacy. J Clin Pharm Ther. 2014;39:343–8.
3. Armijo D, McDonnell C, Werner K. Electronic health record usability: interface design considerations, AHRQ Publication No. 09(10)–0091-2-EF. Rockville: Agency for Healthcare Research and Quality; 2009. October 2009. Available from: https://healthit.ahrq.gov/sites/default/files/docs/citation/09-10-0091-2-EF.pdf.
4. Johnson CM, Johnson TR, Zhang J. A user-centered framework for redesigning health care interfaces. J Biomed Inform. 2005;38:75–87.
5. Kushniruk AW, Patel VL. Cognitive and usability engineering methods for the evaluation of clinical information systems. J Biomed Inform. 2004;37:56–76.
6. Patel VL, Zhang J. Cognition and patient safety. In: Durso FT, editor. Handbook of applied cognition. New York: Wiley; 2007. p. 307–31.
7. Zhang J. Human-centered computing in health information systems. Part 1: Analysis and design. J Biomed Inform. 2005;38:1–3.
8. Zhang J. Human-centered computing in health information systems part 2: evaluation. J Biomed Inform. 2005;38:173–5.
9. Zhang J, Walji MF. TURF unified framework of EHR usability. In: Zhang J, Walji MF, editors. Better EHR: usability, workflow and cognitive support in electronic health records. National Center for Cognitive Informatics and Decision Making in Healthcare; 2014. pp. 29–56. Available from: http://www.researchgate.net/publication/269400453_Better_EHR_Usability_Workflow_and_Cognitive_Support_in_Electronic_Health_Records.
10. Zhang J, Walji MF. TURF: toward a unified framework of EHR usability. J Biomed Inform. 2011;44:1056–67.
11. Jansvier WA, Ghaoui C. Replicating human interactin to support E-Learning. In: Ghaoui C, editor. Encyclopedia of human computer interaction. Hershey: Idea Group; 2006. p. 503.
12. Sittig DF, Wright A, Osheroff JA, Middleton B, Teich JM, Ash JS, et al. Grand challenges in clinical decision support. J Biomed Inform. 2008;41:387–92.

13. AHRQ Patient Safety Network. Patient safety primers: alert fatigue. 2015. Agency for Healthcare Research and Quality (AHRQ). Available at: http://www.psnet.ahrq.gov/primer.aspx?primerID=28.
14. Slight SP, Seger DL, Nanji KC, Cho I, Maniam N, Dykes PC, et al. Are we heeding the warning signs? Examining providers' overrides of computerized drug-drug interaction alerts in primary care. PLoS One. 2013;8(12):e85071.
15. Cadet JV. Clinical decision support: workflow integration is vital for optimizing care. Cardiovascular Business. 2011. http://www.cardiovascularbusiness.com/topics/health-it/clinical-decision-support-workflow-integration-vital-optimizing-care.
16. Karsh B-T. Clinical practice improvement and redesign: how change in workflow can be supported by clinical decision support, AHRQ Publication No. 09-0054-EF. Rockville: Agency for Healthcare Research and Quality; 2009. Available from: https://healthit.ahrq.gov/sites/default/files/docs/page/09-0054-EF-Updated_0.pdf.
17. Gluud C, Nikolova D. Likely country of origin in publications on randomised controlled trials and controlled clinical trials during the last 60 years. Trials. 2007;8:7.
18. Gardner RM. Computerized clinical decision-support in respiratory care. Respir Care. 2004;49:378–86. discussion 386–378.
19. Petersen LA, Orav EJ, Teich JM, O'Neill AC, Brennan TA. Using a computerized sign-out program to improve continuity of inpatient care and prevent adverse events. Jt Comm J Qual Improv. 1998;24:77–87.
20. Zeng Q, Cimino JJ. A knowledge-based, concept-oriented view generation system for clinical data. J Biomed Inform. 2001;34:112–28.
21. Koppel R, Wetterneck T, Telles JL, Karsh B-T. Workarounds to barcode medication administration systems: their occurrences, causes, and threats to patient safety. J Am Med Inform Assoc. 2008;15:408–23.
22. Kowalczyk L. Patient alarms often unheard, unheeded. Boston Globe. Boston. 2011. 13 Feb 2011. Available from: http://www.boston.com/lifestyle/health/articles/2011/02/13/patient_alarms_often_unheard_unheeded/.
23. Baysari M. Finding fault with the default alert. AHRQ Web M&M. October 2013. Available at: http://webmm.ahrq.gov/case.aspx?caseID=310.
24. Shah NR, Seger AC, Seger DL, Fiskio JM, Kuperman GJ, Blumenfeld B, et al. Improving acceptance of computerized prescribing alerts in ambulatory care. J Am Med Inform Assoc. 2006;13(1):5–11.
25. Yuan MJ, Finley GM, Long J, Mills C, Johnson RK. Evaluation of user interface and workflow design of a bedside nursing clinical decision support system. Interact J Med Res. 2013;2:e4.
26. Blumenthal D. Stimulating the adoption of health information technology. N Engl J Med. 2009;360:1477–9.
27. Demiris G, Rantz M, Aud M, Marek T, Tyrer H, Skubic M, et al. Older adults' attitudes towards and perceptions of "smart home" technologies: a pilot study. Med Inform Internet Med. 2004;29:87–94.
28. Rantz MJ, Marek T, Aud M, Tyrer HW, Skubic M, Demiris G, et al. A technology and nursing collaboration to help older adults age in place. Nurs Outlook. 2005;53:40–5.
29. Dowding D, Spilsbury K, Thompson C, Brownlow R, Pattenden J. Nurses' use of computerised clinical decision support systems: a case site analysis. J Clin Nurs. 2009;18:1159–67.
30. Sears A, Jacko JA. Human-computer interaction: designing for diverse users and domains. Boca Raton: CRC; 2009.
31. Norman DA, Draper SW. User-centered system design: new perspectives on human-computer interaction. Hillsdale: Lawrence Earlbaum Associates; 1986.
32. Norman DA, Draper SW. Parallel design. Usability Net. 2015. Available from: http://www.usabilitynet.org/tools/parallel.htm.
33. Bailey B. Paper prototypes work as well as software prototypes. Usability.gov. 2005. Available from: http://www.usability.gov/get-involved/blog/2005/06/paper-prototypes-and-software-prototypes.html.

34. Gong Y, Song H-Y, Wu X, Hua L. Identifying barriers and benefits of patient safety event reporting toward user-centered design. Saf Health. 2015;1:7.
35. Le Reste JY, Nabbe P, Rivet C, Lygidakis C, Doerr C, Czachowski S, et al. The European General Practice Research Network presents a comprehensive definition of multimorbidity in family medicine and long term care, following a systematic review of relevant literature. J Am Med Dir Assoc. 2013;14:319–25.
36. Boyd CM, Darer J, Yu Q, Wolff JL, Leff B. Clinical practice guidelines and quality of care for older patients with multiple comorbid diseases: implications for pay for performance. JAMA. 2005;294:716–24.
37. Stevens LA, Li S, Wang C, Huang C, Becker BN, Bomback AS, et al. Prevalence of CKD and comorbid illness in elderly patients in the United States: results from the Kidney Early Evaluation Program (KEEP). Am J Kidney Dis. 2010;55:S23–33.
38. Yaffe K, Ackerson L, Kurella Tamura M, le Blanc P, Kusek JW, Sehgal AR, et al. Chronic kidney disease and cognitive function in older adults: findings from the chronic renal insufficiency cohort cognitive study. J Am Geriatr Soc. 2010;58:338–45.
39. Zhang X, Decker FH, Luo H, Geiss LS, Pearson WS, Saaddine JB, et al. Trends in the prevalence and comorbidities of diabetes mellitus in nursing home residents in the United States: 1995–2004. J Am Geriatr Soc. 2010;58:724–30.
40. Anderson G. Chronic care: making the case for ongoing care. Princeton: Robert Wood Johnson Foundation; 2010.
41. Taylor AW, et al. Multimorbidity – not just an older person's issue. Results from an Australian biomedical study. BMC Publ Health. 2010;10:718.
42. Roshanov PS, Misra S, Gerstein HC, Garg AX, Sebaldt RJ, Mackay JA, et al. Computerized clinical decision support systems for chronic disease management: a decision-maker-researcher partnership systematic review. Implement Sci. 2011;6:92.
43. Yourman L, Concato J, Agostini JV. Use of computer decision support interventions to improve medication prescribing in older adults: a systematic review. Am J Geriatr Pharmacother. 2008;6:119–29.
44. Jafarpour B, Abidi S. Merging disease-specific clinical guidelines to handle comorbidities in a clinical decision support setting. In: Artificial intelligence in medicine. Murcia, Spain: Springer; 2013 pp. 28–32.
45. Carter JH. Design and implementation issues. In: Berner ES, editor. Clinical decision support systems. New York: Springer; 2007. p. 64–98.
46. Gruber TR. A translation approach to portable ontology specifications. Knowl Acquis. 1993;5:199–220.
47. Kanehisa M, Goto S, Hatori M, Aoki-Kinoshita KF, Itoh M, Kawashima S, et al. From genomics to chemical genomics: new developments in KEGG. Nucleic Acids Res. 2006;34:D354–7.
48. Maedche A, Motik B, Stojanovic L, Studer R, Volz R. Ontologies for enterprise knowledge management. IEEE Intell Syst. 2003;18:26–33.
49. Moja L, Kwag KH, Lytras T, Bertizzolo L, Brandt L, Pecoraro V, et al. Effectiveness of computerized decision support systems linked to electronic health records: a systematic review and meta-analysis. Am J Public Health. 2014;104:e12–22.
50. Noble Z. DoD awards massive health records contract. 29 July 2015. FCW. Available at: https://fcw.com/articles/2015/07/29/dod-dhmsm-award.aspx.
51. Centers for Disease Control and Prevention. Preventing infections in cancer patients. Available at: http://www.cdc.gov/cancer/preventinfections/.
52. Kang H, Gong Y. Developing a self-learning patient safety event reporting system. Innovations in cancer prevention and research conference. Austin; 2015.
53. Karsh BT. Beyond usability: designing effective technology implementation systems to promote patient safety. Qual Saf Health Care. 2004;13:388–94.
54. Visual Design Glossary Terms. Usability.gov. Available at: http://www.usability.gov/what-and-why/glossary/tag/visual-design/index.html.

55. Lowry SZ. Technical evaluation, testing, and validation of the usability of electronic health records. Gaithersburg: National Institute of Standards and Technology; 2012.
56. Ratwani R, et al. EHR vendor usability practices. In: Zhang J, Walji MF, editors. Better EHR: usability, workflow and cognitive support in electronic health records. Houston, TX: National Center for Cognitive Informatics and Decision Making in Healthcare; 2014. pp. 103.
57. Walji MF, Franklin A, Kannampallil T, Zhang Z, Graves K, Li Y, et al. Rapid usability assessment of commercial EHRs. In: Zhang J, Walji MF, editors, Better EHR: usability, workflow and cognitive support in electronic health records. Houston, TX: National Center for Cognitive Informatics and Decision Making in Healthcare; 2014. pp. 91–109.
58. Gong Y, Zhang J. Toward a human-centered hyperlipidemia management system: the interaction between internal and external information on relational data search. J Med Syst. 2011;35:169–77.
59. John BE, Kieras DE. The GOMS family of user interface analysis techniques: comparison and contrast. ACM Trans Comput Hum Interact (TOCHI). 1996;3:320–51.
60. Nielsen J. Guerilla HCI: discount usability engineering to penetrate intimidation barrier. In: Bias RG, Mayhew DJ, editors. Cost-justifying usability. San Diego: Academic; 1994.
61. Zhang J, et al. Using usability heuristics to evaluate patient safety of medical devices. J Biomed Inform. 2003;36:23–30.
62. Thyvalikakath TP, Schleyer TK, Monaco V. Heuristic evaluation of clinical functions in four practice management systems: a pilot study. J Am Dent Assoc. 2007;138(209–210):212–8.
63. Chan J, et al. Usability evaluation of order sets in a computerised provider order entry system. BMJ Qual Saf. 2011;20:932–40.
64. Tang Z, et al. Applying heuristic evaluation to improve the usability of a telemedicine system. Telemed J E Health. 2006;12:24–34.
65. Graham MJ, et al. Heuristic evaluation of infusion pumps: implications for patient safety in Intensive Care Units. Int J Med Inform. 2004;73:771–9.
66. Gong Y, Zhang J. A human-centered design and evaluation framework for information search. AMIA Annual Symposium proceedings. 2005. pp. 281–5. http://www.ncbi.nlm.nih.gov/pubmed/16779046.
67. Johnson CM, et al. Can prospective usability evaluation predict data errors? AMIA Annu Symp Proc. 2010;2010:346–50.
68. Thyvalikakath TP, et al. Comparative study of heuristic evaluation and usability testing methods. Stud Health Technol Inform. 2009;143:322–7.
69. Usability.gov. Usability testing. Available at: http://www.usability.gov/how-to-and-tools/methods/usability-testing.html. 2015.
70. Hua L, Gong Y. Design of a user-centered voluntary patient safety reporting system: understanding the time and response variances by retrospective think-aloud protocols. Stud Health Technol Informat. 2013;192:729–33.
71. Usability.gov. Card sorting. Available at: http://www.usability.gov/how-to-and-tools/methods/card-sorting.html. 2015.
72. Usability.gov. Online surveys. Available at: http://www.usability.gov/how-to-and-tools/methods/online-surveys.html. 2015.
73. Osheroff JA, et al. Improving outcomes with clinical decision support-an implementer's guide. Chicago: HIMSS; 2012.

Chapter 5
Newer Architectures for Clinical Decision Support

Salvador Rodriguez-Loya and Kensaku Kawamoto

Abstract In recent years, the general IT community has been moving from a monolithic-type of software architecture to a service-oriented architecture that involves developing systems using independent, well-defined software services that are then coordinated to meet business needs. The main benefit of a service-oriented architecture is the ability to more easily and more rapidly implement needed business capabilities using independent software services. While lagging behind many industries, the healthcare industry has been moving towards a service-oriented architecture, including in the space of clinical decision support. In this chapter, we describe notable efforts in service-oriented clinical decision support and speculate on its potential evolution in the future.

Keywords Clinical decision support systems • Service oriented architecture • Software architecture • Service-oriented design • Service oriented computing • Medical information systems

Clinical decision support Systems (CDSS) were originally based on a stand-alone architecture, in which the system was fully self-contained and required direct user input for obtaining data. A number of early CDSS were built using this architectural style, for example MYCIN (1975). MYCIN provided advice on antimicrobial therapy for patients with bacterial infections after the physician answered a set of yes-no questions [1]. Similarly, the INTERNIST-I (1982) [2] and DXplain (1987) [3] systems accepted a wide variety of patient findings (e.g., history, physical, laboratory data) as the input and returned a ranked list of possible diagnoses, also known as a differential diagnosis. DXplain is still available and is in continuous development [4]. Although this approach provides a straight-forward mechanism for obtaining the required CDS functionality, it relies on manual entry of the input data to obtain the desired results. Using these systems can therefore be time consuming. For example, entering the relevant data for a complex patient case in the INTERNIST-I system can take about an hour [5].

S. Rodriguez-Loya, Ph.D. (✉) • K. Kawamoto, M.D., Ph.D., M.H.S.
Biomedical Informatics, University of Utah,
421 Wakara Way Suite 208, Salt Lake City, UT 84108, USA
e-mail: salvador.rodriguez@utah.edu; kensaku.kawamoto@utah.edu

E.S. Berner (ed.), *Clinical Decision Support Systems*, Health Informatics,
DOI 10.1007/978-3-319-31913-1_5

As electronic health record (EHR) systems matured, CDS capabilities began to be integrated with EHR systems and other health information technology (IT) systems. This was typically done in a system-specific manner. One of the first integrations between clinical data and CDS capabilities was implemented in 1967 at the LDS Hospital in Salt Lake City, Utah. This EHR system was named HELP, and it was first introduced in the cardiac catheterization laboratory. Since then, the HELP system has been extended to various other clinical areas such as respiratory therapy, intensive care, and pharmacy, to name a few [6]. Subsequently, other similar integrated CDS systems have been developed by different research groups and hospitals [7, 8]. Chapters 13, 14, and 15 describe the HELP system and some of the other systems. However, it soon became clear that a major challenge with these integrated CDS solutions was the difficulty of sharing CDS content developed for one EHR system with another EHR system.

Over the years, as the evidence of CDS effectiveness and the scope of CDS implementations increased, there was a desire to scale CDS across systems and institutions. However, stand-alone CDS architectures were limited by their need for extensive manual data entry, and integrated CDS architectures were limited in their ability to be scaled. At the same time, there was a growing trend in the general IT industry to move towards software architectures that allowed for more reusable components that could be scaled across institutions. In particular, of these so-called component-based architectures, service-oriented architectures (SOA) quickly became predominant. The CDS space has also started to adopt this approach. In this chapter, we aim to address some of the fundamental questions related to the use of Service Oriented Architecture for CDSS, namely:

- What is a service-oriented architecture?
- Is SOA a preferred architecture for enabling scalable CDSS?
- What are notable efforts in the space of service-oriented CDS?

5.1 Service-Oriented Architecture: Definition, Benefits, Challenges, History

Before SOA became the preferred approach for the design, development and integration of distributed systems, most distributed software solutions were based on Remote Procedure Calls (RPC). The most important RPC models were the Common Object Request Broker Architecture (CORBA) and the Distributed Computing Object Model (DCOM). For various reasons, the use of CORBA and DCOM over the Internet proved to be problematic, and none of these technologies took control of the market. With the widespread adoption of the Internet and more specifically the use of the Hypertext Transfer Protocol (HTTP), the notion of SOA started to materialize. In the field of software architecture, the concept of SOA can be defined as a "paradigm for organizing and utilizing distributed capabilities that may be under control of different ownership domains" [9]. The needs of a distributed

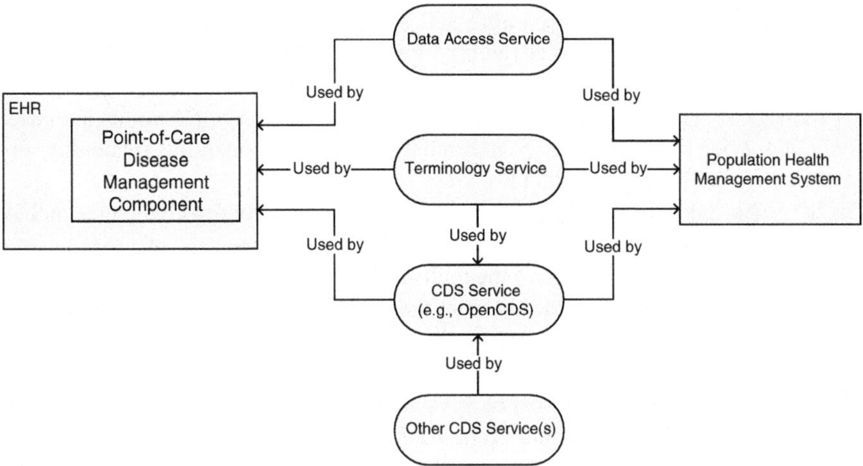

Fig. 5.1 Sample CDS system architecture [10]

computer program may be met by the capabilities of another program that is maintained by a different owner. These needs may be satisfied by combining multiple capabilities, and these capabilities may be designed to address various needs. In the context of SOA, services are the "mechanism by which needs and capabilities are brought together" [9]. The access to these capabilities is provided through well-defined services interfaces. While not required, SOA is commonly implemented using Web services that are accessible over the Internet.

An important feature of SOA is that distributed capabilities can be used without having to know the implementation details. For example, a CDSS that exposes its functionality through a Web service can be used without the client system having to know which technology or platform is being used to implement the service. Figure 5.1 provides an overview of an example SOA-based CDS environment [10]. In this example, a CDS service is used by the point-of-care disease management component of an EHR system and by a population health management system. Figure 5.1 also shows other services that facilitate CDS [10]. A data service that retrieves relevant clinical information from different databases, and other CDS services, such as commercial medication CDS services, are leveraged by the primary CDS service. A terminology service is also leveraged to map between vocabularies. For example, an EHR system may define patient problems in terms of ICD-10 [11] whereas a CDS system may only accept concepts in terms of ICD-9 [11] and SNOMED-CT [12]. In this case, a terminology service can be used by the CDS service to translate the EHR system's problem concepts from ICD-9 to SNOMED-CT to allow for processing.

SOA is well-suited for the development of low cost, large scale systems, as it allows various business functionalities to be implemented and maintained independently in a distributed manner. Additionally, SOA supports software component reusability, scalability and interoperability. Complex applications can be implemented by assembling reusable, self-contained units of functionality, thereby reducing the time and resources required for implementation. Applications scale as the computing infrastructure (e.g., Amazon Elastic Compute Cloud [13]) is grown or reduced according to the service demand. Usually, SOA applications are based on Web service standards (e.g., SOAP and REST), thereby enabling greater interoperability with other systems that use these standards.

SOA can present several challenges, however, with common challenges including security and service discovery [14]. Validating the security of a SOA-based system can be challenging due of the multi-tenant and distributed nature of its components. Discovering services that meet the requirements of the service consumer may also be challenging if there is limited support for the automatic discovery of service semantics.

A number of the key concepts of SOA are exercised at the Service Composition level, namely choreography and orchestration. In service choreography, each participating service defines its part in the interaction, with the details typically described using choreography languages such as the Web Services Choreography Description Language (WS-CDL). In service orchestration, the logic is defined by a single participant, which is referred to as the orchestrator. Service orchestration resembles a process (i.e., sequence of tasks), and it is commonly achieved through the use of process execution languages such as Business Process Management and Notation (BPMN) and Business Process Execution Language (BPEL). Both approaches can have associated challenges. For example, in service orchestration, all data passes through a centralized point (i.e., the orchestrator), which may result in unnecessary data transfer and the orchestrator becoming a bottleneck. On the other hand, choreography models can be harder to design and implement than orchestration models. The decentralized control logic in choreography can bring significant challenges resulting from issues such as control-flow (e.g., which interaction comes after another), time constraints, and asynchronous and concurrent interactions. In service choreography, it is necessary to design an agreement between a set of services in order to define roles and how the collaboration should take place while maintaining SOA principles including service reusability.

5.2 Benefits and Challenges of SOA for Health IT Systems in General and CDSS in Particular

The U.S. Department of Health and Human Services' (HHS) Office of the National Coordinator for Health IT (ONC) defines health IT (HIT) as "the application of information processing involving both computer hardware and software that deals with the storage, retrieval, sharing, and use of health care information, data, and knowledge for communication and decision making" [15]. Using the ONC definition, a variety of applications can be considered health IT including electronic health records, picture archiving and communication systems (PACS), laboratory information systems (LIS) as well as CDS systems [15].

Because healthcare delivery is often fragmented across systems and providers, SOA has been proposed as a promising solution for the integration of healthcare related data across these various types of health IT systems. The decomposition of functionalities or capabilities into relatively autonomous units (i.e., services) simplifies the design and implementation of software solutions to complex problems in health care. SOA supports the strategic reuse of legacy applications, while allowing adoption of new technologies. This enables healthcare organizations to adapt more quickly to the complexity and constant evolution of medical knowledge and health care. Healthcare organizations are also subject to regulations and supervision by authorities and government agencies. In combination with other technologies such as Business Process Management and Business Rules, SOA can enable the implementation of audit controls that allow healthcare organizations to demonstrate that their processes comply with regulations.

For the reasons mentioned above, SOA promises a significant reduction in the cost and time required for HIT implementation and maintenance. These advantages have been identified by governments and organizations worldwide, which strongly promote the adoption of SOA-based health care systems. For example, Canada Health Infoway, a non-profit organization funded by the Canadian government, defines an HIT implementation model based on SOA [16]. The Infoway model connects provincial networks of health care systems to form a national network where electronic health care records can be accessed from different places. Another important initiative is the Healthcare Services Specification Project (HSSP), which is a collaborative effort between Health Level 7 (HL7) and the Object Management Group (OMG). The HSSP focuses on the specification of HIT service standards based on SOA principles [17].

Because health data relevant for CDS may exist in multiple physical locations, SOA can serve as a useful architectural approach for integrating disparate data sources. Additionally, SOA can enable CDSS to be implemented through the assembly of various services providing required functionality, such as for data retrieval, terminology mapping, and patient data evaluation. For example, a SOA can be used to provide personalized care recommendations that combine whole genome sequence information with clinical data and a centralized knowledge repository [18].

Despite the potential benefits of using the SOA paradigm to implement CDS capabilities, Kawamoto et al. describe several challenges to the adoption of this approach to enabling CDS [10]. One of the important challenges they identify is that developing and maintaining generalized CDS services that can be used by multiple applications require considerably more effort than doing so for similar CDS services designed for specific systems [10]. There is also a need for CDS interfaces to be standardized in order to facilitate and encourage component reuse, and the CDS content may need to be customized to meet the unique needs of individual client organizations [10]. Furthermore, defining the optimal service granularity (i.e., scope of service function) can be challenging. Some of the problems that can arise

Table 5.1 Services and capabilities desired for scalable, standards-based, service-oriented CDSS as described by the HL-7 CDS Work Group [19]

Services hosted by CIS that enable a SOA for CDS	Capabilities provided by a CIS that enable a SOA for CDS
Event subscription and notification service	Use of appropriate, standard information models and terminologies
Cohort identification service	Ability to leverage a decision support service
Entity identification service/identity cross-reference service	Ability to leverage a terminology service
Clinical data query service	Ability to leverage a unit conversion service
Resource query service	Ability to leverage a data transformation service
Data acquisition service	Ability to leverage a data presentation service
Data addition/update service	Ability to populate a data warehouse in real-time
Order placement service	Maintenance of audit logs
User communication service	
Task management service	

from inappropriate service granularity include service duplication (several services for similar functions), a proliferation of services, and services that cannot be easily reused in different contexts [10]. In addition, the black-box nature of a CDS service may not be acceptable for some organizations that want to know exactly how a clinical decision has been reached [10]. Finally, healthcare organizations may insist on a CDS service to be locally hosted, which can make it more difficult to achieve economies of scale and enable real-time content updates [10].

5.3 SOA Services and Capabilities Needed for CDS

The HL7 CDS Work Group has identified and published key capabilities and requirements for a Clinical Information System (CIS) to provide SOA-based CDSS [19]. These capabilities and services are shown in Table 5.1.

An important requirement for interoperable, SOA-based CDSS is the development of standard definitions for required services, so that services can be re-leveraged in a scalable manner across organizations. Also needed are resources to facilitate the implementation of such standards-based, SOA-enabled CDS. Described below are notable efforts in this area with regard to service standardization and resource development.

5.4 Healthcare Services Specification Project

The HSSP is a collaboration effort between HL7 and OMG that addresses interoperability challenges by developing SOA service specifications [20]. The specifications focus on the functionality, semantics and technology needed to support interoperability between systems. The goal is to reduce the complexity of implementation, promote effective integration and lower implementation costs. Specifications developed by HSSP include the Retrieve, Locate, Update Service (RLUS) for data retrieval and update, the Decision Support Service (DSS) for evaluating patient data to generate patient-specific care assessments and recommendations, and the Common Terminology Services (CTS2) for providing commonly required terminology functions.

5.5 OpenCDS

OpenCDS is "a multi-institutional, collaborative effort to develop open-source, standards-based CDS tools and resources that can be widely adopted to enable CDS at scale" [21]. An important resource developed by this effort is a knowledge authoring, management, and execution platform that supports relevant HL7 standards including the HL7 Virtual Medical Record (vMR) and HL7 DSS standards. OpenCDS encapsulates knowledge into reusable components that can be shared with different medical systems. Some of the areas where OpenCDS has been leveraged include immunization forecasting, [22] CDS for whole genome sequence information, [18, 23] multimorbidity case management, [24] and CDS-based quality measurements, [25] among others.

5.6 CDS Consortium

The CDS Consortium (CDSC) was established by researchers from Brigham and Women's Hospital, Harvard Medical School, and Partners HealthCare Information System in partnership with the Regenstrief Institute, Kaiser Permanente Northwest Research Group, the Veterans Heath Administration, Masspro, GE Healthcare, Siemens Medical Solutions, and other organizations. The aim of the CDSC is "to asses, define, demonstrate, and evaluate best practices for knowledge management and clinical decision support in healthcare information technology at scale – across multiple ambulatory care settings and EHR technology platforms" [26]. CDSC focuses on several CDS areas such as the development of standards for CDS knowledge representation and demonstrations of CDS implementations at different sites across the United States.

5.7 Health eDecisions and Clinical Quality Framework

The Health eDecisions (HeD) project and the Clinical Quality Framework (CQF) project are part of the Standards & Interoperability framework (S&I) framework sponsored by the U.S. Office of the National Coordinator for Health Information

Technology (ONC) [27]. The goal of HeD was to define and validate standards that enable CDS sharing at scale [28]. The main achievements of HeD include the further development, refinement, and validation of the HL7 vMR data model standard for CDS; the development and validation of the HL7 CDS Knowledge Artifact Specification for representing standard rules, order sets, and documentation templates; and the HL7 DSS Implementation Guide. The CQF project is based on the work accomplished by the HeD, with a focus on harmonizing the standards for CDS and electronic clinical quality measurement [29].

5.8 Healthcare Services Platform Consortium

The Healthcare Services Platform Consortium (HSPC) is a nonprofit community of healthcare providers, software vendors, educational institutions and individuals committed to increasing the quality and reducing the costs of health care [30]. The HSPC's goal is to create a framework for, and facilitate the widespread adoption of, SOA-based architectures for health care that incorporate open data models and terminology standards. Some of the functions of HSPC include the selection of standards for the development of interoperable SOA-based services, as well as the evaluation, testing and certification of software solutions proposed by its members. Some of the standards that have been selected by HSPC include SNOMED CT, LOINC, and RxNorm for terminology; HL7 FHIR for data exchange; and SMART [31] for EHR integration.

5.9 Other Individual Efforts

Beyond these specific efforts, there are a number of other efforts completed or underway. In a systematic review of SOA for CDS, we found 44 studies on this topic [32]. For example, a prominent implementation standard for SOA is Service Component Architecture (SCA). SCA is a set of OASIS specifications designed for building distributed applications based on SOA, and it is the result of the collaboration of major software vendors such as IBM and Oracle [33]. SCA has been adopted by various industries in conjunction with Business Process Management tools and techniques, with a primary goal of addressing the complexity issues that arise with large scale SOA implementations. SCA has been successfully applied to provide guideline-based CDS to physicians within the context of EHR systems [34, 35]. Further details on this and other relevant individual efforts can be found in this aforementioned systematic review of SOA for CDS [32].

5.10 Future Directions

Here, we speculate on the future directions of CDS architectures based on previous and current efforts underway. First, we believe that the trend towards service-oriented CDS will continue. The pace at which it will do so is unclear, but keys to the facilitation of this movement include standardization and the availability of robust content and services to support the approach. Second, just as the general IT industry is moving towards more cutting-edge approaches to SOA and to approaches that go beyond SOA, we anticipate this trend will also start appearing in HIT and in CDS. An example of potential evolution includes movement towards use of SCAs and other advanced architectural approaches, such as the combination of SOA with event-driven and workflow-driven approaches such as Business Process Management. Finally, we anticipate that CDS architectures will also begin to incorporate other trends in the general industry, such as a focus on mobile devices (e.g., smart phones and tablets) and an increasing adoption of Cloud computing.

5.11 Conclusions

CDS implementations have been moving towards SOA, similar to other fields, with a particular focus on standards-based scalability. We anticipate that this movement will continue to gain momentum. Moreover, we anticipate that implementations in this area will continue to follow general trends in HIT and the broader IT marketplace, such as a focus on mobile technologies and Cloud computing.

References

1. Shortliffe EH, Davis R, Axline SG, Buchanan BG, Green CC, Cohen SN. Computer-based consultations in clinical therapeutics: explanation and rule acquisition capabilities of the MYCIN system. Comput Biomed Res. 1975;8(4):303–20.
2. Miller RA, Pople HE, Myers JD. Internist-I, an experimental computer-based diagnostic consultant for general internal medicine. N Engl J Med. 1982;307(8):468–76.
3. Barnett GO, Cimino JJ, Hupp JA, Hoffer EP. Dxplain: an evolving diagnostic decision-support system. JAMA. 1987;258(1):67–74.
4. MGH Laboratory of Computer Science. dxplain project [Internet]. Cited 2015 Apr 30. Available from: http://www.mghlcs.org/projects/dxplain.
5. Wright A, Sittig DF. A four-phase model of the evolution of clinical decision support architectures. Int J Med Inform. 2008;77(10):641–9.
6. Gardner RM, Pryor TA, Warner HR. The HELP hospital information system: update 1998. Int J Med Inform. 1999;54(3):169–82.
7. McDonald CJ, Overhage JM, Tierney WM, Dexter PR, Martin DK, Suico JG, et al. The regenstrief medical record system: a quarter century experience. Int J Med Inform. 1999;54(3):225–53.

8. Miller RA, Waitman LR, Chen S, Rosenbloom ST. The anatomy of decision support during inpatient care provider order entry (CPOE): empirical observations from a decade of {CPOE} experience at Vanderbilt. J Biomed Inform. 2005;38(6):469–85.
9. Advancing Open Standards for the Information Society (OASIS). Reference model for service oriented architecture 1.0 [Internet]. 2006. Available from: http://docs.oasis-open.org/soa-rm/v1.0/soa-rm.pdf.
10. Kawamoto K, Del Fiol G, Orton C, Lobach DF. System-agnostic clinical decision support services: benefits and challenges for scalable decision support. Open Med Inform J. 2010;4:245–54.
11. World Health Organization. International Classification of Diseases (ICD) [Internet]. Cited 28 Jul 2015. Available from: http://www.who.int/classifications/icd/en/.
12. International Health Terminology Standards Development Organisation. Systematized Nomenclature of Medicine-Clinical Terms (SNOMED CT) [Internet]. Cited 28 Jul 2015. Available from: http://www.ihtsdo.org/snomed-ct/.
13. Amazon. Amazon Elastic Compute Cloud (Amazon EC2) [Internet]. Cited 28 Jul 2015. Available from: http://aws.amazon.com/ec2/.
14. Papazoglou MP, Traverso P, Dustdar S, Leymann F. Service-oriented computing: state of the art and research challenges. Computer (Long Beach Calif). 2007;40(11):38–45.
15. U.S. Department of Health and Human Services. What is health IT? [Internet]. Available from: http://www.hrsa.gov/healthit/toolbox/oralhealthittoolbox/introduction/whatishealthit.html.
16. Canada Health Infoway Inc. Emerging technology series, cloud computing in health, white paper [Internet]. 2012. Available from: https://www.infoway-inforoute.ca/index.php/resources/technical-documents/emerging-technology/doc_download/660-cloud-computing-in-health-white-paper-executive-summary.
17. Kawamoto K, Honey A, Rubin K. The HL7-OMG healthcare services specification project: motivation, methodology, and deliverables for enabling a semantically interoperable service-oriented architecture for healthcare. J Am Med Inform Assoc. 2009;16(6):874–81.
18. Welch BM, Rodriguez-Loya S, Eilbeck K, Kawamoto K. Clinical decision support for whole genome sequence information leveraging a service-oriented architecture : a prototype. AMIA 2014 annual symposium. Washington, DC; 2014.
19. Kawamoto K, Jacobs J, Welch BM, Huser V, Paterno MD, Del Fiol G, et al. Clinical information system services and capabilities desired for scalable, standards-based, service-oriented decision support: consensus assessment of the Health Level 7 clinical decision support Work Group. AMIA. Annual symposium proceedings/AMIA symposium AMIA symposium. 2012. pp. 446–455.
20. Health Level Seven (HL7) and the Object Management Group (OMG). Healthcare Services Specification Program (HSSP) [Internet]. Cited 2015 Jun 6. Available from: http://hssp.wikispaces.com/.
21. Kawamoto K. OpenCDS [Internet]. Available from: http://www.opencds.org/.
22. Immunization Calculation Engine (ICE) [Internet]. Cited 2015 Jun 24. Available from: https://cdsframework.atlassian.net/wiki/display/ICE/Home.
23. Welch BM, Loya SR, Eilbeck K, Kawamoto K. A proposed clinical decision support architecture capable of supporting whole genome sequence information. J Pers Med. 2014;4(2):176–99.
24. Martínez-García A, Moreno-Conde A, Jódar-Sánchez F, Leal S, Parra C. Sharing clinical decisions for multimorbidity case management using social network and open-source tools. J Biomed Inform. 2013;48(6):977–84.
25. Kukhareva PV, Kawamoto K, Shields DE, Barfuss DT, Halley AM, Tippetts TJ, et al. Clinical decision support-based quality measurement (CDS-QM) framework: prototype implementation, evaluation, and future directions. AMIA Annu Symp Proc Am Med Inf Assoc. 2014;2014:825–34.
26. CDS Consortium. Clinical decision support consortium [Internet]. Cited 2015 Jul 28. Available from: http://www.cdsconsortium.org/.

27. S&I Framework [Internet]. Cited 2015 Jun 21. Available from: http://siframework.org/.
28. Health eDecision Closing Ceremony Final as posted and presented [Internet]. Cited 21 Jun 2015. Available from: http://wiki.siframework.org/file/view/Closing+Ceremony+Final+as+posted+and+presented1.pptx.
29. Kawamoto K, Hadley MJ, Goodrich K, Reider J. The clinical quality framework initiative: harmonizing clinical decision support and clinical quality measurement standards to enable interoperable quality improvement. Panel presentation at AMIA 2014 annual symposium. 2014.
30. The Healthcare Services Platform Consortium [Internet]. Cited 30 Jun 2015. Available from: https://healthservices.atlassian.net/wiki/display/HSPC/Healthcare+Services+Platform+Consortium.
31. SMART (Substitutable Medical Apps & Reusable Technology) [Internet]. Cited 30 Jun 2015. Available from: http://smarthealthit.org/.
32. Loya S, Kawamoto K, Chatwin C, Huser V. Service oriented architecture for clinical decision support: a systematic review and future directions. J Med Syst. 2014;38(12):1–22.
33. OASIS. Service Component Architecture Assembly Model Specification, Version 1.1, Committee Specification Draft 08 /Public Review Draft 03 31 May 2011 [Internet]. OASIS; Available from: http://docs.oasis-open.org/opencsa/sca-assembly/sca-assembly-spec-v1.1-csprd03.pdf.
34. Rodriguez-Loya S, Aziz A, Chatwin C. A service oriented approach for guidelines-based clinical decision support using BPMN. Stud Health Technol Inform. 2014;205:43–7.
35. Aziz A, Rodriguez S, Chatwin C. From guidelines to practice: improving clinical care through rule-based clinical decision support at the point of care. In: Bikakis A, Fodor P, Roman D, editors. Rules on the web. From theory to applications. Cham: Springer International Publishing; 2014. p. 178–85.

Chapter 6
Best Practices for Implementation of Clinical Decision Support

Richard N. Shiffman

Abstract Implementation of clinical decision support (CDS) is the process by which knowledge about appropriate practice is integrated with systems that are designed to influence provider behavior. We describe a systematic and replicable approach to implementation of knowledge that proceeds from knowledge synthesis that defines ideal care through a knowledge formalization phase in which that knowledge is transformed so it can be processed by computers. Next the knowledge is fitted to local needs, capabilities, and constraints. Finally, new knowledge gained from the implementation completes a feedback loop to inform future decision support activities.

Keywords Decision support • Implementation • Knowledge synthesis • Knowledge formalization • Knowledge localization

Implementation of clinical decision support (CDS)is the process by which knowledge about appropriate practice is integrated with systems that are designed to influence provider behavior. CDS design and implementation considerations are closely interrelated [1]. CDS implementation requires attention to the socio-technical and cognitive aspects of care delivery, as well as organizational function, human-computer interaction, and workflow analysis and reengineering. Implementation is increasingly regarded as a science in its own right that borrows from and contributes to these disciplines.

We describe three phases of CDS development and implementation—knowledge synthesis, knowledge formalization, and knowledge localization—in which knowledge about best clinical practice is captured, transformed into computable format, and embedded in health care systems (Fig. 6.1) [2]. Clinicians and policy makers increasingly speak of a "learning healthcare system" in which a cycle is created by feeding back the results of using CDS to promote advances in patient care, health care delivery processes, and implementation science [3].

R.N. Shiffman, M.D., M.C.I.S. (✉)
Yale School of Medicine, 300 George Street, Suite 501, New Haven, CT 06511, USA
e-mail: Richard.shiffman@yale.edu

E.S. Berner (ed.), *Clinical Decision Support Systems*, Health Informatics,
DOI 10.1007/978-3-319-31913-1_6

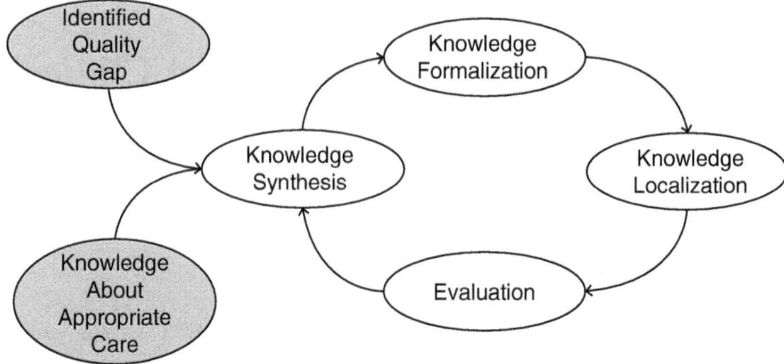

Fig. 6.1 Phases of CDS development and implementation in a learning healthcare system

6.1 Knowledge Synthesis

CDS is intended to improve the quality and safety of health care. Therefore, implementation begins with recognition and acknowledgement of a gap between current processes (and outcomes) of care and ideal care. Raw knowledge about appropriate care is derived from journal articles, monographs, book chapters, meta-analyses of individual studies, and the experience and expertise of subject matter experts. To be useful, this knowledge must be captured, organized, codified, and represented in a manner that can be manipulated by computers.

Knowledge synthesis is the process of combining the results of systematic review of the biomedical literature with the experience and expertise of experts to create recommendations about best practice [2]. *Clinical practice guidelines* represent a particularly rich source of knowledge about best practice. Current, evidence-based practice guidelines are developed and sanctioned by trusted professional societies, government entities, and healthcare delivery organizations. Guideline authoring teams strive to identify and organize unstructured knowledge into a narrative format that includes recommendations about appropriate care.

The 2011 Institute of Medicine report *Clinical Practice Guidelines We Can Trust* provides standards for development of guidelines [4]. According to the IOM, "trustworthy guidelines" should:

- Be based on a systematic review of the existing evidence;
- Be developed by a knowledgeable, multidisciplinary panel of experts from key affected groups;
- Consider important patient sub-groups and patient preferences;
- Be based on an explicit and transparent process that minimizes distortions, biases, and conflicts of interest;
- Be informed by an assessment of anticipated benefits and harms of alternative care options;

- Provide a clear explanation of the logical relationships between alternative care options and health outcomes, and provide ratings of both the quality of evidence and the strength of recommendations; and
- Be reconsidered and revised as appropriate when important new evidence warrants modification of recommendations [4].

To date, there has been considerable variability in the processes employed to develop practice guidelines. Some organizations apply consistent and rigorous methodologies to their development activities with careful evaluation of the evidence-base, while others rely on imprecise capture of expert opinion—sometimes referred to as GOBSAT (Good Old Boys Sitting Around the Table). In an effort to codify successful approaches and make the guideline development process more systematic and replicable, we developed BRIDGE-Wiz (Building Recommendations In a Developer's Guideline Editor), a software application that leads guideline authors through a series of steps intended to improve the clarity and transparency of guidelines and help assure that the guidelines can be implemented [5]. BRIDGE-Wiz focuses first on clearly specifying the recommended actions to be undertaken and the precise circumstances under which these actions are to occur. Next, it asks authors to document anticipated benefits, risks, harms, and costs that may be expected if the recommendation is executed. Finally, it standardizes the language of obligation in which the recommendations are articulated commensurate with the quality of evidence that supports each recommendation and the authors' judgment about the balance of anticipated benefits and harms. Additional tools have been used to help measure guideline quality and implementability of guideline statements, including COGS, [6] AGREE II, [7] NEATS (personal communication, Jane Jue), and eGLIA [8]. The COGS (Conference on Guideline Standardization) and AGREE (Appraisal of Guidelines for Research and Evaluation) are instruments intended to measure guideline quality based on longstanding indicators. The NEATS instrument (National Guideline Clearinghouse Extent Adherence to Trustworthy Standards) is more current and based on the IOM standards for trustworthy guidelines. eGLIA (Electronic Guidelines Implementability Appraisal) examines individual guideline recommendations to highlight potential obstacles to successful implementation.

The product of the Knowledge Synthesis phase of CDS development is an unstructured narrative document containing recommendations about appropriate care and meta-information about how those recommendations were derived and how they should be applied.

6.2 Knowledge Formalization

*Knowledge formalization*is the process of translating narrative guidelines into structured knowledge that can be implemented consistently in CDS applications [2]. Early work in CDSS design showed that knowledge engineers tasked with transforming guideline knowledge into CDSS developed idiosyncratic systems that provided different advice when tested against the same standardized patients [9, 10]. This unfortunate finding emphasizes the importance of transparency of knowledge transformation. Ideally an audit trail should be available to help assure fidelity of the decision support to the original knowledge source.

To help assure accuracy of knowledge translation and auditability of the formalization process, we translate the narrative guideline documents into an intermediate knowledge representation expressed in the eXtensible Markup Language (XML). XML is a multiplatform, Web-based, open standard. Users parse the text of a document (such as a guideline) into chunks delineated by meaningfully labeled "tags", for example:

<guidelineTitle>Hypertension Management</guidelineTitle>.

XML is human-readable, yet can be processed by computers. The process of parsing guideline content into XML can be performed by non-programmers.

The Guideline Elements Model (GEM) schema is a standard model of the content of clinical practice guidelines in XML. It includes 167 tags to describe and characterize textual components of narrative guidelines. The model is hierarchical with the following top-level elements [11]:

- Identity (containing information about title, release date, companion documents, status)
- Developer (including sponsoring organization, names of committee members, funding, conflict of interest declarations)
- Purpose (including focus, objective, and rationale for creating a guideline)
- Intended audience (including users and care settings in which the guideline may be implemented)
- Target Population (including inclusion and exclusion criteria)
- Method of Development (including description of evidence collection and combination, rating schemes for evidence quality and recommendation strength)
- Testing and Revision plans
- Implementation Plan
- Knowledge Components [11]

GEM works well as a knowledge representation intermediate between a narrative guideline and a formally specified CDSS. Most valuable to CDS implementers are the elements in the Knowledge Components hierarchy. In GEM, these elements include definitions of terms used in the guideline, algorithms (flowchart representations of procedural logic), and the guideline's recommendations about appropriate care. The <recommendation> subtree of the GEM hierarchy includes the <conditional> element, which, in turn, comprises:

- <decisionVariable>: the condition(s) under which a recommendation is appropriate, and
- <action>: the appropriate activities to be carried out.

Decision variables and actions together can be used to create IF…THEN rules to represent guideline recommendations.

Other elements in the <KnowledgeComponents> subtree provide tags for the <reason> (why the recommendation was developed and what it is intended to accomplish), <evidenceQuality>, and <recommendationStrength>, among others.

GEM Cutter is an XML editor (available from http://gem.med.yale.edu) that facilitates markup of guideline documents and their transformation from narrative text to a semi-structured format. The user interface provides three side-by-side panels. A user imports the narrative guideline into the leftmost panel. The middle panel provides an expandable list view of the GEM hierarchy. The rightmost panel provides a window for editing and iterative refinement of the guideline text. The user selects relevant text from the leftmost panel, determines where it belongs in the GEM hierarchy, and clicks a button that moves the text into the middle panel visually and adds the text to an evolving XML file.

In many cases, the decision variables and actions are stated in a vague and underspecified manner; occasionally they are frankly ambiguous. To achieve a semi-formal representation, relevant concepts are iteratively clarified and appropriate codes are identified in relevant standardized vocabularies, e.g., diagnosis codes in SNOMED-CT or ICD-10, laboratory results codes in LOINC, drug codes in RxNorm. Further, the logical relationships between and among decision variables and actions are defined using ANDs, ORs, NOTs, and grouped with parentheses. As these refinements are undertaken, the Guideline Elements Model maintains the original text of the recommendation statement to provide an audit trail against which the final edited recommendation may be compared with the original knowledge source.

Several proposals for a semi-formal representation are being developed by standards development organizations, which include Arden Syntax, HQMF, FHIR, and Health eDecisions. The product of knowledge formalization is one or more IF-THEN rules with decidable conditions and executable actions. In addition, concepts are represented in a standardized vocabulary.

There is a limit to how far centralized guideline development teams, such as those supported by professional societies or healthcare delivery organizations, can go in implementing CDS. Ideally, one would wish that a transformed module could simply be plugged into a local electronic health record system and shared. Unfortunately, many site-specific considerations must be addressed before a recommendation can be instantiated in a CDSS.

6.3 Knowledge Localization

The next step in the development of a decision support rule is one of the more complex ones. Once the recommendations have been expressed in statement logic (IF… THEN format) using structured vocabulary, those statements need to be translated into actionable decision support [12].

Knowledge localization encompasses the activities in which formalized knowledge about appropriate care is introduced into the systems that influence care [2]. Knowledge localization takes into account local resource constraints, workflow analysis, functional capabilities of the electronic health record, and the choice of CDS modality. Localization, by its very nature, cannot be fully standardized. Nonetheless, many implementation considerations may be generalized.

6.3.1 Resource Constraints

Implementation often takes a backseat to design and development of a CDSS. Failure to budget for implementation is common and in many cases, implementation makes use of resources that are left over, rather than allocated when the system is first specified. Clearly, early consideration of implementation needs is critical to project success.

A CDS governance structure that can assure the availability of necessary resources and help to prioritize an implementation plan is critical to CDSS success. Clinical leadership must provide support for introduction of all new technology, including CDS. In planning for adoption, implementers should consider incentives to use the systems, having champions on the ground, and integration of performance measurements. An example of an incentive includes having a form autopopulated that allows school and child care to administer medications when those medications are determined to be appropriate by the CDSS [12]. Likewise, a tablet-based device that collects information relevant to decision making in Spanish or Arabic and transmits its English equivalent into the CDSS facilitates use of the CDS and saves time for providers.

6.3.2 Workflow

Effective deployment and integration of CDSS requires analysis and understanding of current and anticipated workflows. Personnel roles and responsibilities vary greatly from facility to facility. Also, the sequence of activities to achieve a goal is often site-specific as are the resources available. Optimal implementation of CDSS requires careful attention to how and by whom information is collected, processed, and acted upon. Often, reengineering of workflow results in enhanced CDS function. Likewise, failure to optimize workflow can result in project failure.

It is also important to use multiple methods to analyze workflow. Individuals may not always be aware of their own processes or may choose not to share "workarounds" when asked to describe their workflow. Direct observation of processes, though time-consuming, can often provide valuable information. For instance, when implementing CDS that was intended to be used at the point-of-care, we found that documentation necessary to trigger the CDS often did not occur until the end of the clinic session when the patient had gone home. We addressed that problem by encouraging patients to directly enter relevant data into the CDS. In order to avoid having to repeat data gathering, the clinician would have to open the CDS while the patient was present.

6.3.3 EHR Functionality

Wright et al. have demonstrated that the technical capability of commercial EHRs to deliver CDS varies widely [13]. Triggers to invoke decision support and the types of data that can be used to make inferences may work well in one system but may be unavailable in another.

Even though formalization represents critical CDS elements in standardized vocabularies, many EHR vendors maintain their own proprietary coding systems into which concepts must be re-coded. This recoding provides opportunities to subvert the intent of the original knowledge sources.

6.3.4 CDSS Design

Careful attention to human factors design principles can help to assure that information is presented in a manner that optimizes information transfer and user acceptance. A set of best practices for CDS design is emerging [14, 15]. These standards call for design consistency, concise and unambiguous language, careful selection of modes for providing advice, and organization of information by problem and clinical goal. Since access to appropriate data for evaluation is a key challenge, implementers should plan to incorporate these elements during design.

In 2009 researchers analyzed more than one thousand randomly selected guideline recommendations and found that the actions could be reliably classified into the following 13 categories: "test, inquire, examine, monitor, conclude, prescribe, perform procedure, refer/consult, educate/counsel, prevent, dispose, advocate, and prepare facility/modify structure of care" [16]. They described how these categories of action types for guideline statements can be used to provide design strategies for implementation. For example, design of systems to implement a "test" action might consider presentation of test options/alternatives, test costs, scheduling options, interpretation aids, patient education about the test, requirements for preparation for the test, and a "tickler" follow-up system. Likewise, a "prescribe" recommendation might be supported by presenting the clinician with drug information, safety alerts (drug-allergy, drug-drug interaction), dosage calculation, pharmacy transmission, and corollary orders. Attention to these recurring themes can enhance CDSS design [16].

Strategies for delivery of decision support differ. While primary care clinicians dealing with an unfamiliar problem may welcome a prescriptive approach to CDS delivery (e.g., "The patient has moderate to severe Condition X for which Drug Y is indicated"), specialists managing a condition with which they are familiar often prefer a critiquing approach in which advice is only provided when a clinician's proposed care differs from actions recommended by the CDSS.

6.3.5 CDS Modalities

CDS can be provided by several modalities. Perhaps the most familiar modality is the *alert or reminder*. If one or more conditions are satisfied, the alert fires within the CDSS. Recent work has indicated that many alerts are perceived as distracting noise by busy clinicians and contribute to a condition known as "alert fatigue" [17]. These users are liable to bypass alerts without heeding the information they contain which has the potential to compromise effective care or patient safety. Care should be taken in employing interruptive alerts and in display of reminders to maximize user acceptance and safe use. Implementers should avoid intrusive CDSS designs wherever possible.

Order sets comprise another frequently used CDS modality. Order sets group information for display and facilitate appropriate choices as CDS users are formulating plans and writing orders. This type of CDS can be highly interactive and display information conditionally based on the user's actions. Order sets have been demonstrated in numerous studies to improve processes and outcomes of care [18]. There is usually a need to get agreement among clinician users as to what orders should be part of an order set. Although this can be time-consuming, it is worth the effort as the order sets can make subsequent use of the system more efficient. For instance, in our GLIDES project, we chose highly respected guidelines published by the National Heart Lung and Blood Institute and in other work, we chose guidelines from trusted professional associations [12].

Visual summaries of recent relevant findings help to organize complex data. Tierney et al. showed that simply presenting physicians with the results of previous tests reduced the ordering of those tests [19]. Likewise, *documentation templates* cue the user to collect and record appropriate information. *Hypertext links* to additional information serve an educational purpose. The *Infobutton* is an HL7 standard that facilitates user-initiated requests for additional information in a context-sensitive manner [20]. *Calculators* can be used to promote accuracy of numeric operations, e.g., calculating a drug dosage in mg/kg or intravenous drip rate. Alternatively, calculators can calculate scores on survey instruments and categorize disease severity based on symptom scores.

6.3.6 Level of Enforcement

The level of enforcement of an alert should be tied to the importance of the information being delivered. Guideline-specified *recommendation strength* can be useful to implementers in determining appropriate levels of enforcement. For example, prescribing a drug to a patient known to be allergic to that drug might result in an alert with a high level of enforcement—a hard stop in which further progress is not possible without burdensome data entry or communication with an authorizer. Hard stops should be reserved for uncommon and potentially serious situations. Lower levels of enforcement might simply require the user's acknowledgement of the alert in order to move forward. Finally, some reminders might simply be informational not requiring any activity on the part of the user.

6.3.7 Participatory Design

End users should participate in CDSS design and development activities from the outset. Importantly, they should recognize that they represent a class of users and should serve as a bilateral communication medium, bringing subject matter expertise to the implementers and explanation of the evolving CDSS to stakeholders.

Providing users with a benefit for using the CDS helps to gain their acceptance. For example, an asthma decision support system was designed to automatically create and populate a permission form for the use of a rescue inhaler at school or camp. Likewise, we developed decision support for improving prescription of opioids for chronic pain. Once a provider indicates an intent to prescribe an opioid, s/he is reminded about non-pharmacologic interventions (e.g., physical therapy, acupuncture, cognitive behavioral therapy, etc.) and referral is facilitated. In addition, the CDSS provides a link to the guidelines that provide the evidence base for the recommendations and another to the state Prescription Drug Monitoring Program, "Making it easy to do it right" is a useful mantra for implementers to follow [21].

6.4 Evaluation and Learning

CDSS success should be measured against the goals originally identified during Knowledge Synthesis. Once tested and deployed, the implementation team should collect data regarding effectiveness, usefulness,and usability of the CDSS. Use of CDS to guide care results in the generation of new data about how adhering to existing recommendations affects health and healthcare. CDSS evaluation helps to shape new recommendations about appropriate care.

Implementers also learn about the usability of the CDSS by planned evaluation activities. Evaluation can include formal or informal observation of users interacting with the CDSS as well as user surveys to assess system usefulness, ease of use, ease of learning and general satisfaction. Chapter 9 discusses other strategies for CDSS evaluation.

A learning health system effectively captures this information and loops it back to be synthesized with indicators of effectiveness [3]. These new data inform future CDSS design and deployment decisions.

6.5 Summary and Conclusions

Clinical decision support has great promise to improve the health of individuals and to improve the delivery of healthcare across populations. In order to do so, CDSS must be based on the best knowledge available systematically and replicably transformed into formats that computers can process. Careful consideration of local needs and resource constraints determines the ultimate success or failure of the system. Knowledge about best clinical practice must be combined with knowledge about effective implementation.

References

1. Berner ES. Clinical decision support systems: state of the art. Rockville, MD: Publication number 09-0069EF. Rockville: Agency for Healthcare Research and Quality; 2009.
2. Shiffman RN, Wright A. Evidence-based clinical decision support. Yearb Med Inform. 2013;8(1):20–7.
3. Institute of Medicine. Best care at lower cost: the path to continuously learning health care in America. Washington, DC: National Academies Press; 2013.
4. Institute of Medicine. Clinical practice guidelines we can trust. Washington, DC: National Academies Press; 2011.
5. Shiffman RN, Michel G, Rosenfeld RM, Davidson C. Building better guidelines with BRIDGE-Wiz: development and evaluation of a software assistant to promote clarity, transparency, and implementability. J Am Med Inform Assoc. 2012;19(1):94–101.
6. Shiffman RN, Shekelle P, Overhage JM, Slutsky J, Grimshaw J, Deshpande AM. Standardized reporting of clinical practice guidelines: a proposal from the Conference on Guideline Standardization. Ann Intern Med. 2003;139:493–8.
7. Brouwers M, Kho M, Browman G, Burgers J, Cluzeau F, Feder G, et al. AGREE II: advancing guideline development, reporting and evaluation in healthcare. Can Med Assoc J. 2010;182:E839–42.
8. Shiffman RN, Dixon J, Brandt C, Essaihi A, Hsiao A, Michel G, et al. The GuideLine Implementability Appraisal (GLIA): development of an instrument to identify obstacles to guideline implementation. BMC Med Inform Decis Mak. 2005;5:23.
9. Patel VL, Allen VG, Arocha JF, Shortliffe EH. Representing clinical guidelines in GLIF: individual and collaborative expertise. J Am Med Inform Assoc. 1998;5:467–83.

10. Ohno-Machado L, Gennari JH, Murphy SN, Jain NL, Tu SW, Oliver DE, et al. The guideline interchange format: a model for representing guidelines. J Am Med Inform Assoc. 1998;5:357–72.
11. ASTM International. Standard specification for Guideline Elements Model version 3 (GEM III)-document model for clinical practice guidelines. Conshohocken, PA, 2012.
12. Guidelines Into Decision Support (GLIDES) (Connecticut). Available from: https://healthit.ahrq.gov/ahrq-funded-projects/guidelines-decision-support-glides. Accessed 9 Dec 2015.
13. Wright A, Sittig DF, Ash JS, Sharma S, Pang JE, Middleton B. Clinical decision support capabilities of commercially-available clinical information systems. J Am Med Inform Assoc. 2009;16(5):637–44.
14. Horsky J, Schiff GD, Johnston D, Mercincavage L, Bell D, Middleton B. Interface design principles for usable decision support: a targeted review of best practices for clinical prescribing interventions. J Biomed Inform. 2012;45(6):1–10.
15. Shobha P, Edworthy J, Hellier E, Segar DL, Schedlbauer A, Avery A, et al. A review of human factors principles for the design and implementation of medication safety alerts in clinical information systems. J Am Med Inform Assoc. 2011;17:493–501.
16. Shiffman RN, Lomotan E, Michel G. Using action-types to design guideline implementation systems (Abstr). Presented at the 6th Conferencia Internacional da Guidelines International Network, Lisbon, 1 Novembro 2009. Abstract published in Acta Medica Portuguesa Volume 22:15; 2009.
17. Payne T, Hines L, Chan R, et al. Recommendations to improve the usability of drug-drug interaction clinical decision support alerts. J Am Med Inform Assoc. 2015;Epub ahead of print.
18. Bobb AM, Payne TH, Gross PA. Viewpoint: controversies surrounding use of order sets for clinical decision support in computerized provider order entry. J Am Med Inform Assoc. 2007;14:41–7.
19. Tierney W, McDonald C, Martin D, Hui S, Rogers M. Computerized display of past test results. Ann Intern Med. 1987;107:569–74.
20. HL7 International. Context-aware knowledge retrieval application (Infobutton), Release 4. HL7 International; 2014.
21. James BC. Making it easy to do it right. N Engl J Med. 2001;345:991–3.

Chapter 7
Impact of National Policies on the Use of Clinical Decision Support

Jacob M. Reider

Abstract The United States federal government has contributed strategic guidance and funding toward the development of a mature national infrastructure for clinical quality improvement. These efforts, aligned with the National Quality Strategy, have created technical foundations, policy levers, and content artifacts that have accelerated the development of clinical decision support in the United States. Legislative and regulatory activities will continue to create opportunity for both technical and content experts in this domain. This chapter explores the major efforts of the US government to promote the effective use of clinical decision support.

Keywords National Quality Strategy (NQS) • Federal health policy • Office the National Coordinator (ONC) • Centers for Medicare and Medicaid Services (CMS) • Agency for Healthcare Research and Quality (AHRQ)

Clinical decision support (CDS) has long been a part of the United States federal government's strategy toward reaching the Triple Aim of better health, better care and lower cost [1]. This chapter will review the federal contributions in this domain beginning in 2008, when a major CDS initiative was launched by the Agency for Healthcare Research and Quality (AHRQ) [2]. As this chapter will describe, the AHRQ projects created a foundation for nearly all of the work that followed, and created both the technical and policy framework that would be required to reach the Triple Aim. While the United States Department of Defense (DoD), the Indian Health Service (IHS), and the Veterans Health Administration (VHA) are also federal entities, this chapter will not address their CDS work. Rather, the emphasis here is on AHRQ, the Centers for Disease Control and Prevention (CDC), the Centers for Medicare and Medicaid Services (CMS), the Office of the National Coordinator for Health Information Technology (ONC) and the US Congress, organizations that have created programs or policies with broad national impact. While DoD, IHS and

J.M. Reider, M.D., F.A.A.F.P. (✉)
Department of Family and Community Medicine, Albany Medical College, 47 New Scotland Ave, Albany, NY 12208, USA
e-mail: jacob@reider.us

E.S. Berner (ed.), *Clinical Decision Support Systems*, Health Informatics,
DOI 10.1007/978-3-319-31913-1_7

VHA certainly have national impact, it is their impact as very large care delivery organizations rather than as defining or implementing policy with national downstream consequences.

7.1 United States Federal Government Clinical Decision Support Initiatives

Today, the basis for federal engagement in CDS is the National Quality Strategy (NQS) which was mandated by the Affordable Care Act and updated annually [3]. First published in 2011, the NQS defines three aims, six priorities and nine levers that will be used to improve health quality in the United States [4]. The National Quality Strategy pursues three broad aims. These aims will be used to guide and assess local, state, and national efforts to improve health and the quality of health care. To advance these aims, the National Quality Strategy focuses on six priorities (see Table 7.1).

Table 7.1 Summary of NQS's aims and priorities

Aims		Priorities	
1.	Better care: improve the overall quality, by making health care more patient-centered, reliable, accessible, and safe	1.	Making care safer by reducing harm caused in the delivery of care
2.	Healthy people/healthy communities: improve the health of the U.S. population by supporting proven interventions to address behavioral, social and, environmental determinants of health in addition to delivering higher-quality care	2.	Ensuring that each person and family is engaged as partners in their care
3.	Affordable care: reduce the cost of quality health care for individuals, families, employers, and government	3.	Promoting effective communication and coordination of care
		4.	Promoting the most effective prevention and treatment practices for the leading causes of mortality, starting with cardiovascular disease
		5.	Working with communities to promote wide use of best practices to enable healthy living
		6.	Making quality care more affordable for individuals, families, employers, and governments by developing and spreading new health care delivery models

Adapted from: Report to Congress, National Quality Strategy, March 2011. Available from http://www.ahrq.gov/workingforquality/nqs/nqs2011annlrpt.pdf

Table 7.2 Summary of NQS's levers

Levers			
1.	Measurement and feedback: provide performance feedback to plans and providers to improve care	6.	Payment: reward and incentivize providers to deliver high-quality, patient-centered care
2.	Public reporting: compare treatment results, costs and patient experience for consumers	7.	Health information technology: improve communication, transparency, and efficiency for better coordinated health and health care
3.	Learning and technical assistance: foster learning environments that offer training, resources, tools, and guidance to help organizations achieve quality improvement goals	8.	Innovation and diffusion: foster innovation in health care quality improvement, and facilitate rapid adoption within and across organizations and communities
4.	Certification, accreditation, and regulation: adopt or adhere to approaches to meet safety and quality standards	9.	Workforce development: investing in people to prepare the next generation of health care professionals and support lifelong learning for providers
5.	Consumer incentives and benefit designs: help consumers adopt healthy behaviors and make informed decisions		

Adapted from: Report to Congress, National Quality Strategy, March 2011. Available from http://www.ahrq.gov/workingforquality/nqs/nqs2011annlrpt.pdf

Each of the nine National Quality Strategy levers (see Table 7.2) represents a core business function, resource, and/or action that stakeholders can use to align to the Strategy. In many cases, stakeholders may already be using these levers but have not connected these activities to National Quality Strategy alignment.

While CDS is not explicitly referenced in this guiding framework for the NQS, CDS is a powerful enabler of all three aims, most of the priorities, and many of the levers. Given this dependence, the federal government has made deep investments in both quality measurement and CDS, and has been working hard to converge these efforts – in both technical and policy domains – toward a unified quality improvement work effort that forms an umbrella for both CDS and clinical quality measures (CQM).

7.2 Technical Foundations

In August 2007, AHRQ solicited proposals for "the development, implementation and evaluation of demonstration projects that advance understanding of how best to incorporate clinical decision support into the delivery of health care … with the overall goal of exploring how the translation of clinical knowledge into CDS can be routinized in practice and taken to scale in order to improve the quality of health care delivery in the U.S." [5]. The successful grantees were Yale University's Guidelines Into Decision Support (GLIDES) project, and Brigham and Women's Hospital's Clinical Decision Support Consortium (CDSC).

better health, and lower cost, two parallel communities had formed to work toward this goal. One, the CDS community, developed methods of intervening in care decisions toward improving them. The other, the quality measurement community, developed clinical quality measures or CQM, with the implicit prediction that measurement will cause improvement. Within and beyond the federal government, CQM and CDS reference different domain models, different standards, and different syntax – even though the majority of the logic is identical. The key difference is one of timeframe: with CDS, one focuses on decisions at the point-of-care and say "for THIS sort of individual, we should offer THAT sort of treatment," while those who focus on CQM look at the same situation retrospectively and say: "for THIS sort of individual, did we offer THAT sort of treatment?"

As HeD evolved in parallel with the quality measures work and the evolution of the Health Quality Measures Format (HQMF), which is the HL7 normative standard that defines an XML expression syntax for clinical quality measures, it became clear that the federal government needed to align these projects toward one domain model, one semantic framework, one services syntax, and one standards work stream. Toward such a unification, the Clinical Quality Framework initiative was launched to converge the work of CDS and CQM into a clinical quality improvement (CQI) initiative. The activity is hosted by the ONC Standards and Interoperability framework where readers can find links to (a) pilot initiatives, (b) draft versions of QUICK, the Quality Improvement and Clinical Knowledge model, (c) the merged successor to the Virtual Medical Record (vMR), as well as (d) the domain model for HeD, (e) the Quality Data Model (QDM), and (f) HQMF [16]. As QUICK and its new syntax, CQL (Clinical Quality Language), evolve, the goal will be to unify artifacts provided by the federal government for both CDS and CQM into this common format. Just as the government currently provides CQMs in HQMF, the long-term goal is that the government will ultimately provide publicly available CDS knowledge artifacts and CQMs in CQF. Then this could be subscribed to by health IT systems and incorporated into workflow without human translation.

7.5 Clinical Decision Support and the HITECH Act

HITECH created the authority and funding for ONC and CMS to create policies and programs that were engineered to improve care and care quality in the United States. As initially designed by ONC and CMS, the programs were created to evolve in three stages: Stage 1 focused on adoption of health IT, Stage 2 focused on exchange of information, and Stage 3 focused on care quality improvement. Each iteration, initially planned to take 2 years, would provide incentives for care providers to adopt health information technology and incorporate it meaningfully into their practices. This is the genesis of the term "meaningful use," as the goal was to incentivize the use of health IT, rather than just the purchase of it. The definition of "meaningful" has been a matter of serious debate, as there remains a great deal of variability in how care delivery organizations operate. What may be meaningful to a pediatric ophthalmologist may or may not be meaningful to a geriatrician and vice versa. The mirror image of the CMS incentive programs (separate programs for Medicare and Medicaid providers) is the ONC's certification program, formally called the Standards and Certification Criteria for Health Information Technology. The first iterations of these regulations were published in 2009, with an effective date of January, 2011.

The regulations for Stage 1 of the EHR incentive programs, as well as the 2011 Standards and Certification criteria, included a clinical decision support requirement. To satisfy the meaningful use expectations, providers and care delivery organizations were required to "[i]mplement one clinical decision support rule relevant to specialty or high clinical priority along with the ability to track compliance with that rule" [17]. HHS defined CDS as "HIT functionality that builds upon the foundation of an EHR to provide persons involved in care processes with general and person-specific information, intelligently filtered and organized, at appropriate times, to enhance health and health care" [17]. The regulations also created certification criteria that defined the functional capabilities that would need to be used in order for the meaningful use requirements to be met. For 2011 certification, the certification requirements were:

(1) Implement rules. Implement automated, electronic clinical decision support rules (in addition to drug-drug and drug-allergy contraindication checking) based on the data elements included in: problem list; medication list; demographics; and laboratory test results.
(2) Notifications. Automatically and electronically generate and indicate in real-time, notifications and care suggestions based upon clinical decision support rules.[18]

Unfortunately, many health IT developers and care delivery organizations interpreted this requirement to mean that programmatic rules would need to be developed that would always result in alerts – raising deep concern that alert fatigue would eliminate the value of the CDS altogether. Furthermore, questions were raised about the definition of "real-time": if a batch process were run overnight to identify patients eligible for a screening colonoscopy or influenza vaccine, would that violate the certification requirement? What if a system provided enhancement of visual display to clearly indicate a patient's need for a given intervention, and it was appropriately based on lab results, medications, and medical problems, but not demographics? Would the omission of demographics mean that the system could not be considered certified CDS? And if a care provider used that capability would he/she be ineligible for meaningful use incentives?

Subsequently, the Stage 2 requirements/2014 certification criteria (published in 2012) and the Stage 3 requirements/2015 certification criteria (published in 2015) addressed many of these questions. Both requirements/criteria expanded the meaningful use requirement to the implementation of five interventions from one, and emphasized that at least four interventions needed to be associated with clinical quality measures. The certification criteria were also modified and expanded, as demonstrated in Table 7.3 [19]. It is important to fully understand each of these requirements in detail, as they form the functional basis for all certified health IT products in the US going forward.

Table 7.3 2015 Certification criteria related to clinical decision support (CDS)

<table>
<tr><th colspan="4">2015 Certification criteria: Clinical decision support (CDS)</th></tr>
<tr><td colspan="4">(i) CDS intervention interaction. Interventions provided to a user must occur when a user is interacting with technology</td></tr>
<tr><td rowspan="8">(ii) CDS configuration</td><td rowspan="8">(A) Enable interventions and reference resources specified in paragraphs (a)(9)(iii) and (iv) of this section to be configured by a limited set of identified users (e.g., system administrator) based on a user's role</td><td colspan="2">(B) Enable interventions:</td></tr>
<tr><td>1. Based on the following data:</td><td rowspan="7">2. When a patient's medications, medication allergies, and problems are incorporated from a transition of care/ referral summary received and pursuant to paragraph (b)(2)(iii)(D) of this section</td></tr>
<tr><td>(i) Problem list;</td></tr>
<tr><td>(ii) Medication list;</td></tr>
<tr><td>(iii) Medication allergy list;</td></tr>
<tr><td>(iv) At least one demographic specified in paragraph (a)(5)(i) of this section;</td></tr>
<tr><td>(v) Laboratory tests; and</td></tr>
<tr><td>(vi) Vital signs</td></tr>
<tr><td colspan="4">(iii) Evidence-based decision support interventions. Enable a limited set of identified users to select (i.e., activate) electronic CDS interventions (in addition to drug-drug and drug-allergy contraindication checking) based on each one and at least one combination of the data referenced in paragraphs (a)(9)(ii)(B)(1)(i) through (vi) of this section</td></tr>
<tr><td rowspan="3">(iv) Linked referential CDS</td><td>(A) Identify for a user diagnostic and therapeutic reference information in accordance at least one of the following standards and implementation specifications:</td><td colspan="2" rowspan="3">(B) For paragraph (a)(9)(iv)(A) of this section, technology must be able to identify for a user diagnostic or therapeutic reference information based on each one and at least one combination of the data referenced in paragraphs (a)(9)(ii)(B)(1)(i), (ii), and (iv) of this section</td></tr>
<tr><td>1. The standard and implementation specifications specified in § 170.204(b)(3)</td></tr>
<tr><td>2. The standard and implementation specifications specified in § 170.204(b)(4)</td></tr>
</table>

(continued)

Table 7.3 (continued)

2015 Certification criteria: Clinical decision support (CDS)		
(v) *Source attributes*. Enable a user to review the attributes as indicated for all CDS resources:	(A) For evidence-based decision support interventions under paragraph (a)(9)(iii) of this section:	(B) For linked referential CDS in paragraph (a)(9)(iv) of this section and drug-drug, drug-allergy interaction checks in paragraph (a)(4) of this section, the developer of the intervention, and where clinically indicated, the bibliographic citation of the intervention (clinical research/guideline)
	1. Bibliographic citation of the intervention (clinical research/guideline);	
	2. Developer of the intervention (translation from clinical research/guideline);	
	3. Funding source of the intervention development technical implementation; and	
	4. Release and, if applicable, revision date(s) of the intervention or reference source	

Adapted from Federal Register [Internet]. 2015. 2015 Edition Health Information Technology (Health IT) Certification Criteria, 2015 Edition Base Electronic Health Record (EHR) Definition, and ONC Health IT Certification Program Modifications: 45 CFR 170.314.(9). 2015 [cited 2015 Nov 14] Available from: https://www.federalregister.gov/articles/2015/10/16/2015-25597/2015-edition-health-information-technology-health-it-certification-criteria-2015-edition-base#p-277

7.6 2015 CDS Certification Criteria

Federal regulations are specified by where in the code of federal regulations (CFR) they can be found. The 2015 certification criteria are in section 170.315, and the CDS criterion is section 9. Therefore this section is referenced as CFR 170.314(9) and there are five elements of this criterion, as shown in Table 7.3.

7.6.1 CDS Intervention Interaction

In the new criteria, CDS is no longer referenced as a "rule" but as an "intervention." The selection of this term was deliberate as "rule" invokes notions of logic, programming and algorithms, while the term "intervention" focuses on the outcome of such methods. ONC sought to direct focus on the activity rather than the method and to allow for innovation wherever possible. ONC also clarifies that CDS interventions must be presented when the user is interacting with the technology.

The regulation therefore does not consider functional capabilities to be CDS unless these capabilities interact with an end user. It is important to note that for ONC's certification, it is not specified that the user needs to be a clinician – just that someone needs to be interacting with the technology itself – presumably as part of an appropriate workflow. Paper byproducts of CDS interventions are therefore not acceptable, but any technology (e.g., smartphone, computer, watch, technically augmented glasses, heads-up data displays, or tactile interfaces such as dynamic Braille) that is certified to perform this capability, would be acceptable.

7.6.2 CDS Configuration

CDS capabilities require configuration, maintenance, optimization, and in many cases, personalization. This criterion specifies first that a certified system is required to include the capability of such configuration by the user. The intent of this requirement is to clarify that some users may require different interventions, and that a system administrator must be able to apply/manage these interventions on the users' behalf.

The section further clarifies that the capabilities such an administrator can enable include interventions based on patient medications, problems, medication allergies, vital signs, lab tests and at least one demographic element: sex, race and ethnicity, preferred language, or sexual orientation and gender identity (SO/GI). Second, this criterion specifies that a system needs to be capable of enabling CDS interventions to be based on medications, problems, or medication allergies that are incorporated into the patient's record as a product of a user acting on a care summary record that is received from another care provider. For example, if a user has incorporated a care summary record that includes a new medication allergy, the system must be capable of informing the user of a potential contraindication to that medication.

7.6.3 Evidence-Based Decision Support Interventions

This criterion dovetails with the "configure" requirement, and expresses that some users need to have the capability of activating CDS interventions, based on each of the "configuration" elements (i.e. medications, problems, etc.) and at least one combination of these elements. For example, a user needs to be able to turn on a CDS intervention that recommends breast cancer screening, based on gender and age, or diabetes screening, based on BMI and lab values. Furthermore, this criterion makes it clear that drug-drug and drug-allergy checking are not considered CDS for the purposes of this criterion, but are addressed in separate certification criteria.

7.6.4 Linked Referential CDS

Linked referential CDS is a link, such as an HTML hypertext link, or other software connection, to a knowledge resource that uses the HL7 Context Aware Knowledge Retrieval Application or "infobutton" standard. The certified technology must be able to leverage the patient's problems, medications, and demographics to connect the user to relevant diagnostic or therapeutic information. For example, based on a patient's problem list, a system might use the infobutton standard to query a knowledge repository for reference information about one of the patient's problems, and offer references or information about that problem that may be of value toward more optimal management.

7.6.5 Source Attributes

This criterion specifies that for any CDS intervention, the science upon which the guidance is based must be made available to the end user in the form of a bibliographic reference. Furthermore, the identity (person or organization) of the developer of the intervention and the funding source of the intervention should also be made available. In some cases, a bibliographic reference may not be available or necessary. For example, a self-evident CDS intervention, such as a suggestion to avoid prescribing a medication to which the patient is allergic, may not require a bibliographic reference. The developer and funding source are important because these may represent biases that the user may want to understand. ONC made no effort to regulate or even define where or how bias may contribute to CDS that is incorporated into a health IT system. Rather, ONC worked to make sure that there would be ways that users could make judgments of bias on their own. For example, if drug company ABC were to pay health IT company XYZ $3,000,000 to include CDS interventions suggesting that every patient with a given condition be prescribed ABC's new medication for that condition, the developer of the intervention (XYZ) would be visible to the user, as would the funding source (ABC). The certification requirement is that the system must be capable of this functionality, and not that every CDS intervention in the system leverages it. This is an important distinction, because "home-grown" CDS interventions that a clinician may create for themselves would not need to incorporate these attributes.

These certification criteria are important because every federal program that invokes the use of certified health IT will reference these capabilities, definitions, and terminology. It is therefore important to understand that while CDS "rules," "artifacts" and "interventions" may be used in some circles interchangeably, the federal programs will generally refer to "interventions" and will invoke iterations of the certification criteria described above and in Table 7.3.

7.7 Implementation and Optimization Guidance

In addition to the policy and standards work, HHS has sought to provide guidance to care delivery organizations so that best practices in CDS implementation and optimization can be defined and leveraged nationwide. Presently, ONC hosts resources on a CDS web page (https://www.healthit.gov/providers-professionals/clinical-decision-support-cds) that provides users with both introductory and advanced resources. These resources include presentations, worksheets, and guidance documents designed to help care delivery organizations capture the right information about CDS opportunities, and then develop thoughtful, well documented CDS interventions.

7.8 The Patient Protection and Affordable Care Act

The Patient Protection and Affordable Care Act, often referred to as "ACA" or "Obamacare," had no explicit references to CDS, but it established the creation of the Patient Centered Outcomes Research Institute (PCORI), and the Patient Centered Outcomes Research (PCOR) Trust Fund [20]. The goal of these initiatives is to leverage health information technology to discover new opportunities for care improvement, and then to disseminate this new knowledge. To facilitate dissemination, AHRQ created the PCOR CDS Learning Network [21], which will:

- Engage clinicians, patients, professional associations, health IT developers, and other stakeholders who can help promote the incorporation of PCOR findings into clinical practice through CDS;
- Identify barriers and facilitators to the use of CDS as a means to disseminate and to implement PCOR findings in clinical practice; and
- Provide consensus-based recommendations to the field of CDS developers, CDS implementers, and other stakeholders about CDS design and implementation best practices [21].

The PCOR CDS Learning Network was launched in Spring 2016, and will be funded through 2020.

7.9 Protecting Access to Medicare Act of 2014 (PAMA)

PAMA, passed in 2014 as a temporary fix to the Sustainable Growth Rate formula by which CMS pays physicians, included a requirement that providers who order advanced diagnostic imaging services consult with appropriate use criteria (AUC) via a clinical decision support mechanism [22]. The rationale for this provision is consensus that AUC would save money and diminish unnecessary patient exposure to radiation by reducing inappropriate imaging services [23]. The law provides a good example of how congressional action imposes a solution on HHS, leaving HHS some (but not infinite) flexibility in making a determination of how, and when, to implement the law's intent through regulation. This is the very first law that explicitly requires ordering providers to use clinical decision support, and therefore may set a precedent for subsequent laws and regulations. An interesting facet of PAMA's provision is that the penalty or 'reimbursement withholding' would be borne by the "furnishing professional" (a term that CMS defines for the purposes of implementing this regulation – meaning the professional that furnishes the services ordered by the ordering professional), while the burden of action, using AUC CDS, would be borne by the ordering provider. This nuance will then require health IT systems to capture which AUC CDS was used by the ordering provider, and have that information transmitted to the furnishing provider so that s/he can, as required by the law, include this information in their bill to CMS, and subsequently have confidence that their services will be reimbursed.

PAMA required CMS to take the first steps toward implementing an AUC CDS mandate in the 2016 Physician Fee Schedule regulation, which was published by CMS on October 20, 2015 [24]. The regulation first describes CMS' experience with AUC, the Medicare Imaging Demonstration (MID) project [25]. It also summarizes experiences from other care delivery organizations that have leveraged AUC and CDS in image ordering, while providing a sound overview of the timeline of how and when CMS will fully implement this program.

CMS appropriately states the CDS mechanisms through which providers access AUC: "…must be integrated into the clinical workflow and facilitate, not obstruct, evidence-based care delivery," and that "the ideal AUC is an evidence-based guide that starts with a patient's specific clinical condition or presentation (symptoms) and assists the provider in the overall patient workup, treatment and follow-up" [26]. The agency therefore set in motion the first of a series of annual regulatory actions that will result in full implementation of this program by 2018.

The first step addresses how CMS will assure that each AUC is evidence-based, but will avoid a framework that would have CMS approve of criteria one-by-one. Rather, they will approve "Provider Led Entities" (PLEs) who will apply to CMS for qualification. Once approved, these entities will develop or endorse AUCs. Only AUCs developed or endorsed by PLEs will be applicable under the program.

The second step of the program will be to certify CDS mechanisms for the delivery of AUCs. While CMS originally planned to begin this process in 2016, they have delayed this until at least 2017 [27]. There is therefore no guidance regarding the form or syntax in which AUCs are delivered, nor specifications for the technical implementations of the CDS that would be used to deliver AUCs. This regulatory process would ideally be aligned with the ONC/CMS CQF standards activities so that when AUCs are created, the interventions are based on QUICK, and logic expressions expressed in CQL. Such a requirement could be incorporated into the PLE application process, such as an agreement to create AUCs in these forms and even an agreement to participate in the CQF initiative. Or it could be incorporated into the definition of the CDS standards that CMS will publish in the future.

In the regulation, CMS has been clear that this will not be in place by the January 1, 2017 deadline that was defined by PAMA: "we fully anticipate that we will be able to finalize rules and requirements around the CDS mechanism and approve mechanisms through rulemaking in 2017. This timeline will significantly impact when we would expect practitioners to begin using those CDS mechanisms to consult AUC and report on those consultations. We do not anticipate that the consultation and reporting requirements will be in place by the January 1, 2017 deadline established in section 218(b) of the PAMA" [28].

This program is important because AUC for imaging is just a category of knowledge artifact. Once there is clarity regarding the specific technical and semantic requirements for the CDS, it is likely that CMS and others will take advantage of this delivery channel for other high priority knowledge artifacts such as immunizations, opioid abuse prevention, antibiotic stewardship, and infectious disease/bioterrorism emergencies.

7.10 Medicare Access and CHIP Reauthorization Act of 2015 (MACRA)

The 2015 passage of MACRA created sweeping changes in how CMS compensates providers and care delivery organizations [29]. Like PAMA, the law defines a broad framework that defines the "what" of the new payment framework, while CMS will, through rulemaking, define the specifics of the program and how it will be implemented. While a thorough review of MACRA is beyond the scope of this chapter, it is important to understand some of the basics, as this law opens the door to a great deal of motivation for care delivery organizations to accelerate their adoption of CDS.

MACRA evolves existing payment structures over several years from ones that are based on fee-for-service to ones that incentivize care quality, and the meaningful use of health IT. The program has two primary components:

- The Merit-Based Incentive Payment System (MIPS), which coalesces the Physician Quality Reporting System (PQRS), the EHR incentive programs ("meaningful use") and the value based modifier program. MIPS will align the quality reporting measures, processes, and technical requirements, and will reward providers who perform well, while penalizing providers who choose not to participate or who perform poorly.
- Alternate Payment Models (APMs) such as ACOs, advanced PCMHs or other innovative value-based programs. Providers who participate in such programs will not have to participate in MIPS or any of its components, but will (after 2020) be required to use certified health IT [29].

These programs will all shift providers' focus from volume and efficiency toward the three aims of the National Quality Strategy (better care, healthy people and communities, affordable care). MIPS incentivizes performance on clinical quality measures and meaningful use of health IT. In order to be successful in achieving high quality scores, CDS will need to be implemented. So while there is no explicit expectation defined for the use of CDS, it is clearly a necessary component of success in MIPS. In the same way, providers participating in APMs will need to leverage health IT and CDS in order to achieve the quality, cost and efficiency goals of many of the APM programs.

7.11 Impact of Federal Programs on CDS

Clinical Decision Support is not the end-point of any of these federal programs, and it is therefore difficult to measure the causality of any federal program on one capability of health IT systems. CDS is a method that is employed toward the goals of the triple aim. Nonetheless, widespread adoption of health IT in the United States from 2009 to 2015 is a clear result of the HITECH act. We will certainly continue to see an expansion of our reliance on health IT as the maturity and usability of systems improve, in part due to the improved specificity of CDS interventions in the context of integrated "big data," machine learning, and genomic research.

The impact of PAMA on imaging facilities, furnishing professionals (and their systems' interoperability with those of ordering providers) and ordering providers cannot be understated. The success or failure of this effort, the first explicit legal requirement for CDS, will define how or whether future CDS requirements will be shaped.

7.12 FDA Regulation of Clinical Decision Support

The Food and Drug Administration has the authority to regulate medical devices in the United States. The 2012 Food and Drug Administration Safety and Innovation Act (FDASIA) required HHS to develop "a report that contains a proposed strategy and recommendations on an appropriate, risk-based regulatory framework pertaining to health information technology, including mobile medical applications, that promotes innovation, protects patient safety, and avoids regulatory duplication" [30]. The report, published in April 2014 [31], outlined a regulatory framework that defines three broad categories, with escalating levels of regulatory oversight: (1) administrative health IT functions, (2) health management health IT functions, and (3) medical device health IT functions. The report proposes that administrative health IT functions would require no additional oversight. Health IT management functions, which includes "most clinical decision support", would require oversight by ONC. It would ultimately be incorporated into a regulatory process that expands beyond ONC's current certification program toward a more proactive engagement, perhaps through the creation of a patient safety center. Finally, medical device health IT functions would be regulated as medical devices by the FDA.

Therefore the two key questions for CDS developers and implementers are: what characteristics define CDS that belongs in the "health IT function" and what are the characteristics of CDS that belongs in the "medical device" category? The report states:

> Clinical decision support (CDS) provides health care providers and patients with knowledge and person-specific information, intelligently filtered or presented at appropriate times, to enhance health and health care. Because its risks are generally low compared to the potential benefits, FDA does not intend to focus its oversight on most clinical decision support. FDA, instead, intends to focus its oversight on a limited set of software functionalities that provide clinical decision support and pose higher risks to patients, such as computer aided detection/diagnostic software and radiation therapy treatment planning software. [31]

Examples of CDSS that FDA would not regulate include order sets, drug-drug and drug-allergy alerts, most drug dosing calculations, duplicate testing alerts, or diagnostic suggestions based on information in the patient's record. The report offers a few examples of higher-risk CDSS that would be regulated by the FDA, and commits to provide more detailed guidance in the future. Higher risk CDSS include:

- Computer aided detection/diagnostic software,
- remote display or notification of real-time alarms (physiological, technical, advisory) from bedside monitors,
- radiation treatment planning,
- robotic surgical planning and control, and
- electrocardiography analytical software [31]

All of the example products share an attribute of autonomy: while lower risk CDSS offer information to a person, and the person will then take action, higher risk CDSS perform complex actions and may in fact represent the "last mile" between the care provider and the patient. For example, robotic surgery planning and control software carries forward the surgeon's intent to cut, staple, or retract. A malfunction in this software could be deadly, and there is no human "safety net" between the software and the patient.

7.13 Clinical Decision Support for Immunizations (CDSi)

The Centers for Disease Control and Prevention (CDC), in collaboration with the ONC, have developed a process that aims to (a) improve the speed with which new immunization recommendations are incorporated into practice, (b) reduce the redundant data entry that is currently required by care providers and health IT companies, and (c) improve the accuracy of immunization forecasting. The project has created a set of knowledge resources including logic specifications (immunization schedule logic) and supporting data (XML representations of all currently available immunizations). The resources and overview information are available at CDC's CDSi resource page [32].

Historically, bi-annual updates to the immunization schedules are published by the Advisory Committee on Immunization Policies (ACIP) in PDF documents and posted to the CDC website. These documents are reviewed, translated into logical expressions, and then implemented in health information technology. The process is slow, error-prone, and redundant.

The long-term goal of the CDSi project is that health IT systems will be capable of subscribing to updated immunization guidance and the moment that guidance is published, would incorporate it into appropriate workflow. Such a model could deliver the guidance to an EHR, a regional immunization information system (IIS), a department of public health, or any other appropriate endpoint.

7.14 Challenges

When government or any authority defines how constituents reach a given goal, rather than just that the goal is reached, there is always a risk that the method prescribed is not actually the best path to success. For example, early Peace Corps volunteers learned that "great ideas" hatched in Washington DC for solving malnutrition in rural African villages were dismal failures, while those who observed the "positive deviants" in the outlier families who seemed to be thriving, and then replicated the methods those families used, were successful. "Healthy family" was therefore the goal. Had the Peace Corps volunteers rigidly maintained that all families adopt imported ideas such as "grow rice" or "adopt a goat," widespread success would have continued to be elusive. Another example: with the emergence of compact fluorescent light bulbs (CFLs), many municipalities outlawed the sale of incandescent bulbs and explicitly named CFLs as the mandatory alternative. Yet, only a few short years after the introduction of CFLs, light emitting diodes (LEDs) are now available. These bulbs are inexpensive, less polluting, and use less energy than CFLs. The regulation lags behind the technology, especially when the technology is explicitly prescribed.

In the same way, there is concern that the EHR incentive programs have been too prescriptive about (a) how care delivery organizations should use them, (b) how health IT developers should implement them, and (c) what should happen in the future. How do we allow for innovation, yet still provide sufficient guidance on standards to allow a broad ecosystem to flourish? It is possible that the usability challenges, alert fatigue complaints, and the slow pace of progress in the Clinical Quality Framework (CQF) will cause the "CDS baby to be thrown out with the bathwater." Without continued focus, and the passionate work of leaders such as the authors of this book, combined with the continued and coordinated support from CMS, AHRQ, CDC and ONC, the evolution of CDS in the United States could slow, and the near-term opportunities to improve health will not be realized. The key is that efforts are coordinated with CQF standards activities, as well as with the emerging regulations to support PAMA and its likely successors.

7.15 Future Initiatives

PAMA represents a model of congressional activism that could either go very well or very badly, depending on how smoothly the regulatory components integrate with existing programs. If it goes well, we will likely see more statutory activism like this from Congress, or similar initiatives as mentioned above in the domains of opioid abuse prevention, antibiotic stewardship, and infectious disease/bioterrorism emergencies. Each of these domains represent a high priority for the U.S. Department of Health and Human Services, and therefore represents great opportunity for the public funding of clinical decision support knowledge artifacts and delivery channels.

7.16 Summary and Conclusion

The federal government's National Quality Strategy has created a sound foundation for focused improvements in care, care quality, and cost. Best practices in health care delivery are discovered and implemented through a cyclic process of research, discovery, guideline development, decision support, care delivery, quality and effectiveness measurement and (starting the cycle over again) research. As we follow a similar path toward the evolution of CDS, different federal agencies are responsible for different parts of the CDS lifecycle. AHRQ is responsible for foundational learning and experimentation, and therefore sponsored the CDSC and GLIDES projects. ONC is responsible for standards policy definition, and coordination of other agencies' use of such standards. CDC and CMS are organizations that have "last mile" responsibilities in delivering content that serves a strategic purpose, and the National Library of Medicine (NLM) is responsible for collaborating with AHRQ and ONC to curate the proper semantic foundation for all of this to occur.

With the migration towards value-based care in the United States between 2015 and 2020, we will see increasing pressure for care delivery organizations to deliver outcomes that align with the National Quality Strategy. Combined with maturing technical standards, improved usability and interoperability of health IT systems, we are approaching a "tipping point" where we will soon see CDS become an essential and expected component of every health IT product.

References

1. Berwick DM, Nolan TW, Whittington. The triple aim: care, health, and cost. Health Aff. 2008;27(3):759–69.
2. Mardon R, Mercincavage L, Johnson M, Finley S, Pan E, Arora D. Findings and lessons from: AHRQ's Clinical Decision Support Demonstration Projects. (Prepared by Westat under Contract No. HHSA 290-2009-00023I). AHRQ Publication No. 14-0047-EF. Rockville, MD: Agency for Healthcare Research and Quality. June 2014 [cited 2015 Nov 14]. Available from: https://healthit.ahrq.gov/sites/default/files/docs/page/findings-and-lessons-from-clinical--decision-support-demonstration-projects.pdf.

3. Congress.Gov [Internet]. H.R.3590 – Patient Protection and Affordable Care Act; 2010 [cited 2015 Nov 14]. Available from: https://www.congress.gov/111/plaws/publ148/PLAW-111publ148.pdf.
4. Agency for Healthcare Research and Quality [Internet]. Rockville MD: AHRQ; 2015. National Strategy for Quality Improvement in Health Care: Report to Congress; 2011 [cited 2015 Nov 16]. Available from: http://www.ahrq.gov/workingforquality/nqs/nqs2011annlrpt.pdf.
5. Agency for Healthcare Research and Quality [Internet]. Rockville MD: AHRQ; 2007 August. Request for Proposals; 2007 [cited 2015 Nov 14]. [Solicitation No.: AHRQ-07-10045]. Available from: http://archive.ahrq.gov/fund/contarchive/rfp0710045.htm.
6. Walker J, Pan E, Johnston D, Adler-Milstein J, Bates DW and Blackford Middleton. The value of health care information exchange and interoperability. Health Aff. 2005 Jan:(10–8).
7. Shiffman RN, Karras BT, Agrawal A, Chen R, Marenco L, Nath S. GEM: a proposal for a more comprehensive guideline document model using XML. J Am Inform Assoc. 2000;7:488–98. doi:10.1136/jamia.2000.0070488.
8. Hajizadeh N, Kashyap N, Michel G, Shiffman RN. GEM at 10: a decade's experience with the guideline elements model. AMIA Ann Symp Proc. 2011;2011:520–8.
9. Rosenfeld RM, Shiffman RN. Clinical practice guideline development manual: a quality-driven approach for translating evidence into action. Otolaryngol Head Neck Surg. 2009;140(6 Suppl 1):S1–43. doi:10.1016/j.otohns.2009.04.015.
10. Health Level Seven International [Internet]. Ann Arbor MI: HLSI; c2007-2015. Arden Syntax v2.10 (Health Level Seven Arden Syntax for Medical Logic Systems, Version 2.10); 2014 Nov [cited 2015 Oct 1]. Available from: http://www.hl7.org/implement/standards/product_brief.cfm?product_id=372.
11. Rand Corporation [Internet]. Santa Monica CA: Rand Corporation. Lewis J, Hongsermeier TM, Blackford Middleton, Bell DS. A prototype knowledge-sharing service for clinical decision support artifacts; 2012 [cited 2015 Oct 1]. Available from: http://www.hl7.org/implement/standards/product_brief.cfm?product_id=372.
12. Raetzman SO, Osheroff J, Greenes RA, Sordo M, Hohlbauch AA, Coffey RM. Final report: structuring care recommendations for clinical decision support. AHRQ Publication No. 11-0025-2-EF. Santa Barbara CA: Thomson Reuters. Sept 2011 [cited 2015 Nov 15]. Available from: https://healthit.ahrq.gov/sites/default/files/docs/citation/SCRCDS%2520FINAL%2520SUMMARY%2520REPORT.pdf.
13. Byrne C, Sherry D, Mercincavage L, Johnston D, Pan E, Schiff G. Technical report: advancing clinical decision support – key lessons in clinical decision support implementation. Task order HHSP23337009T.Wesat. Date Unknown [cited 2015 Nov 15]. Available from: https://www.healthit.gov/sites/default/files/acds-lessons-in-cds-implementation-deliverablev2.pdf.
14. U.S. Government Publishing Office [Internet]. Washington DC: GPO; 2009. American Recovery and Reinvestment Act of 2009: 42 USC 300jj; 2009 [cited 2015 Nov 15]. Available from: http://www.gpo.gov/fdsys/pkg/BILLS-111hr1enr/pdf/BILLS-111hr1enr.pdf.
15. S&I Framework [Internet]. San Francisco CA: Tangient LLC; c2015. Health eDecisions Homepage; 2015 [cited 2015 Nov 14]. Available from: http://wiki.siframework.org/Health+eDecisions+Homepage.
16. S&I Framework [Internet]. San Francisco CA: Tangient LLC; c2015. Clinical Quality Framework Initiative; 2015 [cited 2015 Nov 14]. Available from: http://wiki.siframework.org/Clinical+Quality+Framework+Initiative.
17. Regulations.gov [Internet]. Medicare and Medicaid Programs; Electronic Health Record Incentive Program; 2010 [cited 2015 Nov 14]. Available from: http://www.regulations.gov/#!documentDetail;D=CMS_FRDOC_0001-0520.
18. Federal Register [Internet]. 2015. Health information technology: initial set of standards, implementation specifications, and certification criteria for electronic health record technology: 45 CFR 170.304(e). 2010 [cited 2015 Nov 14] Available from: https://www.federalregister.gov/articles/2010/07/28/2010-17210/health-information-technology-initial-set-of-standards-implementation-specifications-and.

19. Federal Register [Internet]. 2015. 2015 Edition Health Information Technology (Health IT) Certification Criteria, 2015 Edition Base Electronic Health Record (EHR) Definition, and ONC Health IT Certification Program Modifications: 45 CFR 170.314.(9). 2015 [cited 2015 Nov 14] Available from: https://www.federalregister.gov/articles/2015/10/16/2015-25597/2015-edition-health-information-technology-health-it-certification-criteria-2015-edition-base#p-277.
20. HHS.gov [Internet]. 2015. Compilation of Patient Protection and Affordable Care Act. Subtitle D of Title VI - Sec. 6301. Patient-Centered Outcomes Research. 2010 May 1 [cited 2015 Nov 14] Available from: http://www.hhs.gov/sites/default/files/ppacacon.pdf.
21. US Department of Health and Human Services. RFA-HS-15-003. AHRQ Patient-Centered Outcomes Research Clinical Decision Support Learning Network (U18). [cited2015 Dec 7] Available from http://grants.nih.gov/grants/guide/rfa-files/RFA-HS-15-003.html.
22. Congress.Gov [Internet]. H.R.4302 – Protecting Access to Medicare Act of 2014; 2015 [cited 2015 Nov 16]. Available from: https://www.congress.gov/bill/113th-congress/house-bill/4302/text?overview=closed.
23. Boland GW, Weilburg J, Duszak Jr R. Imaging appropriateness and implementation of clinical decision support. J Am Coll Radiol. 2015;12(6):601–3.
24. Federal Register [Internet]. 2015. Medicare Program; Revisions to Payment Policies under the Physician Fee Schedule and Other Revisions to Part B for CY 2016: 80 FR 71102 [cited 2015 Nov 16]. Available from: https://www.federalregister.gov/articles/2015/11/16/2015-28005/medicare-program-revisions-to-payment-policies-under-the-physician-fee-schedule-and-other-revisions#p-1992.
25. Timbie TW, Hussey PS, Burgette LF, Wenger NS, Rastegar A, Brantley I, et al. Medicare imaging demonstration final evaluation: report to congress [Internet]. Santa Monica: Centers for Medicare & Medicaid Services; 2014. [cited 2015 Nov 14], Available from: http://www.rand.org/content/dam/rand/pubs/research_reports/RR700/RR706/RAND_RR706.pdf.
26. Federal Register [Internet]. 2015. Medicare Program; Revisions to payment policies under the physician fee schedule and other revisions to Part B for CY 2016 [cited 2015 Nov 14]. Available from: https://www.federalregister.gov/articles/2015/11/16/2015-28005/medicare-program-revisions-to-payment-policies-under-the-physician-fee-schedule-and-other-revisions#p-1997.
27. Federal Register [Internet]. 2015. Medicare program; Revisions to payment policies under the physician fee schedule and other revisions to Part B for CY 2016 [cited 2015 Nov 14]. Available from: https://www.federalregister.gov/articles/2015/11/16/2015-28005/medicare-program-revisions-to-payment-policies-under-the-physician-fee-schedule-and-other-revisions#p-2009.
28. Federal Register [Internet]. 2015. Medicare Program; Revisions to Payment Policies under the Physician Fee Schedule and Other Revisions to Part B for CY 2016 [cited 2015 Nov 14]. Available from: https://www.federalregister.gov/articles/2015/11/16/2015-28005/medicare-program-revisions-to-payment-policies-under-the-physician-fee-schedule-and-other-revisions#p-2075.
29. Congress.Gov [Internet]. H.R.2 – Medicare access and CHIP Reauthorization Act of 2015; 2015 [cited 2015 Nov 15]. Available from: https://www.congress.gov/bill/114th-congress/house-bill/2/text.
30. U.S. Government Publishing Office [Internet]. Washington, DC: GPO; 2012. Food and Drug Administration Safety and Innovation Act; 2012 [cited 2015 Nov 14]. Available from: http://www.gpo.gov/fdsys/pkg/BILLS-112s3187enr/pdf/BILLS-112s3187enr.pdf.
31. U.S. Food and Drug Administration [Internet]. Silver Spring, MD: FDA; 2015. FDASIA Health IT Report: Proposed Strategy and Recommendations for a Risk-Based Framework; 2014 [cited 2015 Nov 14]. Available from: http://www.fda.gov/downloads/AboutFDA/CentersOffices/OfficeofMedicalProductsandTobacco/CDRH/CDRHReports/UCM391521.pdf.
32. Centers for Disease Control and Prevention [Internet]. Atlanta, GA: CDC; 2015. Clinical Decision Support for Immunization (CDSi); 2015 [cited 2015 Nov 14]. Available from: http://www.cdc.gov/vaccines/programs/iis/cdsi.html.

Chapter 8
Ethical and Legal Issues in Decision Support

Kenneth W. Goodman

Abstract The use of computers to help humans make diagnoses and prognoses in the practice of medicine or nursing is an exciting and unsettling development in the evolution of clinical and hospital practice. Such use engenders ethical and legal challenges paralleling those challenges seen regularly to arise with the introduction of many new technologies in healthcare. In the case of computational decision support systems, the most salient ethical issues involve standards of care, appropriate uses and users and professional relationships. Balancing patient safety against opportunities to improve care constitutes a tension that mirrors the difficulty encountered in debates about whether and how the government should regulate decision support systems. At ground are questions of accountability, responsibility and liability. In most cases, we lack adequate empirical data to arrive at uncontroversial conclusions. In the context of an exciting new technology, the reduction of that ignorance itself becomes an ethical imperative.

Keywords Accountability • Bioethics • Decision support systems • Error • Ethics • Legal issues • Liability • Prognostic scoring systems • Regulation • Responsibility

Contemporary bioethics has evolved in part in response to new technology. Cardiopulmonary resuscitation has become so common that we often do not let patients die without trying it first, but this is a comparatively recent development and it bedevils hospital ethics committees daily. The transplantation of organs was once front-page news, but now that it is quotidian, the greatest ethical challenges lie in finding enough organs. Health information technology is in many respects still in its adolescence, but it will touch more lives than any other technology in the history of the healing sciences. Health IT includes a rich vein of ethical issues, perhaps none so interesting as whether, when and by whom an intelligent machine should be used to render a diagnosis or prognosis.

Nature is generally consistent and dependable. In human biology, discrete maladies or illnesses tend consistently to produce particular signs and symptoms. This

K.W. Goodman, Ph.D. (✉)
Institute for Bioethics and Health Policy, University of Miami Miller School of Medicine, POB 016960 (M-825), Miami, FL 33101, USA
e-mail: kgoodman@med.miami.edu

E.S. Berner (ed.), *Clinical Decision Support Systems*, Health Informatics,
DOI 10.1007/978-3-319-31913-1_8

correlation makes possible the process of diagnosis and prognosis. In fact, so strong is our belief in the regularity of signs and symptoms that the process has long been regarded as straightforward, if not easy: "…there is nothing remarkable," Hippocrates suggested some 2,400 years ago, "in being right in the great majority of cases in the same district, provided the physician knows the signs and can draw the correct conclusions from them" [1].

To be sure, consistency, reliability and reproducibility do not always or even often entail simplicity, and accurate diagnoses and prognoses can be quite difficult, even given the regularity of many signs and symptoms. For one thing, "knowing the signs" requires a great deal of empirical knowledge and experience. For another, there is rarely a unique and isomorphic relationship between symptom and disease. Significantly, Hippocrates smuggles into his account a presumption of the very thing being described. To say that being right is unremarkable when one can draw the "correct conclusions" is to say that it is easy to be right when you know how to be right. Or, making an accurate diagnosis or prognosis is easy if one knows how to make an accurate diagnosis or prognosis.

The need to make accurate diagnoses is not based merely on the personal satisfaction that comes from being right, as gratifying as that is. It is based on the good effects that follow more frequently from accurate diagnoses than from inaccurate diagnoses. It is also based on the bad effects that error often entails.

In the context of trust and vulnerability that shape patient-physician and patient-nurse encounters, there emerges a suite of ethical imperatives: adhere to, or surpass, educational and professional standards; monitor changes in one's domain; know when one is out of one's depth. Decision support systems have great potential to assist clinicians, but their use also raises a number of ethical issues. In fact, this is evidence for the maturity of the science: new health technologies almost always elicit ethical issues, and it should come as no surprise that clinical decision support would provide a number of challenges for those who use, or would use, computers to assist, guide or test clinical decisions. Any comprehensive treatment of computational decision support should include a review of ethical issues. In what follows, we identify a number of such issues that emerge when intelligent machines are used to perform or support clinical decisions, and we survey key legal and regulatory issues.

8.1 Ethical Issues

8.1.1 Background and Current Research

It has been clear for decades that health computing raises interesting and important ethical issues. In a crucial early contribution, a physician, a philosopher and a lawyer identified a series of ethical concerns, not the least of which are several surrounding the questions of who should use a "medical computer program" and under what circumstances [2]. Another early contribution emphasized the challenges raised by threats to physician autonomy [3].

What has emerged since has been called the "Standard View" of computational decision support, including diagnosis [4]. Randolph A. Miller, M.D., a key figure both in the scientific evolution of computational decision support and in scholarship on correlate ethical issues, has argued that "Limitations in man-machine interfaces, and more importantly, in automated systems' ability to represent the broad variety of concepts relevant to clinical medicine, will prevent 'human-assisted computer diagnosis' from being feasible for decades, if it is at all possible." [4] Another way of putting this is to say that computers cannot either in principle or at least for the foreseeable future supplant human decision makers. Here is how we put it elsewhere:

> [T]he practice of medicine or nursing has never been and never will be merely or exclusively about the making of accurate inferences. The rendering of a diagnosis will, except in the simplest of cases, always be probabilistic in one degree or another, and induction alone cannot resolve all uncertainty, incorporate human values, or reveal causal relationships necessary for successful clinical practice. [5]

These observations entail ethical obligations, namely that computers ought not be relied on to do what humans do best, and that a computer's decisions cannot as a matter of course or policy be allowed to trump a human decision or diagnosis. Indeed, more than a quarter-century later, this is still the correct view, even as various forms of decision support are routinely embedded in enterprise-wide electronic health records.

Happily, the Standard View was advanced not by those hostile to the development and use of clinical diagnostic decision support systems, but by leading proponents. The Standard View signals a conservative and cautious approach to application of a new technology, and as such captures important moral intuitions about technological change, risks and standards.

Interest in the three-way intersection of ethics, medicine and computing has increased steadily since initial efforts to explore these issues, and "ethics and informatics" now may be regarded as a subfield deserving of its own research and literature [6]. Although the field admits of many and varied topics, we may identify three core areas of ethical concern as having emerged in discussions of computer systems that are used to remind, provide consultation or advise clinicians: (1) care standards; (2) appropriate use and users; and (3) professional relationships.

8.1.2 Care Standards

We know a great deal about responsibility in medicine and nursing. For instance, we know that practitioners should generally not deceive their patients. We know that patients can be especially vulnerable, and that such vulnerability should be respected. And we know that physicians and nurses have a responsibility to do their best, irrespective of economic (dis)incentives, and that they should not attempt treatments that are beyond their training or expertise.

Learning how to meet these and other responsibilities in the context of a broad variety of social problems is arguably the leading task in bioethics. We must ask first whether computing tools help or hinder attempts to meet responsibilities, and second whether the tools impose new or special responsibilities. The overarching question may be put thus: does the new technology improve patient care? If the answer is affirmative we may suppose we have met an important responsibility. If the answer is negative, it seems clear we should not use the new technology. The problem is, we often do not know how to answer the question. That is, we are sometimes unsure whether care will be improved by the use of new technologies. If we want to meet the responsibility to avoid harm, for instance, we are impotent until we can determine the effects of the technology (see Chap. 9 for a discussion of evaluation). What follows from this is that empirical uncertainty magnifies ethical issues and, in consequence, error avoidance emerges as an ethical imperative to maximize positive, short-term consequences and to ensure that, in the long run, informatics is not associated with error or carelessness or the kind of cavalier stance often associated with high-tech boosterism.

The concept of error avoidance is wed to that of a standard of care. Standards evolve in the health professions because they plot the kinds of actions that are most successful in achieving certain ends. To fail to adhere to a standard is thus to increase the risk of error, at least in a mature science. Because errors or their consequences are generally regarded as harms or evils, the obligation to hew to standards is an ethical one.

But standards are empirical constructs, and so are open to revision. New evidence forces changes in standards. (This demonstrates why clinicians have an ethical obligation to monitor the scientific maturation of their disciplines by reading journals, attending conferences, etc.) To be sure, the precise content of any standard might be open to dispute. The "reasonable person" standard requires the postulation of a vague entity; this is particularly problematic when reasonable people disagree, as is often the case in medicine and nursing. A "community standard" similarly fails to identify a bright line between error and success in all circumstances in which it might be invoked. Note also that it is not always bad to forgo adherence to a practice standard—the standard will generally be invoked in ethical and legal contexts only when there is a bad outcome, or a flagrant disregard for the risk of a bad outcome. Sometimes there are good reasons to violate a standard. This demonstrates how some clinical progress is possible: if everyone in all cases stuck to a rigid standard there would be no internal evidence to support modifications of the standard. In other cases, standards are modified as a result of clinical trial findings, observational studies and serendipitous discoveries.

In the case of computer-assisted decisions, the challenge is perhaps best put in the form of a question: Does use of a decision support system increase the risk of error? Three considerations are noteworthy here. First, while accurate diagnoses and other decisions are often linked to optimal treatment, this is not always the case: some patients are treated appropriately despite an inaccurate diagnosis, and some are treated incorrectly despite an accurate diagnosis. Second, one might still be able to provide an optimal treatment with a vague or imprecise diagnosis [7]. Third, computers can guide decisions (or perform diagnosis-like functions) outside of clinical contexts, as for instance in a variety of laboratory tests and in alarm and alert systems.

To ask if a computer diagnosis increases or decreases the risk of diagnostic or other error is in part to ask whether it will improve patient care. If the answer is that, on balance, the tool increases (the risk of) error, then we should say it would be inappropriate to use it. Significantly, though, what is sought here is an empirical finding or a reasoned judgment—where such a finding is often lacking or even methodologically hard to come by; or where such a judgment is based on inadequate empirical support, at least according to standards otherwise demanded to justify clinical decisions.

This means that we are pressed to answer an ethical question (Is it acceptable to use a decision support system?) in a context of scientific uncertainty (How accurate is the system?). Many challenges in contemporary bioethics share this feature, namely, that moral uncertainty parallels scientific or clinical ignorance.

What we generally want in such cases is a way to stimulate the appropriate use of new technologies without increasing patient risk. One approach to doing this is given the nearly oxymoronic term "progressive caution." The idea is this: "Medical informatics is, happily, here to stay, but users and society have extensive responsibilities to ensure that we use our tools appropriately. This might cause us to move more deliberately or slowly than some would like. Ethically speaking, that is just too bad" [8]. Such a stance attempts the ethical optimization of decision-support use and development by encouraging expansion of the field, but with appropriate levels of scrutiny, oversight and, indeed, caution. The moral imperative of error avoidance is, in other words, not anti-progressive. Rather, it is part of a large and public network of checks and balances that seeks to optimize good outcomes by regulating conflicts between boosters and nay-sayers. The idea of progressive caution is just an attempt to capture the core values of that regulation.

It has been clear since the first efforts to address ethical issues in medical informatics that as computers help the sciences of medicine and nursing to progress, they will also contribute to changes in the standard of patient care. When that happens, however, it increases the likelihood that computer use will come to be required of clinicians. Put differently: In a comparatively short time, there has been a major shift in the availability and use of informatics tools. To the degree that informatics can improve the practice of the health professions, there is a requirement that its tools be used.

This point is often the most disturbing for practitioners. It is troublesome that one might have an obligation to use a tool that has been presented as controversial and in need of further validation. But there is no contradiction here. In fact, it appears that the evolution of health informatics parallels the emergence of other exciting and controversial tools, ranging from organ transplantation techniques and advanced life support to laparoscopic surgical procedures and genetic testing and therapy. It is often the case in history that progress invites this tension. What is wanted is evidence that people of good will can both advance science and safeguard against abuses. Research studies that examine not just the accuracy of the systems, but how they are used, are essential to the process of acquiring that evidence.

8.1.3 Appropriate Use and Users

One way to abuse a tool is to use it for purposes for which it is not intended. Another is to use a tool without adequate training. A third way is to use a tool incorrectly (carelessly, sloppily, etc.) independently of other shortcomings.

There are a number of reasons why one should not use computer applications in unintended contexts. First, a tool designed for one purpose has a greater likelihood of not working, or not working well, for other purposes. To be sure, one might successfully perform an appendectomy with a kitchen knife, or dice vegetables with a scalpel, but it is bizarre to suggest that one should try either, except in an emergency. A hospital computer system may be used inappropriately if, for instance, it was designed for educational purposes but relied on for clinical decision support; or developed for modest decision support (identifying a number of differential diagnoses) but used in such a way as to cause a practitioner to abandon a diagnosis or other decision arrived at by sound clinical judgment.

In ethically optimizing the use of clinical decision support systems, it is perhaps reassuring to know that we have many models and precedents. From advanced life support and organ transplantation to developments in pharmacotherapy and genetics, society regularly has had to cope with technological change in the health sciences. Managing change requires that new tools are used appropriately and by adequately qualified practitioners. Education is at the core of such management. Identifying qualifications and providing training must be key components of any initiative to expand the use of clinical decision support software. Ethical concerns arise when we are unsure of the appropriate or adequate qualifications and levels of training [2, 5].

The fear is that a health care novice or professional ignorant of a system's design or capacity will use a decision support system in patient care. The reason the former is worthy of concern is that, as above, the practice of medicine and nursing remain human activities. A nonphysician or non-nurse cannot practice medicine or nursing, no matter how much computational support is available. This is also a concern in the context of consumer health informatics, or the widespread availability of online health advice to the untrained (see Chap. 10). What this means is that the novice might not know when the system is in obvious error or has produced clearly flawed output, when it is operating on insufficient information, when it is being used in a domain for which it was not designed, and so on.

There are also several reasons we must focus ethical attention on the use of clinical decision support software by computationally naive health professionals: Such professionals might not use such software to good effect (either by over- or underestimating its abilities), might not be using it properly, or, like the novice, might not know when the system is being used in inappropriate contexts. Such fears can be addressed by requirements that decision-support users have appropriate qualifications and be adequately trained in the use of the systems. Unfortunately, it is not yet clear what those qualifications should be, or how extensive a training program would be adequate. It is clear, however, that the use of decision support software cannot in the long run advance ethically without a better sense of where to establish guideposts for qualifications and training. This remains an increasingly important area of research.

A further ethical concern about appropriate use and users emerges from the potential to deploy decision support systems in contexts of practice evaluation, quality assessment, reimbursement for professional services and the like. One can imagine an insurance company or managed care organization using decision support to evaluate, or even challenge, clinical decisions. What makes such use problematic is precisely the same ensemble of concerns that led us to disdain applications in other contexts: the primacy of human cognitive expertise, uncertainty about adequate qualifications, and doubt about the consequences for improved patient care. This is not to say that a machine cannot give a correct answer in a particular case but, rather, that there are inadequate grounds to prefer machine decisions as a matter of general policy.

8.1.4 Professional Relationships

Many patients believe, mistakenly, that their physicians are omniscient. Many physicians believe, mistakenly, that their patients are ignoramuses. Recognition of these mistakes has led in recent years to the development of the idea of "shared decision making," namely that patients and providers are most productively seen as partners [9–11]. If this is so, and there is much to recommend it in many (though not all) instances, then we need to assess the effect of a third partner—the computer.

There are two overriding areas of ethical concern here. The first is that the computer will create conceptual or interpersonal distance between provider and patient. Communicating about uncertainty, especially when the stakes are high, has long been a challenge for clinicians. That a computer might be used to (help) render a diagnosis, for instance, causes us to run the risk of what we will call the "computational fallacy." This is the view that what comes out of a computer is somehow more valid, accurate, or reliable than human output. Providers and patients who take such a view introduce a potentially erosive, if not destructive, element into shared decision making contexts. Anything that increases the likelihood that a patient decision or choice will be perceived as misguided or stupid adds to the problem that shared decision making was supposed to solve.

Now, it might be supposed that a physician or nurse can eliminate at least some of this tension by not disclosing to a patient that clinical decision support software was used in his or her case. But this introduces our second area of ethical concern, namely, the question whether patients should be given this information. The answer to this question must be determined against a background shaped by (1) patient sophistication and understanding of medical and statistical information and (2) clinician sophistication and understanding of communication approaches and strategies. In any case, it is inappropriate to use computer data or inferences to trump hesitant patients, or bully them into agreeing with a health professional [12].

This point has been made most clearly in the discussion of prognostic scoring systems, or software used in critical care medicine in part to predict patient mortality. On the one hand, patients with poor prognoses might still benefit from extensive interventions, and these benefits might be important enough for the patient and/or family to seek them; on the other hand, patients with good survival odds might judge the prolongation of life to be of little value when weighed against the difficulty or burden of extensive interventions [13, 14].

A related issue has arisen with increased frequency as patients gain access to decision support software and use it either for self-diagnosis, treatment decisions or to make demands on physicians, perhaps even to challenge or second-guess them. The difficulties raised by these demands and challenges will multiply as decision-support systems improve. As discussed in Chap. 10, there is a sense in which one might regard such access as an important tool in the process of shared decision making: it will not do to expect patients to become involved in their own care and simultaneously constrain their sources of information. Contrarily, a patient might constitute a paradigm case of an inappropriate system user, especially in those cases in which the system causes someone to forgo appropriate medical care. Additional research is required to gauge the use and effects of online "clinical calculators" and related decision-support tools. For all we know, they will emerge as sources of comfort to hypochondriacs—who then seek clinical attention—as foundations of information with which to challenge clinicians.

We might compare patient use of clinical decision support systems to patient use of medical texts and journals. In years past, there was an inclination to regard such access as risky and hence inappropriate. While a little knowledge can be dangerous, a position that does not go beyond such a view seems to miss an opportunity to educate patients about their illnesses and the relation between health literature on the one hand and medical and nursing knowledge and practice on the other. Much the same point can be made about patient use of decision tools: a physician should respond to such use by making clear that computers are not surrogates for health professionals, and that the practice of medicine or nursing entails far more than statistical induction from signs, symptoms and lab values. To be sure, it would be well if actual practice embodied this insight.

As long as the healing professions are practiced in a matrix of scientific uncertainty and patient values, we err if we appoint computational decision support as a surrogate for compassionate communication, shared decisions, and quality care by competent humans.

8.1.5 Decision Support in Genetics and Genomics

The primacy of human decision making in contemporary clinical practice should be extended to the emerging world of personalized or individualized medicine and pharmacogenomics. The idea that treatments might be customized, drugs titrated or therapies tailored to individual patients is compelling. Such treatments, drugs and therapies will, in principle, work accordingly as clinicians can make use of specific patients' genomes to target interventions. This goal has sparked a new generation of research programs and no little excitement. As discussed in Chap. 12, personalized medicine is an information-intensive affair, and some degree of decision support is already anticipated or under development [15–18].

It might develop that the intersection of clinical decision support systems and pharmacogenomics will raise no new ethical issues, that the issues to appear will parallel those with which we are already familiar; or, conversely, this intersection will be a seeding ground for new and unexpected ethical challenges. Predictions supporting the former might appeal to the idea that many competent clinicians remain uncomfortable with genetic information and so might, at least initially, and until a new generation of gene-savvy clinicians emerges, rely more heavily on decision support. Furthermore, genetic and genomic data and information are less causally certain than more familiar kinds of clinical data and information, and this, too, might lead to greater reliance on intelligent machines that can guide a decision maker. So any new ethical challenges will be a matter of degree, not of kind. Contrarily, the prediction that personalized medicine will present us with novel ethical challenges finds support in the idea that it is not merely clinician ignorance or innocence that will drive genomic decision support but, rather, that there will be so much information and it will be so complex that good decision support will be *necessary* to the new practice. We might, that is, cross a frontier if it becomes clear that in the face of such complexity it is irrational not to use computerized decision support.

Decision support is likely to evolve in any of several settings, for instance:

- Reproductive medicine: Given high risk and uncertainty, exquisitely difficult decisions have long challenged us in the contexts of genetic counseling and preimplantation genetic diagnosis [19]. Automating the application of decision trees for reproductive decisions and therapeutic options will entail the need for careful ethical analysis and policy development. We have not yet conducted adequate analysis to guide the use of computerized decision support tools for genetic counseling.
- Return of results: The management of complex and probabilistic information for the sake of patient education and disclosure is a source of extended debate. The use of decision support software linked to electronic health records presents significant opportunities and challenges regarding the communication of complex and clinically significant information to patients [20].
- Workflow: If, as predicted, the genomic tools of personalized medicine will be incorporated into quotidian medical practice, genomic decision support will

become embedded in that practice [21]. This has implications for privacy, informed consent and the scope of shared decision making by patients and clinicians.

The growth and evolution of pharmacogenomics and personalized medicine should be regarded as an opportunity to incorporate ethical analysis in the use of new technology at the outset—instead of after the fact as is, unfortunately, too often the practice.

8.2 Regulation and the Law

Computers and software raise conceptually fascinating and important practical questions about responsibility, accountability and liability. Further, the question whether a decision support system is a medical device needing governmental regulation is a source of tension and debate. Scientists, clinicians, philosophers, lawyers and government and policy officials must grapple with a variety of knotty problems.

The intersection of medicine, computational decision support and law has been addressed mostly in speculative terms. The use of clinical decision support systems is not widespread enough to have stimulated legislation or illuminating precedent, and, indeed, such systems seem so far to have little influence on clinician practice [22]. Moreover, medicine and computing share little in the way of a common legal history. The following observation is as apt today as it was a quarter-century ago:

> The introduction of computerized decision-making will require the merger of computer science and medical care; two areas with fundamentally different legal traditions. The legal differences between the computer field and medicine are striking. Medicine is tightly regulated at all levels. Most health care providers are licensed, and a rigid hierarchical system is the norm. Yet, computer systems and companies are created in a totally unregulated competitive environment in which "software piracy" is common, standardization is in its infancy, licensing is a method of transferring trade secret software, and companies begin in garages. [23]

8.2.1 Liability and Decision Support

The overriding legal issue related to computational decision support has been and remains liability for use, misuse—or even lack of use—of a computer to make or assist in rendering diagnoses and other decisions [24–28]. In the United States, tort law holds providers of goods and services accountable for injuries sustained by users. Because of legal and regulatory variation, there are similarities and differences in other countries [29–31]. Such accountability is generally addressed by either the negligence standard or the strict liability standard.

The negligence standard applies to services, and strict liability applies to goods or products, although negligence can sometimes also apply to goods, as in cases of negligent product design. Significantly, however, there is no consensus regarding whether decision support systems are services or products, in part because these systems have properties that resemble both services and products [2, 23, 24, 32, 33]. For instance, a physician's diagnosis is clearly a service and any liability for erroneous diagnoses is judged by the negligence standard. If a human diagnosis is considered a service, then, it is argued, a computer diagnosis (or the task of writing the computer code that rendered the diagnosis) should have the same status. Contrarily, commercial decision-support systems are manufactured, mass-marketed, and sold like entities uncontroversially regarded to be products.

An additional complication is that these systems are sold to hospitals, physicians, patients and others, and, indeed, are now available on the World Wide Web. If a patient is injured by a defective system, it remains to be determined who used the system (the physician? the patient?) and whether it was misused. Also, it can be exquisitely difficult to identify the defect in a computer program [24], as well as to answer the important question whether a physician could have intervened and prevented the application of mistaken advice [2, 5].

There has emerged an interesting attempt to make the case that if a clinician is adequately informed about a decision tool and its shortcomings and potential harms, then this clinician can be assigned accountability, blame and liability. The "learned intermediary" doctrine holds that a physician or nurse is a kind of conceptual or intellectual gate keeper such that if the machine were to malfunction, then the clinician *ought* to be able to detect the malfunction. While it is probably true that a competent clinician ought to be able to detect any number of brute errors (by human or machine), it is not clear in a complex case—given the extraordinary intricacy of some software and the size of some databases—that a human in all cases may be assigned blame if something goes wrong. Such a level of accountability requires not a learned intermediary, but an infallible one [5].

There is no clear standard for use of decision support software by clinicians. Physicians or nurses might someday be found negligent either for accepting a mistaken computer decision or, having erred themselves, for failing to have used a decision support system that might have proved corrective. In either case, the determination of negligence will have to be weighed against prevailing community or reasonable-person standards. As with other areas of practice, errors will increase liability accordingly as the practitioner is seen to have fallen behind, or moved too far ahead of, such standards.

There is an urgent need for additional conceptual analysis to assist the law in sorting out these puzzles. Local trial courts and juries will often be out of their depth if called on to adjudicate liability claims that challenge fundamental conceptions of responsibility and accountability. Similar difficulties arise in other areas, such as in the intellectual property domain, when there is a need to determine whether computer software is an invention or a work of art. In one interesting approach to these questions, Professor John Snapper attempted an account of responsibility that would not impede the future—and presumably salutary—development of mechanical decision support. On this account, the attribution of responsibility and duty *to computers* for certain actions will maximize the good that will result from increased use of improved decision support systems. [34] The idea is that use of conceptually inadequate legal tools to punish system designers, owners and users might have a chilling effect on the evolution of decision support technology. Spreading responsibility around, and including computers as agents to which responsibility may be assigned, is said to offer the potential of stimulating system design and the benefits this would entail.

This much is clear: physicians and nurses who disdain computers will be ignorant of machines that can in principle improve their practice, and hence patient care. Zealots who take computers to constitute adequate or even superior human surrogates will have lost touch with the human foundations of their profession. At either extreme the risk is high of falling outside emerging standards. This is a mistake—in ethics and at law.

8.2.2 Regulation of Clinical Decision Support Systems

Although the history of governmental regulation of health care products, at least in the United States, is traceable to the Pure Food and Drug Acts of 1906, the regulation of medical devices was not formalized until the Federal Food, Drug, and Cosmetic Act of 1938. There, medical devices were defined as "instruments, apparatus, and contrivances, including their components, parts and accessories, intended: (1) for use in diagnosis, cure, mitigation, treatment, or prevention of diseases in man or other animals; or (2) to affect the structure or any function of the body of man or other animals" [35, 36]. In 1976, motivated by the increased complexity of devices and by reports of some devices' shortcomings and failures, Congress approved comprehensive Medical Device Amendments to the 1938 regulations; the amendments were to "ensure that new devices were safe and effective before they were marketed" [37, 38]. In 1990, a new regulation replaced that emphasis on premarket approvals with an emphasis on post-market surveillance [39]. More recently:

> The term "device" ... means an instrument, apparatus, implement, machine, contrivance, implant, in vitro reagent, or other similar or related article, including any component, part, or accessory, which is –
>
> (1) recognized in the official National Formulary, or the United States Pharmacopeia, or any supplement to them,
> (2) intended for use in the diagnosis of disease or other conditions, or in the cure, mitigation, treatment, or prevention of disease, in man or other animals, or
> (3) intended to affect the structure or any function of the body of man or other animals, and which does not achieve its primary intended purposes through chemical action within or on the body of man or other animals and which is not dependent upon being metabolized for the achievement of its primary intended purposes. [40]

The question whether a clinical decision support system constitutes a device subject to government regulation remains tricky and controversial and, in consequence, remains an interesting and important policy—and conceptual—issue. In Chap. 11, Miller examines some of the issues associated with FDA regulation.

Answering the question whether software in general or clinical decision support systems in particular should be subject to government regulation will require a delicate policy balancing act between patient safety on the one hand and innovation on the other [41]. Several reasons are commonly offered in opposition to government regulation, including the following:

- Software is most accurately regarded as a mental construct or abstract entity, i.e., the sort of thing not customarily falling within the FDA's regulatory purview.
- Practitioners—not software—have traditionally been subjected to licensing requirements.
- Software evolves rapidly and locally, and any sort of national software monitoring is likely to be ineffective or impossible.
- Software is imperfect, and so improvement and refinement—not perfection—must be the standard to be striven for and met.

Several of these points could be in line with an influential stance held by a former commissioner of the agency, namely that the FDA should "apply the least regulation allowed to remain consistent with the requirements of public health and safety" [42].

At ground is the sometimes tacit assumption that government regulation (like faulty law, as above) will have a chilling effect on innovation. This is an empirical claim. To take it seriously, without adequate evidence, would require that its advocates explain away the fact that most informatics tools as used in most hospitals are not innovative, and continue to suffer from poor quality—without any regulation whatsoever. In the United States, even incentives, as under "meaningful use" requirements, have not yet produced compelling, peer-reviewed documentation of nontrivial improvements in *system* quality. Meanwhile, the putative and undemonstrated benefits of innovation come at the expense of putting patients at unnecessary risk.

There might be a middle ground between hard regulation and laissez faire disinterest. The idea, some two decades old, of chartering "autonomous software oversight committees," not unlike research ethics committees or the institutional review boards, to evaluate software has yet to enjoy testing or trial implementation [43, 44]. This is unfortunate. If we devoted as much effort to identifying creative and progressive ways of ensuring patient safety through responsible software use as we do to selling systems, we would perhaps spark a renaissance of safe and effective system development. This would protect the legitimate interests of system developers while making it clear that, at ground, we are first and properly concerned with the wellbeing of patients.

The debate over medical software regulation represents one of the most important controversies of the Computer Age. The balancing of risks and benefits, as well as public safety and technological progress, means that scientists, clinicians and policy makers have one of civilization's most interesting—and challenging—tasks.

8.3 Conclusion and Future Directions

Clinicians, philosophers, lawyers and policy makers have grappled for decades with social, ethical and legal issues raised by the growth of health informatics, perhaps especially by progress in development of tools for computational diagnosis. What has emerged is a recognition that future scientific growth must be guided by corresponding attention to ethical issues. These issues address the role of error avoidance and standards; of appropriate use and users; and of professional relationships. Scientific programs and publications may be regarded as duty-bound to shape and contribute to environments in which further attention to ethical, legal and social issues is encouraged. Indeed, to the extent that morality guides the law, vigorous programs to identify and debate ethical issues will be of no small service to society as legislatures, courts and government regulators and policy makers attempt to apply the insights of ethics to practical problems in health informatics.

More research on ethical issues in computational decision support is essential for this process. We have, for instance, not yet adequately addressed issues that arise when clinical calculators, diagnostic tools and the like are made available on the World Wide Web; we are not yet clear about the level of ethics education that is appropriate for students in health informatics; and there remains much work to be done at the intersections of ethics and system evaluation and ethics and standards of care.

Elsewhere in the history of science and technology, such challenges are often taken to constitute evidence of the growth and maturation of an applied science. This is certainly the case for computational decision support and, indeed, for all of health informatics.

References

1. Hippocrates. Prognosis. In Lloyd GER, ed. Hippocratic Writings (trans. by Chadwick J, Mann WN). London: Penguin Books; 1983; 170–185.
2. Miller RA, Schaffner KF, Meisel A. Ethical and legal issues related to the use of computer programs in clinical medicine. Ann Intern Med. 1985;102:529–36.
3. de Dombal FT. Ethical considerations concerning computers in medicine in the 1980s. J Med Ethics. 1987;13:179–84.
4. Miller RA. Why the standard view is standard: people, not machines, understand patients' problems. J Med Philos. 1990;15:581–91.
5. Goodman KW. Ethics, medicine, and information technology: intelligent machines and the transformation of health care. Cambridge: Cambridge University Press; 2015.
6. Goodman KW. Addressing ethical issues in health information technology. Guest Editorial. Camb Q Healthc Ethics. 2015;24:252–4.
7. Berner ES, Webster GD, Shugerman AA, et al. Performance of four computer-based diagnostic systems. N Engl J Med. 1994;330:1792–6.
8. Goodman KW. Bioethics and health informatics: an introduction. In: Goodman KW, editor. Ethics, computing and medicine: informatics and the transformation of health care. Cambridge/New York: Cambridge University Press; 1997. p. 1–31.

9. Forrow L, Wartman SA, Brock DW. Science, ethics, and the making of clinical decisions. JAMA. 1988;259:3161–7.
10. Rubin MA. The collaborative autonomy model of medical decision-making. Neurocrit Care. 2014;20(2):311–8.
11. Hall DE, Prochazka AV, Fink AS. Informed consent for clinical treatment. CMAJ. 2012;184(5):533–40.
12. Goodman KW. Outcomes, futility, and health policy research. In: Goodman KW, editor. Ethics, computing and medicine: informatics and the transformation of health care. Cambridge: Cambridge University Press; 1997. p. 116–38.
13. Brody BA. The ethics of using ICU scoring systems in individual patient management. Prob Crit Care. 1989;3:662–70.
14. Knaus WA. Ethical implications of risk stratification in the acute care setting. Camb Q Healthc Ethics. 1993;2:193–6.
15. Kullo IJ, Jarvik GP, Manolio TA, et al. Leveraging the electronic health record to implement genomic medicine. Genet Med. 2013;15:270–1.
16. Ginsburg GS, Haga SB. Translating genomic biomarkers into clinically useful diagnostics. Expert Rev Mol Diagn. 2006;6(2):179–91.
17. Altman RB. Translational bioinformatics: linking the molecular world to the clinical world. Clin Pharmacol Ther. 2012;91(6):994–1000.
18. Abugessaisa I, Saevarsdottir S, Tsipras G, et al. Accelerating translational research by clinically driven development of an informatics platform – a case study. PLoS One. 2014;9(9), e104382.
19. Zuradzki T. Preimplantation genetic diagnosis and rational choice under risk or uncertainty. J Med Ethics. 2014;40(11):774–8.
20. Gottesman O, Kuivaniemi H, Tromp G, et al. The electronic medical records and genomics (eMERGE) network: past, present, and future. Genet Med. 2013;15(10):761–71.
21. Lazaridis KN, McAllister TM, Babovic-Vuksanovic D, et al. Implementing individualized medicine into the medical practice. Am J Med Genet C Semin Med Genet. 2014;166C(1):15–23.
22. Pearson SA, Moxey A, Robertson J, et al. Do computerised clinical decision support systems for prescribing change practice? A systematic review of the literature (1990–2007). BMC Health Serv Res. 2009;9:154. doi:10.1186/1472-6963-9-154.
23. Brannigan VM, Dayhoff RE. Medical informatics: the revolution in law, technology, and medicine. J Legal Med. 1986;7:1–53.
24. Miller RA. Legal issues related to medical decision-support systems. Int J Clin Monit Comput. 1989;6:75–80.
25. Mortimer H. Computer-aided medicine: present and future issues of liability. Comput Law J. 1989;9:177–203.
26. Turley TM. Expert software systems: the legal implications. Comput Law J. 1988;8:455–77.
27. Anderson JG. Social, ethical and legal barriers to e-health. Int J Med Inform. 2007;76(5–6):480–3.
28. Lluch M. Healthcare professionals' organisational barriers to health information technologies-a literature review. Int J Med Inform. 2011;80(12):849–62.
29. Beier B. Liability and responsibility for clinical software in the Federal Republic of Germany. Comput Methods Programs Biomed. 1987;25:237–42.
30. Brahams D, Wyatt J. Decision aids and the law. Lancet. 1918;ii:632–4.
31. Allaërt FA, Dussere L. Decision support system and medical liability. Proc Annu Symp Comput Appl Med Care. 1992;750–753.
32. Birnbaum LN. Strict products liability and computer software. Comput Law J. 1988;8:135–56.
33. Gill CJ. Medical expert systems: grappling with the issues of liability. High Tech Law J. 1987;1:483–520.

34. Snapper JW. Responsibility for computer-based decisions in health care. In: Goodman KW, editor. Ethics, computing and medicine: informatics and the transformation of health care. Cambridge: Cambridge University Press; 1997. p. 43–56.
35. Munsey RR. Trends and events in FDA regulation of medical devices over the last fifty years. Food Drug Law J. 1995;50:163–77.
36. Public Law No. 75-717, 52 Stat. 1040 (1938), as amended 21 U.S.C. Sections 301 et seq. 1988.
37. Kessler DA, Pape SM, Sundwall DN. The federal regulation of medical devices. N Engl J Med. 1987;317:357–66.
38. Public Law No. 94-295, 90 Stat. 539 (1976), codified at 21 U.S.C. Sections 360c et seq. 1982.
39. Brannigan VM. Software quality regulation under the Safe Medical Devices Act of 1990: hospitals are now the canaries in the software mine. Proc Annu Symp Comput Appl Med Care. 1991:238–242.
40. Federal Food, Drug, and Cosmetic Act, 21 U.S.C. § 321 SEC. 201, 2006–2010.
41. Karnik K. FDA regulation of clinical decision support software. J Law Biosci. 2014;1(2):202–8.
42. Young FE. Validation of medical software: present policy of the Food and Drug Administration. Ann Intern Med. 1987;106:628–9.
43. Miller RA, Gardner RM. Summary recommendations for the responsible monitoring and regulation of clinical software systems. Ann Intern Med. 1997;127(9):842–5.
44. Miller RA, Gardner RM. Recommendations for responsible monitoring and regulation of clinical software systems. JAMIA. 1997;4:442–57.

Chapter 9
Evaluation of Clinical Decision Support

David F. Lobach

Abstract The value and financial impact of clinical decision support systems need to be better understood. This understanding can be formulated through evaluations of decision support systems. This chapter discusses a framework for identifying an evaluation strategy and selecting an evaluation type in order to address important questions concerning clinical decision support systems (CDSS). The chapter also summarizes the existing literature regarding what is known about evaluations conducted on CDSS and about the features of systems that are associated with successful implementations. In order to assist the reader with framing an evaluative study of a CDSS, the chapter includes a multistep approach to formulating an evaluation illustrated by a parallel description of an actual CDSS evaluation study. Finally, the chapter concludes with the identification of several challenges and pitfalls that can be specifically associated with CDSS evaluations.

Keywords Clinical decision support systems • Summative evaluation • Formative evaluation • Randomized controlled trial • Clinical outcomes • Evaluation methodology • Study design

This chapter will explore three aspects of evaluating clinical decision support systems (CDSS): a description of a framework for the evaluation of CDSS; a review of evaluations that have been done on CDSS; and an outline of an approach for conducting an evaluation of a CDSS. The objectives of this chapter are: (1) to provide a context for the value of CDSS evaluation and expose the reader to the types of evaluations that can be performed as well as common outcomes from CDSS evaluations; (2) to summarize findings from CDSS evaluations particularly focusing on systematic reviews and meta-analyses looking at the effectiveness of CDSS and at features that are associated with successful CDSS; and finally, (3) to discuss issues related to performing an evaluation of a CDSS along with an example of a CDSS

D.F. Lobach, M.D., Ph.D., M.S., F.A.C.M.I. (✉)
Klesis Healthcare, Durham, NC, USA

Community and Family Medicine, Duke University Medical Center,
Box 3886 DUMC, Durham, NC 27710, USA
e-mail: david.lobach@klesishealthcare.com

E.S. Berner (ed.), *Clinical Decision Support Systems*, Health Informatics,
DOI 10.1007/978-3-319-31913-1_9

evaluation study. The ultimate goal for this chapter is to help the reader to appreciate the scope of CDSS evaluation, the work that has already been done in evaluating CDSS, and the process of conducting an evaluation of a CDSS.

9.1 Strategies for CDSS Evaluation

From the most simplistic vantage point, CDSS evaluation entails the systematic collection of information about one or more specific aspects of a CDSS in order to gain further insight and understanding about the system. The ultimate intent of CDSS evaluation is to inform or influence decisions related to CDSS design, use, implementation, or effectiveness through the use of empirically collected data. Establishing a framework for CDSS evaluation depends on the question(s) the evaluation seeks to resolve. The process involves identifying a specific evaluation strategy model that defines the intent of the evaluation, and then selecting an appropriate evaluation methodology. Evaluation strategy models can focus on scientific/experimental questions, management issues, qualitative attributes, or user experience [1]. While these strategies are separated for the purposes of discussion, many evaluation projects will draw from multiple strategies in order to gain a full understanding of the impact of a CDSS.

The scientific or experimental models often tend to be most familiar. These models rely heavily on the collection of data that enables systematic comparisons through experimental and quasi-experimental research designs. This model strategy can address issues such as the effectiveness of CDSS to impact decision-making, the effect of CDSS on care process measures, the impact of CDSS on clinical outcomes, or the determination of which system components are most effective.

Management-focused evaluation models seek to understand the impact and effects of a CDSS in the larger context of an overall organization. These contextually-oriented evaluations can generate insights related to workflow disruption, productivity impact, and/or process changes. Findings arising from a management-focused evaluation strategy provide awareness regarding the practical implications of CDSS implementation on work practices. Such findings can be used to refine and modify workflow, to identify bottlenecks or disruptions in service, or highlight newly gained efficiencies.

Qualitative strategies rely on observation and generate data through subjective human interpretation. For example, the qualitative strategy can be used to generate observations pertaining to the effect of CDSS on work processes, decision making, and care delivery. In many instances, qualitative data are systematically reviewed and categorized in order to discover recurring themes and identify trends or patterns.

Participant-oriented strategy models seek to gain understanding regarding the CDSS user experience. These strategies can rely on direct user input in the form of validated survey instruments or on interviews and discussions in order to obtain user feedback. For analysis, user feedback is often categorized in order to find common themes across multiple users. These studies are exceedingly valuable for refining CDSS so that they will be user-friendly and effective with the intended recipients of the technology.

9.2 Types of CDSS Evaluations

At the highest level, CDSS evaluations can be divided into one of two categories: formative evaluation and summative evaluation [2]. The category selected depends on the ultimate purpose of the evaluation. Formative evaluation refines and improves attributes of the CDSS technology. As implied by its name, formative evaluation seeks to mold and shape a CDSS in most cases prior to its full implementation. Formative studies can follow several different approaches. Needs assessment determines what need or needs the CDSS should address, the extent of the needs, and what approaches could be used to meet the identified needs. Evaluability assessment explores the feasibility of a CDSS evaluation and how such an evaluation can be structured [1]. A structured conceptualization study establishes the most appropriate target population for the CDSS and can begin the process of identifying potential outcomes from system use. An implementation evaluation explores the fidelity of the CDSS in context and serves to identify potential barriers or pitfalls for actual system use. A process evaluation determines the impact of delivering the CDSS on work processes and procedures. These two latter study types are particularly useful for identifying potential problems with a CDSS implementation before they become disruptive in a production environment.

The techniques used for formative evaluations depend in part on the types of questions that are being addressed. Commonly used techniques that could support several of the formative approaches include brainstorming, focus groups, think-aloud sessions, structured interviews, nominal group techniques, concept mapping, and Delphi polls [1]. With regard to techniques for specific approaches beyond the previously identified general methodologies, needs assessment can be accomplished through surveys, interviews with stakeholders, and gap analysis; implementation evaluation may benefit from model creation or simulation studies; and process evaluation may be informed through qualitative and quantitative monitoring from information systems.

Summative evaluations, in contrast to formative evaluations, seek to assess effects or outcomes resulting from a CDSS. Often summative evaluations are the evaluation type that comes to mind when one thinks about evaluating a CDSS. The most familiar summative evaluations focus on the effect of CDSS on process measures or clinical outcomes. Several different study designs can be used to conduct summative outcome evaluations, including randomized controlled trials (parallel group, crossover, or cluster), quasi-experimental investigations (non-randomized trial, historical before – after trial, or time series trial), and observational studies (cohort, case-control, or case series) [3]. Other less familiar types of summative evaluations include impact evaluations, designed to assess intended or unintended consequences of a CDSS in the production environment; cost-effectiveness or cost-benefit analysis, focusing on the financial consequences of a CDSS implementation; secondary analysis, using existing data to explore new research questions about a CDSS; and meta-analysis, integrating outcome results from multiple studies in order to assess an overall impact from CDSS as a whole.

9.3 Types of Outcomes Assessed in CDSS Evaluations

An important aspect of any CDSS evaluation is the primary metric used to answer the question behind the evaluation. Formative and summative studies reporting evaluations of CDSS have looked at a wide variety of potential outcomes [4]. As Bright et al. indicate, the outcomes identified in published CDSS studies can be grouped into the following seven primary categories:

- Clinical (Length of stay, morbidity, mortality, health-related quality of life, adverse events)
- Health care process (Adoption/implementation of CDS-recommended preventive care/clinical study/treatment, patient adherence to CDSS recommendation, impact on user knowledge)
- Health care provider workload, efficiency, and organization (Number of patients seen/unit time, clinician workload, efficiency)
- Relationship-centered (Patient satisfaction)
- Economic (Cost, cost-effectiveness)
- Health care provider use and implementation (User acceptance, satisfaction, and use and implementation of CDS) [4].

Many studies report on more than one type of outcome, even though one particular outcome may be selected as primary for the purposes of determining the study sample size. Among the 311 CDSS evaluation studies included in a recent review, clinical outcomes were included in 20 % of randomized controlled trials, 35 % of quasi-experimental trials, and 45 % of observational studies. In contrast, healthcare process measures were included in 86 % of randomized controlled trials, 75 % of quasi-experimental studies, and 69 % of observational studies [4].

9.4 Findings from Systematic Reviews of CDSS

Systematic reviews of evaluation studies of CDSS have explored both the effectiveness of CDSS to impact process measures and clinical outcomes and the features of CDSS that are associated with a significant clinical impact. Studies evaluating the effectiveness of CDSS have been reviewed through the Agency for Healthcare Research and Quality-sponsored Evidence-based Practice Center at Duke University [5]. For this review, a CDSS was defined as "any electronic system designed to aid directly in clinical decision making, in which characteristics of individual patients are used to generate patient-specific assessments, recommendations that are then presented to clinicians for consideration." Examples of CDSS included in the Lobach et al. review included the following: alerts, reminders, order sets, drug-dosage calculations, and care summary dashboards that provide performance feedback on quality indicators or benchmarks [5]. A total of 160 manuscripts representing 148 unique studies were identified and abstracted for inclusion in the systematic analysis. This review determined that CDSS evaluations demonstrate "strong evidence that CDSS… are effective in improving health care process measures across diverse settings using both commercially and locally developed systems" [5]. Relatively little evidence was available to show the impact of CDSS on clinical outcomes and health care costs. The evaluative studies from this review showed that CDSS now have demonstrable effectiveness not just at academic medical centers with locally developed CDSS but also across diverse community healthcare settings using commercially developed CDSS tools [5].

In addition to the AHRQ-sponsored review noted above, CDSS evaluation studies have been serially reviewed by Haynes and colleagues [6–8]. These reviews have demonstrated the historical evolution of CDSS and their impact. The initial review from 1994, a systematic analysis of CDSS evaluation studies that included only 28 controlled trials of CDSS evaluations showed that CDSS improved clinician performance through preventive care, reminders and computer-aided quality assurance [6]. Only three of the ten studies that assessed patient outcomes showed significant improvements. The next systematic review of CDSS evaluation studies was published in 1998 [7]. This review included 68 controlled trials. The use of CDSS was found to have beneficial effects on clinician performance in 66 % (43 out of 65) of the studies. Benefits were shown for drug dosing decision support in 9 of 15 studies, diagnostic assistance in 1 of 5 studies, preventive care reminders in 14 of 19 studies, and on general medical care issues in 19 of 26 studies. Benefit of CDSS was found in 6 of 14 studies that assessed patient outcomes. Of the negative eight outcome studies, Hunt et al. determined that only three had sufficient power greater than 80 % to detect a clinically important effect [7]. The next serial review was published in 2005 [8]. This review of CDSS evaluation studies encompassed 100 randomized and nonrandomized trials, including 97 controlled trials assessing clinician performance. In 64 % of the studies, CDSS improved clinician performance for diagnosis, preventive care, disease management, drug dosing, or drug prescribing. Of the 52 trials that assessed patient outcomes, only 7 reported improved outcomes with CDSS and no reports showed benefit on major outcomes such as mortality. Most of the studies focusing on clinical outcomes were insufficiently powered to detect a clinically important difference [8].

Most recently, evaluation studies focusing on CDSS associated with electronic health record systems (EHRs) have been systematically reviewed by Moja et al. [9]. This review identified 28 randomized controlled trials in which rule-or algorithm-based CDSS were integrated with EHRs and outcome measures reflecting morbidity, mortality, or economic impact were assessed. Sixteen trials measured mortality rates, but found no statistically significant impact. In the nine trials that assessed morbidity, defined by the authors as occurrence of illness (such as pneumonia, myocardial infarction, or stroke), progression of diseases, or hospitalizations, a small but statistically significant effect was detected. In the 17 trials that reported economic outcomes, differences in costs and health service utilization were detected, but the magnitude of the effect was small. Across all economic outcomes, Moja et al. concluded that there was no consistent advantage for EHRs with CDSS compared to those without CDSS [9].

In summary, evaluations of the impact of CDSS to date have shown that these systems can improve care process measures using both locally developed or commercial CDSS in academic and community-based care settings. More research is needed to determine the effect of CDSS on clinical outcomes and on the economic consequences of using these systems.

With regard to CDSS features that contribute to success, an initial systematic review of CDSS evaluation studies reporting on 71 comparisons of control versus CDSS and focusing on features of CDSS that are associated with a clinical impact was published by Kawamoto et al. [10]. This study showed that CDSS including five specific features were more likely to improve clinical practice than systems without these features. Kawamoto et al. found that the features associated with an impact on clinical practice included the following: "(1) automatic provision of decision support as part of clinician workflow, (2) provision of decision support at the time and location of decision making, (3) provision of recommendations rather than just an assessment, (4) use of a computer to generate decision support, and (5) provision of decision support as part of clinician workflow" [10].

CDSS evaluation studies that identified features associated with successful CDSS implementations were also included in the AHRQ-sponsored review of CDSS evaluation studies [5]. This report confirmed the effectiveness of three features previously identified by Kawamoto et al. namely automatic provision of decision support as part of clinician workflow, provision of decision support at the time and location of decision making, and provision of a recommendation and not just an assessment. The Lobach et al. review also identified six additional features that correlated with successful CDSS systems. These features included:

- Integration with charting or order entry system to support workflow integration,
- No need for additional clinician data entry,
- Promotion of action rather than inaction,
- Justification of decision support via provision of research evidence,
- Local user involvement in the development process, and
- Provision of decision support results to patients as well as providers [5].

Lobach et al. noted that many of the evaluation studies included CDSS with more than one feature, and thus it was difficult to determine the importance or impact of any one individual feature [5].

A more extensive systematic review reporting on 148 CDSS evaluation studies was published by Roshanov et al. [11] This review found that CDSS were associated with success when (1) the system was developed by the authors of the study, (2) the system provided advice to both patients and clinicians, and (3) the system required a reason for overriding advice. Roshanov et al. also found that "advice presented in electronic charting or order entry systems showed a strong negative association with success" [11]. In contrast to the findings reported by Kawamoto et al. [10], Roshanov et al. found that neither advice automatically provided in workflow nor advice provided at the time of care were associated with successful CDSS [11].

To date, efforts to identify the most critical features associated with successful CDSS have been inconclusive in that the largest studies have reported conflicting results. The findings do imply that features that integrate CDSS into existing workflows and justify the CDSS recommendations lead to greater success; however, more evaluations deliberately focusing on the impact of specific CDSS features are needed.

9.5 Approach to Conducting an Evaluation of a CDSS

There is no "one-size fits all" approach for evaluating CDSS since each system has nuances about its operation and use, and every implementation environment has unique differences and challenges related to evaluation. Accordingly, the following section does not provide specifics for formulating a CDSS evaluation, but instead offers seven guiding questions to facilitate planning an evaluation that accommodates the implementation environment. These guiding questions have been used over the years to assist informatics graduate students with developing thesis and dissertation projects as well as for the formulation of plans for several successful research grants for CDSS development and evaluation. One of the studies resulting from a research grant funded by the Agency for Healthcare Quality and Research will be used as an illustrative example [12]. This project assessed a CDSS that was in use for population health management among 20,000 Medicaid beneficiaries in Durham County, North Carolina. This project was possible in part because every Medicaid enrollee was included in a care management network so that every patient had an assigned medical home and an assigned care manager. Care managers were allocated to a specific population by clinic site, patient age (i.e., pediatric or adult), and native language (i.e., English or Spanish). The decision support tool was designed to detect missing care services such as regular hemoglobin A1c assays for patients with diabetes and potentially inappropriate use of healthcare resources such as emergency department visits for low severity indications or ambulatory care-sensitive conditions. The CDSS tool received administrative claims and enrollment data from the North Carolina Medicaid office monthly and daily admission, discharge, and transfer (ADT) data through a Health Level 7 (HL7) interface from the hospitals and emergency departments in the region [13]. When sentinel events, defined in this context as notable activities that deviate from expected or optimal care pathways such as hospitalizations for ambulatory care sensitive conditions, low severity emergency department visits, missing recommended laboratory tests or services, were detected by the system, notifications for each index patient were communicated to the appropriate care manager via secure email. Sentinel events were prioritized and filtered so that each care manager would receive only the top 20 most important events each day for his/her patient population.

Question #1: *What will be the impact if the CDSS is successful*? Since every CDSS is designed with an intended purpose, this first question seeks to define what the anticipated result would be if the CDSS worked optimally. After "success" is defined, the corollary question is whether or not this success can be measured directly. If direct measurement is not possible, what surrogate measures could be used to reflect the desired success? In the example study, the goal of the CDSS was to increase the completion rates of recommended care services, and decrease potentially inappropriate emergency department (ED) use and hospitalizations [12]. In addition, success would also result in decreased overall medical costs because expensive ED visits and hospitalizations would be converted to primary care visits [12].

Question #2: *What data are needed to show/measure success or the surrogate outcome*? In order to determine whether or not success has been achieved, empirical data need to be collected and analyzed to assess whether or not the CDSS fulfilled its intended purpose. The data for measuring success need to be defined and characterized. As a reference, the types of outcomes that have been measured in published CDSS studies were summarized above in section 9.3. For the example study, the primary measure was to be emergency department utilization rates. In addition, we also included secondary measures such as low severity ED rates, hospitalization rates, the completion of appropriate medical services, and medical costs in total and broken down across categories of emergency department services and ambulatory care [12].

Question #3: *How can these data be obtained*? One issue to decide is what the ideal dataset would be for measuring a desired outcome; however, obtaining the needed data for all potential study subjects can be challenging. It is important that the evaluation data be available from a common source across both intervention and control subjects. In many instances, supplemental data are collected for the intervention group as part of the research protocol. These data, however, cannot be used to determine the primary study outcome since they are not available for the control group. If the data needed to measure the primary outcome are not available, a different primary outcome or a surrogate for the primary outcome may need to be selected. For the example study, emergency department utilization rates could be readily calculated from Medicaid claims data as could hospitalization rates, completion of medical services, and even medical costs. These data were available for both intervention and control subjects in the target study population [12].

Question #4: *What type of evaluation is possible in the environment of the CDSS*? Now that the desired outcome for measuring the impact of the CDSS has been defined and the necessary data for calculating this metric have been identified, several pivotal issues need to be addressed that determine the type of study that can be performed in the CDSS environment. As discussed above, the likely study type would be a summative evaluation in order to quantitate the impact of the CDSS on the primary outcome. Within the summative evaluation type, a researcher needs to select an appropriate study design. As a general rule, the most rigorous study design possible is desirable. The next step is to define precisely who the study participants should be. For CDSS evaluation studies, this step can be challenging in that the CDSS content is often delivered to a clinician, but the desired impact is assessed on patients. Whichever study subject group is selected, this group needs to serve as the unit of randomization if a randomized controlled trial design is selected. For the example study, a randomized controlled trial was selected as the study design since the research team had complete control over the distribution of the CDSS recommendations [12]. We opted to use patients as our unit of randomization since the data from the study outcomes would be based on data pertaining to individual patients (i.e., ED utilization rates). As is common with randomized controlled trials involving CDSS evaluations, we then needed to ascertain whether significant contamination would occur since the individuals receiving the CDSS notifications, the care managers, could have contact with patients assigned to both the control and intervention groups. The issue of contamination is addressed below in Question #6.

Question #5: *How should the outcome data from the study groups be compared*? This question seeks to determine what type of data analysis will be necessary in order to ascertain whether or not the impact of the CDSS intervention was significant. The answers to this question will define the analytical approach for comparing the primary outcome measure between study groups. These answers will also dictate what the study sample size and duration need to be in order to achieve an appropriate level of statistical power for the primary outcome. The sample size and study duration are ultimately dictated by the event rate of the primary outcome measure. At this juncture, the researcher needs to determine what a clinically significant difference in the primary measure would be between the intervention and control groups. A sufficient number of primary outcome events needs to occur in order to provide an opportunity to establish a statistically significant difference. For the example project, [12] we were able to determine that the rate of ED utilization within the population was 42.7 visits per month per 1,000 Medicaid beneficiaries. From preliminary studies, we concluded that a change in emergency utilization rates of 20 % would be feasible and would be clinically significant. We estimated that we would be able to enroll approximately 80 % of the available study subjects in the trial. With this number of subjects, we determined that the study duration would need to be 9 months and the power to detect a significant difference would exceed 80 % for an odds ratio for event reduction of 0.80 based on a two-sided test of proportions with a significance level of 0.05. For making comparisons between study groups, estimates for intervention impact on study outcomes were based on generalized estimating equations with a working correlation matrix to account for clustering within families [12].

Question #6: *How can contamination be avoided or controlled*? As mentioned above, under Question #4, the challenge of contamination is prevalent in many randomized controlled trials of CDSS since the patients are often the unit of randomization, but the CDSS intervention is conveyed to clinicians. Clinicians often have contact with patients who have been randomized to the intervention as well as with patients randomized to the control arm. In some instances, it is possible to randomize clinicians and assign all of the clinician's patients to a particular study arm. The challenge with this approach is that patients are sometimes seen by different clinicians and can then crossover between study groups, leading to a new type of contamination. A cluster randomized trial design in which entire clinician groups or clinic sites are randomized as a unit can control for crossover contamination; however, this approach can significantly limit sample size because the sample size lies somewhere between the number of clusters randomized and the number of patients for whom outcome measures will be determined. In the example study, [12] the contamination question was whether or not a care manager would have contact with subjects randomized to the intervention group and subjects randomized to the control group, and if so, whether this contact would have significant effects on the study outcomes. We determined that the care managers could have contact with both intervention and control subjects; however, this contact with both groups was felt to invoke minimal contamination since the recommendations for intervention were highly patient specific (e.g., pediatric patient X had a low severity emergency department encounter for fever yesterday) and care managers would not know to initiate contact with control subjects without receiving the CDSS guidance. Of note, we did make one adjustment in our unit of randomization such that the randomization was actually based on family units since receipt of an intervention for one family member could potentially impact health behaviors of other family members [12].

Question #7: *What is the economic impact or return on investment (ROI) from the CDSS*? With the increasing emphasis on controlling healthcare costs, inclusion of measures that will reflect the economic impact of a CDSS intervention are becoming increasingly important [14]. In general, the economic measures can be tied to the changes anticipated in the primary outcome. Basically, if the desired impact is achieved, what are the cost implications? For the sample study, [12] we were seeking to decrease emergency department utilization rates. A decrease in emergency department utilization should contribute to significant cost savings. For this study, we opted to look at total costs for patients in each study arm recognizing that saving costs in one area could lead to increased costs in a different area. For our study, we hypothesized that decreased emergency department utilization rates could lead to increased visits at primary care clinics. In addition, other hypothetical cost implications resulting from our CDSS interventions could be increased rates of testing and potentially increased pharmaceutical costs because intervention subjects would be likely to have more contact with the healthcare system [12].

As mentioned above, these seven questions are intended to assist with the formulation of a CDSS evaluation study. They are not prescriptive with regard to how an evaluation should be conducted for a given CDSS and system environment. Table 9.1 summarizes the seven evaluation questions.

As the "rest of the story" regarding the sample CDSS evaluation project, we did not show a decrease in total emergency department utilization rates or costs across the entire population as our primary study outcomes. However, when we drilled down and looked at the impact of the intervention on low severity ED utilization

Table 9.1 Questions to guide the formulation of a CDSS evaluation

1. Define result if system is successful
Can this success be measured directly?
If not, what surrogate measure can be used to reflect success?
2. What data are needed to show/measure success or surrogate outcome?
3. Where can these data be obtained?
4. What type of evaluation is possible in system environment?
Define study design (historical control, randomized controlled trial)
Identify study participants
5. How should these data be compared?
Define analytical approach
Estimate sample size
Determine statistical power
6. How can contamination be avoided or controlled?
7. What is the economic impact/ROI?

rates, we found a statistically significant reduction in the intervention group relative to the control subjects (8.1 vs. 10.6/100 enrollees, $p<0.001$). In further sub-analysis focusing specifically on the pediatric population, we discovered a statistically significant reduction in total ED utilization rates (18.3 vs. 23.5/100 enrollees, $p<0.001$), translating to a reduction in utilization rate from 28 % to 23 % in the intervention arm. We also demonstrated a statistically significant total cost savings of $500 per pediatric intervention subject during the 9-month study. When the cost saving results were extrapolated across the entire pediatric population, we determined that the annual cost savings for Medicaid would be the on the order of $1.5 million in a single county [12].

9.6 Challenges Associated with Evaluation of CDSS

While evaluation is critical for developing, implementing, assessing impact, and establishing ROI for CDSS, conducting studies of CDSS is fraught with unique challenges. To begin with, performing a rigorous study of CDSS with a simultaneous control arm is often difficult because CDSS tools tend to be components of larger systems. In many instances, it is difficult to allow access to CDSS for some users and not for others. This challenge has increased further with the integration of CDSS capabilities into EHRs. Rarely can an individual site or investigator control the access to CDSS resources within a commercial EHR product thus limiting opportunities for a simultaneous control arm. In almost no instances can the intervention subject be blinded to the intervention. As a consequence, evaluators of

CDSS systems often need to settle for historical controls with a before-after clinical trial study design.

As a second challenge, even when the CDSS can be provided to one group of users, but not another, contamination becomes a problem as illustrated above. As already described, the direct user of CDSS advice is frequently the clinician, even though the impact of the CDSS is assessed on patient outcomes. In clinical settings, it is not unusual for patients to receive care from several clinicians within a practice and for clinicians to care for patients of their colleagues. As a result, non-intervention patients can be exposed to clinicians receiving a CDSS intervention and intervention clinicians can have encounters with patients from both the intervention and control arms of the study.

A further consequence of the discordance between the clinician as the recipient of the CDSS intervention and the patient as the unit of randomization and focal point for the outcome measures is the challenges that arise for data analysis. Special analytic techniques are frequently needed in order to unravel the potential dependencies and co-variation that can arise in these settings. Experienced statisticians are needed on the team in order to navigate the analytic quagmire.

An additional difficulty is that definitive randomized controlled trials are often large studies and can be quite expensive and difficult to organize [15]. As a consequence, many evaluations of CDSS rely on less rigorous study designs and thus tend not to supply the best evidence for CDSS impact.

Another challenge with CDSS evaluation is ensuring adequate exposure to the intervention. In many systems, clinical decision support is an adjunct to the primary workflow and can be easily overlooked or neglected by busy clinicians. In order to have a definitive study of a CDSS, high use rates of the CDSS are required. Over the years, many studies have failed to show impact because the "dose" of CDSS that was "consumed" by the target clinician study subjects was too low. Most of these studies are assessed with an intention-to-treat framework and show no impact for the overall effect. When sub-analyses are conducted and the results for substantive CDSS users are isolated, a positive impact is often detected.

A sixth challenge for evaluating CDSS also relates to problems concerning CDSS usage. In many studies the targeted outcome is a relatively infrequent event such as an adverse drug event for a specific pharmaceutical. In order to have sufficient instances in which the CDSS intervention is activated, the CDSS needs to be regularly used by clinicians so that the CDSS is engaged when the infrequent event occurs [15].

A final and often unanticipated challenge is receiving institutional review board (IRB) approval for CDSS evaluation studies, especially randomized controlled trials. Many CDSS evaluation studies are conducted using computerized information systems in clinical settings that may serve large populations of patients. At the outset, it is often unknown which patients will prompt a CDSS-driven recommendation. In many instances, all patients serviced by the information system need to be included in the study population and thus randomized in the event a CDSS recommendation is generated (or, could be generated, but is withheld for control subjects) for one of these patients. It becomes unrealistic and impractical to consent all of the

Table 9.2 Special challenges arising from evaluation studies on CDSS

Special challenges
Difficulty conducting randomized controlled trials due to limited capacity to selectively turn the system on and off for subsets of users
Contamination in randomized controlled trials
Discordance between CDSS target users (e.g., clinicians) and the target for CDSS impact measurement (e.g., patients)
RCTs of CDSSs are expensive and difficult to conduct
CDSS sometimes have limited use by clinicians mitigating their impact
Need for widespread use of CDSS to generate sufficient power especially for relatively infrequent event outcomes such as adverse drug events
Obtaining Institutional Review Board approval

patients who are receiving care through the information system associated with the CDSS. In these scenarios, IRB review boards may find it difficult to allow a study to be performed on subjects who have been randomized into a clinical trial without the subjects' consent. In such instances, a waiver of consent will need to be justified in order to conduct the study. Such waivers can be justified because these studies promote an evidence-based standard of care and involve minimal risk to the study subjects. As an illustration of this challenge, the example study described above [12] required 9 months in order to obtain Institutional Review Board approval. Many conversations and meetings were necessary to help the IRB understand the nature of a technology clinical trial. Ultimately, a waiver of consent was granted for the trial. Table 9.2 summarizes the challenges for evaluation of CDSS.

9.7 Conclusions/Observations

The rapid expansion of biomedical knowledge and the desire to utilize this knowledge expeditiously at the bedside necessitate the use of tools to support decision making in the delivery of healthcare. Evaluation of these decision supporting systems is becoming increasingly important in order to demonstrate the impact these systems have on the health care triple aim of increased quality, improved health, and lower costs [16]. CDSS evaluations also provide insights regarding how to make systems more effective and efficient for seamless integration into the care delivery process.

Multiple strategies exist for pursuing evaluation of CDSS depending on the particular issues that need to be explored. Strategies can focus on scientific or experimental questions, management concerns, qualitative system attributes, or user experience. After an evaluation strategy has been identified, the type of evaluation to be conducted needs to be determined. In general, evaluations can be formative, focusing on the development and refinement of the CDSS, or summative, exploring the impact of the system on selected outcomes. The types of outcomes that have been reported in the biomedical literature include clinical parameters, healthcare process measures, workload and efficiency metrics, stakeholder satisfaction, economic impact, and implementation factors.

Published evaluations of CDSS have shown that these tools can improve clinician performance of care processes such as ordering appropriate tests, making correct diagnoses, selecting effective medications, and complying with preventive service recommendations. Initially these benefits were only seen with locally developed systems in academic medical centers. The research evidence now demonstrates that commercial systems can also achieve these benefits and that the benefits can be obtained in community-based settings. The available data on clinical outcomes such as morbidity and mortality is less compelling. A few studies have demonstrated reduced morbidity and decreased length of stay with the use of decision support. Some studies have also shown economic benefits from the use of decision support, but in most instances, the benefits have been relatively small.

Direct evaluation of CDSS has led to the identification of system features that are associated with a positive impact. While the findings from these studies are somewhat inconsistent across studies, there is evidence to suggest that providing decision support for both clinicians and patients, integrating decision support into the clinical workflow, and requiring justification when decision support recommendations are not followed, are all associated with system success.

Conducting an evaluation of a decision support system requires identification of the most salient impact expected from the system, identifying a source of data from which to measure this impact, and designing a study that will generate these data empirically. CDSS evaluations present some unusual challenges in that the systems are often used by clinicians, but the system impact is assessed on patients. This dissonance between the system user and the unit for measuring impact has ramifications for study design, sample size calculations, subject randomization, data analysis, and controlling contamination. In addition, conducting randomized controlled trials to assess decision support is challenging because creating a study environment in which a simultaneous control can be available is often impossible since systems are used across entire enterprises and cannot be selectively turned on and off for a subset of users or patients.

In spite of the challenges associated with evaluating CDSS, these evaluations are critical for the advancement of the field. Multiple types of approaches can be used for evaluating CDSS. A growing body of evidence is becoming available that shows the value of these systems for impacting care processes. More evaluative studies are needed to assess the impact of CDSS on clinical outcomes and economic measures. In addition, evaluations are needed to determine how to create tools that can more efficiently and effectively be integrated seamlessly into the clinical workflow.

References

1. Trochim WMK. Research methods knowledge base: introduction to evaluation. 2006. http://www.socialresearchmethods.net/kb/intreval.php. Accessed 03 July 2015.

2. Spaulding DT. Program evaluation in practice: core concepts and examples for discussion and analysis. San Francisco: Wiley; 2014.
3. Mitchell K. Study design and statistical analysis: a practical guide for clinician. New York: Cambridge University Press; 2006. p. 11–32.
4. Bright TJ, Wong A, Dhurjati R, Bristow E, Bastian L, Coeytaux RR, et al. Impact of clinical decision support systems: a systematic review. Ann Intern Med. 2012;157:29–43.
5. Lobach D, Sanders GD, Bright TJ, Wong A, Dhurjati R, Bristow E, et al. Enabling health care decisionmaking through clinical decision support and knowledge management. Rockville (MD): Agency for Healthcare Research and Quality (US); 2012 Apr. (Evidence Report/ Technology Assessments, No. 203.) Available from: http://www.ncbi.nlm.nih.gov/books/ NBK97318/. Accessed 15 Sept 2015.
6. Johnston ME, Langton KB, Haynes RB, Mathieu A. Effects of computer-based clinical decision support systems on clinician performance and patient outcome. A critical appraisal of research. Ann Intern Med. 1994;120(2):135–42.
7. Hunt DL, Haynes RB, Hanna SE, Smith K. Effects of computer-based clinical decision support systems on physician performance and patient outcomes: a systematic review. JAMA. 1998;280(15):1339–46.
8. Garg AX, Adhikari NK, McDonald H, Rosas-Arellano MP, Devereaux PJ, Beyene J, et al. Effects of computerized clinical decision support systems on practitioner performance and patient outcomes: a systematic review. JAMA. 2005;293(10):1223–38.
9. Moja L, Kwag KH, Lytras T, Bertizzolo L, Brandt L, Pecoraro V, et al. Effectiveness of computerized decision support systems linked to electronic health records: a systematic review and meta-analysis. Am J Public Health. 2014;104(12):e12–22.
10. Kawamoto K, Houlihan CA, Balas EA, Lobach DF. Improving clinical practice using clinical decision support systems: a systematic review of randomized controlled trials to identify system features critical to success. BMJ. 2005;330:765–8.
11. Roshanov PS, Fernandes N, Wilczynski JM, Hemens BJ, You JJ, Handler SM, et al. Features of effective computerised clinical decision support systems: meta-regression of 162 randomised trials. BMJ. 2013;346:f657.
12. Lobach DF, Kawamoto K, Anstrom KJ, Silvey GM, Willis JM, Johnson FS, et al. A randomized trial of population-based clinical decision support to manage health and resource use for Medicaid beneficiaries. J Med Syst. 2013;37:9922.
13. Lobach DF, Kawamoto K, Anstrom KJ, Kooy KR, Eisenstein EL, Silvey GA, et al. Proactive population health management in the context of a regional health information exchange using standards-based decision support. AMIA Annu Symp Proc. 2007; 473–7.
14. Eisenstein EL, Anstrom KJ, Macri JM, Crosslin DR, Johnson FS, Kawamoto K, Lobach DF. Assessing the potential economic value of health information technology interventions in a community-based health network. AMIA Annu Symp Proc. 2005;221–5.
15. Berner ES. Clinical decision support systems: state of the art. AHRQ Publication No. 09-0069-EF. Rockville: Agency for Healthcare Research and Quality (US); 2009 June. Available from https://www.healthit.ahrq.gov/sites/default/files/docs/page/09-0069-EF_1.pdf. Accessed 15 Sept 2015.
16. Berwick DM, Nolan TW, Whittington. The triple aim: care, health, and cost. Health Aff. 2008;27:759–69.

Chapter 10
Decision Support for Patients

Holly B. Jimison and Christine M. Gordon

Abstract Research studies have shown that access to health information and decision support can enable patients to be more active participants in the treatment process, leading to better medical outcomes. Decision support may take the form of health risk appraisals, understanding symptoms and when to see a doctor, as well as support for treatment choices and health management in the home. Many systems are designed to improve shared decision making, blending the expertise of clinicians in areas of diagnosis and prognosis with patients' knowledge of their preferences and values on potential health outcomes. Technologies designed to provide clarity and improved access to decision support tools for patients have the potential to improve the quality of health care decisions and health outcomes more generally.

Keywords Decision aid • Empowerment • Shared decision making • Patient preferences • Usability

10.1 Introduction

This chapter introduces the concept of technology-based decision support systems for patients. With the rapid growth in smart phones, sensor technologies, and more ubiquitous Web access for patients of all demographics, we have an opportunity to empower patients to be active participants in their health management and decision making. The field of consumer health informatics deals with "developing and evaluating methods and applications to integrate consumer needs and preferences into information management systems in clinical practice, education, and research" [1]. This technology ranges from systems providing background information on wellness, symptoms, diseases, and possible treatments to more comprehensive and interactive systems that support the management of chronic diseases. There are also

H.B. Jimison, Ph.D. (✉) • C.M. Gordon, M.P.H.
College of Computer and Information Science, Bouvé College of Health Sciences, Northeastern University, 360 Huntington Ave., 202 WVH, Boston, MA 02115, USA
e-mail: h.jimison@neu.edu; c.gordon@neu.edu

E.S. Berner (ed.), *Clinical Decision Support Systems*, Health Informatics,
DOI 10.1007/978-3-319-31913-1_10

systems that support a patient's shared decision making with a clinician for important medical issues. Today more than ever, consumers and patients are using information technology as an important component of their medical care.

10.2 Role of Consumer Health Informatics in Patient Care

Research studies have shown that access to health information can enable patients to be more active participants in the treatment process, leading to better medical outcomes [2–5]. Health education is an important aspect of doctor-patient communication. Patients report that they want to be informed about their medical condition [6, 7], and the process of sharing information enhances the doctor-patient relationship. In Pew Internet's Health Online 2013 Survey, they found that 72 % of U.S. adults reported having looked online for health information in the past year, and that 35 % reported having looked online to determine what medical condition they or someone else might have [8]. Of those seeking health information online, 46 % said that it led them to think they needed to seek medical care, while 38 % found it was something they could take care of at home, and 11 % reported that it was both or in-between. Clearly, the Web is a common source of health information. However, many people still consult with family and friends in addition to seeing a clinician. In fact, the Pew Health Online Survey found that, for serious conditions, 70 % sought information, care, or support from) a health care professional, 60 % consulted with family and friends, and 24 % discussed it with patients with a similar diagnosis [8].

Materials for patients and consumers on the Web run the gamut from generic patient education materials and background information presented in an electronic format to interactive decision aids. Most consumers (77 %) begin looking online for health information using a search engine (e.g., Google, Bing, Yahoo). Others (13 %) limit their search to known specialty sites, such as WebMD.com or MayoClinic.org. Often, search engines will return links to these specialty sites or to a general reference site like Wikipedia. The vast majority of people looking online for health information end up on these specialty sites [8].

Websites that specialize in health information usually organize the material so that it is accessible by both symptoms and condition/diagnosis. Each condition or diagnosis will contain background information on causes and symptoms, information on how the disease or condition is diagnosed, and possible treatment options. A key feature of these sites is letting the user know when and how soon to see a clinician or if the condition can be managed at home. Many health websites offer wellness information and information on other health topics, such as aging. One of the clear advantages of being able to search for information on these sites is that photographs (especially useful for skin conditions), diagrams, and videos can be readily accessed and used both educationally and to help clarify symptoms.

Additionally, many health websites offer interactive tools for patients. These range from simple calculators of BMI (body mass index) to health risk appraisals and checks for drug-drug interactions. The rapid growth of consumer health software and materials on the Web, as well as new sensor developments and the rapid uptake of mobile communication devices have facilitated patient participation in their health care and decision making. These interactive systems have been developed to assist patients with informed consent [9, 10], health management [11], as well as coping and decision-making skills [9–11].

Interactive tools for patient decision support or health management include the following:

- Support algorithms for when to see a clinician or when to manage at home
- Health risk assessments, health metric calculators
- Interactive systems for health management (e.g., fitness, weight loss, smoking cessation)
- Interactive systems for disease management (e.g., heart failure, diabetes, asthma)
- Online forums on health topics for social support and condition management advice
- Patients' access to their electronic health record, patient/physician email, tailored discharge summaries
- Decision support tools for patients to make treatment or care choices
- Decision support tools to prepare patients for shared decision making in a clinical visit

Interactivity and tailoring of health materials has been shown to improve health outcomes [12–15] and is an important aspect of the more intensive tools for patients. The remaining topics in this chapter will relate to computer tools, sensors and communication devices that interface with the patient directly with interactivity and tailoring to facilitate their decisions and management of their health.

10.2.1 Empowerment and Self-efficacy

Involvement in one's medical care also involves the concepts of patient empowerment and self-efficacy. Empowerment and self-efficacy are closely linked concepts. In general, empowerment can be thought of as the process that enables people to "own" their lives and have control over their destiny. It is closely related to health outcomes in that powerlessness has been shown to be a broad-based risk factor for disease. Studies demonstrate that patients who feel "in control" in a medical situation have better outcomes than those who feel "powerless" [16–18].

Similarly, self-efficacy is a patient's level of confidence that he or she can perform a specific task or health behavior in the future. Several clinical studies have shown self-efficacy to be the variable most predictive of improvements in patients' functional status [19–26]. For example, in a study of functional status after bypass surgery, self-efficacy explained more variability in functional status outcomes than did measures of disease severity, functional capacity, comorbidity, or preoperative functioning [27]. Additionally, in a study on patients with rheumatoid arthritis, the degree of perceived self-efficacy was correlated with reduced pain and joint inflammation and improved psychosocial functioning [21]. In cancer patients, a strong positive correlation was found between self-efficacy and quality of life and mood [28]. In the prevention area, perceived self-efficacy was shown to play a significant role in smoking cessation relapse rate, control of eating and weight, and adherence to general preventive health programs [29].

Given the strong influence of empowerment and self-efficacy on health outcomes, it is important to incorporate a focus on these concepts when designing systems for patient use. The feeling of empowerment and self-efficacy can be enhanced, for instance, by online support groups where patients are able to connect, communicate, and engage in problem solving with others who have similar medical problems. This has been investigated and demonstrated with several life-changing health conditions, such as breast cancer and HIV/AIDS [12, 30–34]. An important measure of the success of health information systems is how well they promote empowerment and self-efficacy for patients.

10.2.2 Incorporating Patient Preferences

As medical care increasingly focuses on chronic disease, it is especially important that patient preferences regarding the long-term effects of their medical care be taken into account. For patients to be adequately informed to make decisions regarding their medical care, it is important that they obtain information about the quality of life associated with the possible medical outcomes of these decisions. Yet the reliable assessment of a patient's preferences and risk attitudes for clinical outcomes is probably the weakest link in most clinical decision making. Efforts to explore the use of computers in communication about health outcomes, and in assessing patients' preferences for various health outcomes, have addressed these issues [13, 14, 35]. Information on patient preferences is important for tailoring information to patients and for providing decision support [13]. Tailored information has been found to be more effective in providing consumer information [36] and is preferred by patients [37]. In addition to differences in preferences for health outcomes, patients differ in the degree to which they choose to be involved in decision making. Research confirms that age (younger), gender (females), and education level (higher) are strong predictors of the desire to be involved in medical decisions. There is also a higher desire to be involved in medical decisions that appear to require less medical expertise, such as a knee injury, as opposed to a cancerous growth [37].

10.3 Interactive Tools for Patient Decision Support

The number of commercial computer and Web-based products to support patients' health information needs is growing rapidly. The information and decision aids range from general home healthcare reference information to symptom management and diagnostic decision support. There has been a dramatic surge in consumers' use of the Web to acquire health information [8]. Physicians, clinics, hospitals, and insurers are all redefining their business practices to incorporate the Internet and Web delivery systems. The following sections describe the various types of health information and decision support applications available for patients and their families.

10.3.1 Patient Decision Support for Diagnosis

Some of the health portals that offer general reference and drug information also offer interactive tools to assist patients in health assessment, symptom management, and limited diagnostic information (usually in preparation for shared decision making in an office visit). Health risk assessments usually take the form of a questionnaire with questions on family history and health behaviors. After completion, patients receive a tailored report with a summary of results that may help them prioritize their health goals. There are many vendors providing health risk appraisal instruments [38] with most having certification from the National Committee for Quality Assurance [39]. The tailored information identifies an individual's health risk factors and researchers have shown that this information alone may improve health behaviors and outcomes [40]. In some cases, the health risk assessment information may then be linked to a personal health record and shared with one's clinician.

Many health portals on the Web also offer various health screening tools. For example, several sites have depression screening self-assessments using a questionnaire style format (e.g., Web MD's depression test embedded in a page with links to further information on depression) [41]. These types of assessments allow the patient to know when to pursue diagnostic advice from a health care professional and when to seek treatment. Other types of self-assessments include screening for childhood and adult attention disorder [42, 43], Alzheimer's disease [44], eating disorders [45], etc.

Several health portals also offer calculator style tools to help patients manage their health. For example, after entering height and weight, patients can obtain their body mass index. Pregnancy calculations and target heart rate calculations are also amenable to this approach. Websites such as HealthStatus.com{healthstatus.com} additionally offer "calculators" to estimate blood alcohol level, basal metabolic rate, body fat, ideal weight, and recommended calories per day to achieve goal weight.

Occasionally, the health websites will offer diagnostic aids for patients. However, there has been some reluctance to offer advice that is overly specific. The usual approach on the health sites that offer symptom-based diagnosis is to assess a symptom or two and then present a list of possible causes, with links to further reading. As an example, WebMD [46] has an integrated Symptom Checker. The patient first enters a symptom and then selects related factors, such as frequency or "triggered by." Possible causes/diagnoses are then presented to the user with links to associated reading material. The next step for many individuals is to decide when to see a clinician. For symptoms like shortness-of-breath, rectal bleeding, or even cough, the sites will generally offer guidelines on "when to see a doctor," distinguishing between emergency care, making an appointment, or self-care.

10.3.2 Support for Patients' Treatment Decisions

Most of the interactive decision aids that have been developed recently have focused on the patient's role in participating in treatment decisions. As noted above, optimal decisions incorporate not only quality information about the diagnosis and prognosis (areas of a clinician's expertise) but also information on a patient's preferences with regard to the potential health and treatment outcomes. To varying degrees and depending on the condition, the process of shared decision making, whereby the patient and physician jointly contribute background information to generate a treatment decision, becomes an important element of health care management. The Robert Wood Johnson Foundation report on Shared Decision-Making and Benefit Design [47] points out that eight out of ten adults over the age of 40 make health decisions on a regular basis. This includes surgical decisions, whether to have screening tests, or what medication to take. Yet many patients report a lack of involvement in these decisions. Conditions such as breast cancer, early stage prostate cancer, and chronic stable angina are examples of situations where various treatment options are available, including "watchful waiting", but also where the decision on treatment choice is sensitive to patient values and preferences. Researchers have found that when patients discuss preferences with their physicians, they are more likely to get the care they want [48], and that patients who are more engaged in their health and health care have better outcomes [49]. The Cochrane Review led by Stacey et al. looked at the effectiveness of decision aids for patients' treatment decisions [49]. They found that these tools improved patients' knowledge about their treatment options and reduced decisional conflict related to feeling uninformed or unclear about their preferences and values. They also found moderate quality evidence that the decision aids promoted patients to take a more active role in decision making and have a better understanding of risk.

Many of these treatment decision aids can be found on health portals, such as WebMD.com or MayoClinic.org. The Agency for Health Care Research and Quality offers shareable decision aids [50] for a limited number of diseases and conditions.

The guides consist of background material on the condition, how the condition is diagnosed, treatment options with thorough descriptions, and the pros and cons of each option. The background material is supplemented with video clips on the Web. The goal of this approach is not to provide the patient with a diagnosis or specific recommendation, but to prepare the patient to be an informed participant in making treatment decisions during the next visit to the clinician. Their tools often offer supplementary video education and patient testimonials, as well as questionnaires with printable results that reflect the patient's submitted values, questions and concerns. These can then be taken to an office visit with a clinician in preparation for shared decision making regarding a test or treatment.

The largest selection of links to patient treatment decision aids (at least 300) can be found at the Ottawa Hospital Research Institute (OHRI) Web page on decision aids for patients [51]. Most of the decision tools are produced and maintained by Healthwise, Inc. [52], which then serves as a provider of content for Web-based health portals, such as WebMD.com [53]. These decision aids typically list the relevant treatment options, provide background information, and describe the various risks, benefits, and why a doctor might recommend a particular treatment or procedure versus "watchful waiting". Although available online, they are typically paper based and printable for the patient to take to a clinic visit. A key contribution with these is that the probability of success or risk associated with treatment is displayed in a graphical format for the patient. Assistance with understanding side effects and a method for describing patient values (using a scale from Not Important to Very Important) is provided.

Researchers associated with the International Patient Decision Aids Standards (IPDAS) Collaboration have created a framework [52, 53] for evaluating each of the identified patient decision aids on the OHRI website [51]. They classify the decision aids according to health condition, options available, appropriate audience, developer, year of last update/review, format, language, and provide a link to the source. They then evaluate each decision aid on 11 content criteria, 9 development process criteria and 2 effectiveness criteria. Table 10.1 summarizes the guidelines and evaluation criteria they developed using a two-stage Web-based Delphi process.

The goal of having a process to define the quality of decision aids for patients is to influence developers in creating more usable and effective tools for patients and to help providers and patients in finding, selecting, and using the best tools available to support shared decision making.

10.3.3 Other Areas of Decision Support for Patients

In addition to decision support tools for health risk appraisal, diagnosis, screening tests and treatment decisions, support is required for many areas of patient self-management and decision support in the home environment. Self-management is important for a number of chronic conditions, including diabetes, heart failure, and

Table 10.1 Criteria developed by the International Patient Decision Aids Standards Collaboration to judge the quality of patient decision aids [54, 55]

Information	Health condition
	Decision
	Options
	Potential benefits
	Potential harms
Probabilities	Potential outcomes – general
	Potential outcomes – subpopulation
	Ability to compare (e.g., same denominator)
	Multiple ways to view probabilities (e.g., words and diagram)
Test interpretation	If test, description of false positive and false negative
	Estimated chances of false positive and false negative
Values	Description of potential outcomes (positive and negative)
	Method to clarify and state personal values for outcomes
Guidance	How to make the decision
	Topics to discuss with a clinician
Development	Needs assessment with patients and professionals
	Reviewed by patients and professionals
	Field tested with patients and professionals
Evidence	Description of evidence from previous research
	Description of quality of evidence
Disclosure	Author/developers' credentials and affiliation
Plain language	Report of readability level from standard scale
Evaluation	Demonstrate improvement in patient's knowledge
	Correspondence between patient values and treatment choice

asthma. These conditions require vigilant monitoring and self-care on the part of patients and/or family members. For example, patients with diabetes must monitor blood glucose levels on a regular basis, as well as manage diet and exercise. For patients with heart failure, it is important to monitor weight and symptoms of shortness of breath or fatigue, along with careful medication management. Patients with asthma must also regulate medications with symptoms and environmental triggers. Especially for newly diagnosed patients, these care regimens can be quite daunting. There are many forms of technology support for patients with chronic conditions, ranging from mobile phone applications directly available to a patient to sophisticated disease management interventions delivered by a clinic or health insurer.

Monitoring technologies include a variety of blood glucose meters, wireless weight scales, peak flow meters for asthma, wireless blood pressure cuffs, bed sensors to measure sleep quality, wireless ECG leads for heart rate, heart rate variability, and arrhythmia monitoring, as well as the new wrist-worn devices with accelerometers (activity), and measures of electrodermal activity (stress), and heart rate. Disease management systems typically share the data both with the patient and with a nurse care manager at a remote facility who can then respond to system generated alerts (e.g., to change the diuretic medication dose for a patient who retained too much water weight in the past 3 days).

With the recent increase in popularity of wearable sensors and coaching technologies, many patients and consumers interested in wellness interventions are directly purchasing sensors and services to promote health behavior change. Many of the devices with accelerometers and heart rate detectors offer real time and summary feedback on activity levels and sleep. Many have accompanying goal setting modules and feedback to encourage users to achieve their health behavior change goals.

In some cases, decision support and advice on care management solutions comes from other patients who have similar conditions. There are a variety of online support groups or discussion boards available for nearly every disease imaginable. Some are formally organized through a health delivery system, such as Kaiser Permanente [56]. Others are accessible through health portals, such as WebMD [53]. Quite often, with chronic conditions where most of the health care actually happens in the home and environment and is related to self-care, patients become the experts in how best to manage and implement care plans. Sites such as WebMD [53] have also found it useful to have a separate section with information for newly diagnosed patients. More detailed information on specific diseases or conditions is often available from societies or groups specializing in a topic. Online medical dictionaries, disease-specific discussion boards, and "ask-an-expert" services are also often found as components of health portal sites. The vast array of health resources available to patients' mobile phone applications and on the Web that provide support in care management also include tools to educate patients about their medications, such as RxList [57], DrugInfoNet [58], and RxMed [59]. Systems available on websites such as Drugs.com [60] can be used to detect drug-drug interactions, similar to systems used in hospitals and clinics, but using pictures and lay language.

10.4 Usability of Patient Decision Support Tools

One of the most important factors in the success of patient decision aids has to do with the usability of the interface and method in which the information is conveyed. General guidelines for developing useable and meaningful decision support for patients are listed below:

10.4.1 Intuitive Interface

- Graphical metaphors easily understood by the general populace
- Designed for use by naïve, untrained users

- Online help available at every stage
- Immediate word definitions available in every application

10.4.2 Complete Coverage/Coordination

- Single location for information on disease and health concerns
- Coordinated with routine medical care

10.4.3 Hierarchical Presentation

- Simple summary information presented first
- More detail and complexity available as desired
- Guided movement through databases
- User requests anticipated, pre-searched to improved speed

10.4.4 Presentation of Materials Tailored to the Individual

- Appropriate for the assessed reading level
- Appropriate for education and medical expertise
- Culturally sensitive
- In the appropriate language
- Tailored to history and assessed patient-specific health risks
- Patient preferences incorporated

10.4.5 Facilitate Quality Decision Making

- Health outcomes information included
- Patient preferences on health outcomes incorporated
- Summary of tailored decision support information

These guidelines are important for the developers of decision aids, as well as for patients and providers as they choose systems to use or recommend to others.

10.5 Helping Patients Judge the Quality of Health Information

Judging the quality of health materials on the Web or as part of decision tools is particularly challenging for patients/consumers. Not all sites are "peer reviewed," published, or created by professionals with expertise in the covered topics. Because the quality of health information is so critical for consumers, several organizations have created guidelines for judging the quality of information on the Web for consumers [61–63]. Some of the criteria included in all of these guidelines are topical relevance, currency of the information, accuracy, and authoritativeness or objectivity.

From the consumer's point of view, topical relevance is certainly important when assessing the usefulness and quality of a website or computer application. The relevance of a site is context-specific and depends on the particular question an individual consumer has in mind. To find appropriate materials, sites must be clearly organized and/or have intelligent search functions. In addition, the relevance of the material depends on the degree to which it is tailored to the individual and is appropriate to their specific needs. Most health material on the Web is generic and not interactively tailored to individuals, basically replicating what could be found in a textbook or brochure. The final aspect of relevance to an individual has to do with whether the material is action-oriented and either helps the consumer make a healthcare decision that may lead to an action or promotes health behavior change.

The currency or timeliness of information is an important consideration. It is often difficult to have a generalized policy on how often health materials need to be updated. However, most professional sites ensure at least quarterly review of all materials. Consumers may judge the currency of website information by looking for date stamps or a notice of date of creation and/or update. It is important to note that some websites use algorithms to automatically update their time stamp even if the material has not been changed or even reviewed, giving the impression that the information is current. Responding to the difficulty that consumers are likely to have in judging these aspects of website quality, the Health on the Net (HON) Foundation [63] has promoted an ethical code of conduct and a set of standards for website developers to ensure the reliability of medical and health information available on the Internet. Consumer health sites that display an HON certificate signify that they are in compliance with the HON code of conduct and standards. Providing health information and interventions over the Internet is becoming an increasingly important component of health care. Ensuring that the materials are unbiased, accurate, relevant, and timely is fundamental to providing quality health care.

10.6 Patient Access, Literacy and Numeracy

As the demand for more health information and decision support grows, the need for wider availability of these systems becomes even more important. Today, these systems can be found in a variety of settings and forms. In addition to consumers searching the Web at home, public access computer systems can be found in public libraries, health resource centers, worksites, schools, and community centers. Different systems may require quite different physical locations. For instance, many patients are uncomfortable exploring sensitive health information in a public space.

There are many factors that influence the health information seeking behavior of patients. As documented by several researchers, these factors include demographic divisions such as age, gender, disability, race and ethnicity, and socioeconomic status [64–68]. Research indicates that these demographic variables can predict differences in the amount and type of health information that patients want. Whereas some patients may not seek much information, for many of those who desire information, serious barriers to the use of these systems still exist.

A lack of reading ability is a functional barrier affecting use of computer systems. According to the U.S. Department of Education's National Institute of Literacy's 2015 survey [69], 32 million adults in the U.S. are unable to read – 14 % of the population. Surprisingly, 21 % of adults in the U.S. read below a fifth grade level and 19 % of high school graduates are unable to read. Most studies on the comprehension of health education handouts typically show that only half of the patients are able to comprehend written health materials [70–72]. Studies confirmed that patients' reading levels were well below what was needed to understand standard health brochures [73]. In developing health information for patients, one cannot assume that a patient who has completed a certain grade level in school can read at the corresponding level. Numerous studies on literacy and readability confirm the widespread problem of low literacy skills [74–76]. Health materials should be written at least three grade levels lower than the average educational level of the target population [77]. Text characteristics also play an important role in comprehension and retention of material. Organization and clarity need to be considered in creating educational materials [78]. Computers with multimedia capabilities can correct some of these problems by conveying information through video, audio and graphics that would normally be presented as written text. These systems can also be adapted for multiple foreign languages.

In addition to language and literacy issues, an area that is often overlooked relates to the cultural issues associated with health information-seeking behavior and the willingness to use computers to access health information. Most developers have not invested the time to develop systems that are culturally and linguistically relevant to diverse populations. Finally, the question of who will pay for the access and use of technologies for consumer health information is still an unresolved issue. Educational and socioeconomic factors still determine access to computers and information technologies. Younger, wealthier, and well-educated patients are more likely to have access to home computers, diagnostic software, and Internet services.

The poor and socioeconomically disadvantaged already have worse health outcomes and worse access to medical care. Special effort is required to ensure ease of access and ease of use of health information systems so as to not further disadvantage the very people who have the greatest need for these resources.

10.7 The Future of Decision Support Systems for Patients

Advances in communications, sensors, data analytics and information processing technology are changing the way in which medicine is practiced, with dramatic impact on how patients are beginning to receive their health information and interact with the medical care system. There has also been a shift toward consumers becoming empowered participants and assuming a more active role in their medical care decisions through increased and more effective access to healthcare information and decision tools. The developers of computer applications for patients have pushed the field of consumer health informatics forward with many innovative systems.

However, to achieve significant improvements in the quality of care and health outcomes, researchers and system developers need to focus on bringing the knowledge gained from previous work in health education and behavior change into the design of new systems. This is a rapidly developing field, with significant innovations in the commercial sector, but research in several areas is still needed to move the field forward in providing real benefits to patients' health outcomes and in showing the effectiveness of the systems to purchasers of health care. The criteria for evaluating computer-based decision support systems for patients are similar to the criteria for physician systems, namely accuracy and effectiveness [79]. However, the rapid deployment of these systems in an ever changing medical care environment makes critical evaluation of consumer health information systems extremely difficult. Websites and smart phone applications change daily, and access to one system usually means increased access to many others. It is important to understand the potential effectiveness of investments in this area. Careful needs assessment before system development, usability testing during development, clinical trials, and studies of use and outcomes in natural settings are all critical to our understanding of how to best provide health information and decision assistance to patients.

References

1. Eysenbach G. Consumer health informatics. BMJ. 2000;320(7251):1713–6.
2. Brody DS, Miller SM, Lerman CE, Smith DG, Caputo GC. Patient perception of involvement in medical care: relationship to illness attitudes and outcomes. J Gen Intern Med. 1989;4(6):506–11.
3. Greenfield S, Kaplan S, Ware Jr JE. Expanding patient involvement in care. Effects on patient outcomes. Ann Intern Med. 1985;102(4):520–8.

4. Korsch BM. What do patients and parents want to know? What do they need to know? Pediatrics. 1984;74(5 Pt 2):917–9.
5. Mahler HI, Kulik JA. Preferences for health care involvement, perceived control and surgical recovery: a prospective study. Soc Sci Med. 1990;31(7):743–51.
6. Ende J, Kazis L, Ash A, Moskowitz MA. Measuring patients' desire for autonomy: decision making and information-seeking preferences among medical patients. J Gen Intern Med. 1989;4(1):23–30.
7. Waitzkin H. Doctor-patient communication. Clinical implications of social scientific research. JAMA. 1984;252(17):2441–6.
8. Fox S, Duggan M. Health online 2013. In: Pew Research Center's Internet & American Life Project. 2013. Pew Research Center.
9. Cordasco KM. Obtaining informed consent from patients: brief update review, in making health care safer II: an updated critical analysis of the evidence for patient safety practices. Rockville: Agency for Healthcare Research and Quality (US); 2013.
10. Jimison HB, Sher PP, Appleyard R, LeVernois Y. The use of multimedia in the informed consent process. J Am Med Inform Assoc. 1998;5(3):245–56.
11. Murray E. Web-based interventions for behavior change and self-management: potential, pitfalls, and progress. Medicine 20. 2012;1(2):e3.
12. Gustafson DH. The use and impact of a computer-based support system for people living with AIDS and HIV infection. Proc Annu Symp Comput Appl Med Care. 1994;604–8.
13. Jimison HB, Henrion M. Hierarchical preference models for patients with chronic disease. Med Decis Making. 1992;7:351.
14. Goldstein MK, Clarke AE, Michelson D, Garber AM, Bergen MR, Lenert LA. Developing and testing a multimedia presentation of a health-state description. Med Decis Making. 1994;14(4):336–44.
15. Krebs P, Prochaska JO, Rossi JS. A meta-analysis of computer-tailored interventions for health behavior change. Prev Med. 2010;51(3–4):214–21.
16. Peterson C, Stunkard AJ. Personal control and health promotion. Soc Sci Med. 1989;28(8):819–28.
17. Cassileth BR, Zupkis RV, Sutton-Smith K, March V. Information and participation preferences among cancer patients. Ann Intern Med. 1980;92(6):832–6.
18. Israel BA, Sherman SJ. Social support, control and the stress process. In: Glanz K, Lewis FM, Rimer BK, editors. Health behavior and health education: theory, research and practice. San Francisco: Jossey-Bass; 1990.
19. Mullen PD, Laville EA, Biddle AK, Lorig KR. Efficacy of psychoeducational interventions on pain, depression, and disability in people with arthritis: a meta-analysis. J Rheumatol Suppl. 1987;14 Suppl 15:33–9.
20. Maibach E, Flora J, Nass C. Changes in self-efficacy and health behavior in response to a minimal contact community health campaign. Health Commun. 1991;3:1–15.
21. Lorig K, Chastain RL, Ung E, Shoor S, Holman HR. Development and evaluation of a scale to measure perceived self-efficacy in people with arthritis. Arthritis Rheum. 1989;32(1):37–44.
22. Holman H, Lorig K. Patient education in the rheumatic diseases – pros and cons. Bull Rheum Dis. 1987;37(5):1–8.
23. Bandura A. Self-efficacy: toward a unifying theory of behavioral change. Psychol Rev. 1977;84(2):191–215.
24. O'Leary A, Shoor S, Lorig K, Holman HR. A cognitive-behavioral treatment for rheumatoid arthritis. Health Psychol. 1988;7(6):527–44.
25. Feste C, Anderson RM. Empowerment: from philosophy to practice. Patient Educ Couns. 1995;26(1–3):139–44.
26. Anderson RM, Funnell MM, Butler PM, Arnold MS, Fitzgerald JT, Feste CC. Patient empowerment. Results of a randomized controlled trial. Diabetes Care. 1995;18(7):943–9.
27. Allen JK, Becker DM, Swank RT. Factors related to functional status after coronary artery bypass surgery. Heart Lung. 1990;19(4):337–43.

28. Cunningham AJ, Lockwood GA, Cunningham JA. A relationship between perceived self-efficacy and quality of life in cancer patients. Patient Educ Couns. 1991;17(1):71–8.
29. O'Leary A. Self-efficacy and health. Behav Res Ther. 1985;23(4):437–51.
30. Gustafson DH, Bosworth K, Hawkins RP, Boberg EW, Bricker E. CHESS: a computer-based system for providing information, referrals, decision support and social support to people facing medical and other health-related crises. Proc Annu Symp Comput Appl Med Care. 1992;161–5.
31. Pingree S, Hawkins RP, Gustafson DH, Boberg EW, Bricker E, Wise M, Tillotson T. Will HIV-positive people use an interactive computer system for information and support? A study of CHESS in two communities. Proc Annu Symp Comput Appl Med Care. 1993;22–6.
32. Mo PKH, Coulson NS. Empowering processes in online support groups among people living with HIV/AIDS: a comparative analysis of 'lurkers' and 'posters'. Comput Hum Behav. 2010;26(5):1183–93.
33. van Uden-Kraan CF, Drossaert CHC, Taal E, Shaw BR, Seydel ER, van de Laar MAFJ. Empowering processes and outcomes of participation in online support groups for patients with breast cancer, arthritis, or fibromyalgia. Qual Health Res. 2008;18(3):405–17.
34. van Uden-Kraan CF, Drossaert CH, Taal E, Seydel ER, van de Laar MA. Participation in online patient support groups endorses patients' empowerment. Patient Educ Couns. 2009;74(1):61–9. doi:10.1016/j.pec.2008.07.044.
35. Lenert LA, Sturley A, Watson ME. iMPACT3: internet-based development and administration of utility elicitation protocols. Med Decis Making. 2002;22(6):464–74.
36. Skinner CS, Strecher VJ, Hospers H. Physicians' recommendations for mammography: do tailored messages make a difference? Am J Public Health. 1994;84(1):43–9.
37. Thompson SC, Pitts JS, Schwankovsky L. Preferences for involvement in medical decision-making: situational and demographic influences. Patient Educ Couns. 1993;22(3):133–40.
38. Alexander G. Health risk appraisal. Int Electron J Health Educ. 2000;3(Special):133–7.
39. NCQA. Wellness and health promotion report card. 2009. Accessed 11/3/2015. Available from: http://reportcard.ncqa.org/WHP/External/.
40. Ozminkowski RJ, Goetzel RZ, Wang F, Gibson TB, Musich S, Bender J, Edington DW. The savings gained from participation in health promotion programs for medicare beneficiaries. J Occup Environ Med. 2006;48(11):1125–32.
41. WebMD. Depression assessment. Available from: http://www.webmd.com/depression/depression-assessment/. Accessed 12 Mar 2015.
42. Adult Attention Deficit Disorder Center of Maryland. Online screening test. Available from: http://www.addadult.com/getting-help/for-you/online-screening-test/. Accessed 11 Jan 2015.
43. Psych Central. Attention deficit disorder (ADD/ADHD) test. Available from: http://psychcentral.com/quizzes/addquiz.htm. Accessed 12 Mar 2015.
44. Alzheimer's Association. Tests for Alzheimer's disease and dementia. 2015 11/1/2015]; Available from: http://www.alz.org/alzheimers_disease_steps_to_diagnosis.asp. Accessed 12 Mar 2015.
45. National Eating Disorders Association. Online eating disorder screening. 11/1/2015. Available from: http://www.nationaleatingdisorders.org/online-eating-disorder-screening.
46. WebMD. WebMD symptom checker. 11/3/2015. Available from: http://symptoms.webmd.com/.
47. American Institutes for Research. Shared decision-making and benefit design. Princeton: Robert Wood Johnson Foundation; 2013. Available from: http://www.rwjf.org/en/library/research/2013/04/shared-decision-making-and-benefit-design.html. Accessed 12/3/2015.
48. AGS Choosing Wisely Workgroup. American Geriatrics Society identifies five things that healthcare providers and patients should question. J Am Geriatr Soc. 2013;61(4):622–31.
49. Stacey D, Bennett CL, Barry MJ, Col NF, Eden KB, Holmes-Rovner M, Llewellyn-Thomas H, Lyddiatt A, Légaré F, Thomson R. Decision aids for people facing health treatment or screening decisions. Cochrane Database Syst Rev. 2011;10:CD001431.

50. Agency for Healthcare Research and Quality. Effective health care program: patient decision aids. Available from: http://effectivehealthcare.ahrq.gov/index.cfm/tools-and-resources/patient-decision-aids/. Accessed 12 Mar 2015.
51. Ottawa Hospital Research Institute. Patient decision aids. 6/22/2015 11/1/2015. Available from: https://decisionaid.ohri.ca/azlist.html.
52. Healthwise. Boost shared decision making. 11/1/2015. Available from: http://www.healthwise.org/products/decisionaids.aspx.
53. WebMD. 11/3/2015. Available from: www.webmd.com.
54. Elwyn G, O'Connor A, Stacey D, Volk R, Edwards A, Coulter A, Thomson R, Barratt A, Barry M, Bernstein S, Butow P, Clarke A, Entwistle V, Feldman-Stewart D, Holmes-Rovener M, Llewellyn-Thomas H, Moumjid N, Mulley A, Ruland C, Sepucha K, Sykes A, Whelan T. Developing a quality criteria framework for patient decision aids: online international Delphi consensus process. BMJ. 2006;333(7565):417.
55. Joseph-Williams N, Newcombe R, Politi M, Durand MA, Sivell S, Stacey D, O'Connor A, Volk RJ, Edwards A, Bennett C, Pignone M, Thomson R, Elwyn G. Toward minimum standards for certifying patient decision aids: a modified Delphi consensus process. Med Decis Making. 2013;34(6):699–710.
56. Kaiser Permanente. Programs & classes. 11/1/2015. Available from: https://healthy.kaiserpermanente.org/health/care/consumer/health-wellness/programs-classes.
57. Rx List The Internet Drug Index. 11/3/2015. Available from: http://www.rxlist.com.
58. DrugInfoNet.com. 11/3/2015. Available from: http://www.DrugInfoNet.com.
59. Rx Med. 11/3/2015. Available from: http://www.rxmed.com.
60. Drugs.com. 11/3/2015. Available from: http://www.drugs.com/drug_interactions.html.
61. DISCERN Online. Quality criteria for consumer health information. 9/17/15. Available from: http://www.discern.org.uk/.
62. Agency for Healthcare Research and Quality. Assessing the quality of internet health information. 2014 Dec 2014 11/3/2015. Available from: http://www.ahrq.gov/research/data/infoqual.html.
63. Health on the Net Foundation. Health on the Net Foundation Code of Conduct (HONcode) for medical and health web sites. 8/25/14 9/17/15. Available from: http://www.hon.ch/HONcode/.
64. Cline RJW, Haynes KM. Consumer health information seeking on the internet: the state of the art. Health Educ Res. 2001;16(6):671–92. doi:10.1093/her/16.6.671.
65. Harris RM, Wathen CN, Fear JM. Searching for health information in rural Canada. Where do residents look for health information and what do they do when they find it? Inf Res, 2006:12(1) paper 274. Available at http://InformationR.net/ir/12-1/paper274.html.
66. European Centre for Disease Prevention and Control. TECHNICAL REPORT. A literature review on health information-seeking behaviour on the web: a health consumer and health professional perspective: insights into health communication. Available at: http://ecdc.europa.eu/en/publications/Publications/Literature%20review%20on%20health%20information-seeking%20behaviour%20on%20the%20web.pdf.
67. Jimison HB, Sher PP. Presenting clinical and consumer data to patients. In: Chapman GB, Sonnenberg FA, editors. Decision making in health care: theory, psychology, and applications. New York: Cambridge University Press; 2000.
68. Jimison H, Gorman P, Woods S, Nygren P, Walker M, Norris S, Hersh W. Barriers and drivers of health information technology use for the elderly, chronically Ill, and underserved. Evidence Report/Technology Assessment No. 175 (Prepared by the Oregon Evidence-based Practice Center under Contract No. 290-02-0024). AHRQ Publication No. 09-E004. Rockville: Agency for Healthcare Research and Quality. Nov 2008.
69. Statistics Brain Research Institute. Illiteracy statistics. How many American adults can't read? Statistics on adult illiteracy rates in the U.S.? What percent of U.S. adults can't read? [cited 11/3/2015; Available from: http://www.statisticbrain.com/number-of-american-adults-who-cant-read/.

70. Davis TC, Crouch MA, Wills G, Miller S, Abdehou DM. The gap between patient reading comprehension and the readability of patient education materials. J Fam Pract. 1990;31(5):533–8.
71. Doak CC, Doak LG, Root IH. Teaching patients with low literacy skills. Philadelphia: J. B. Lippincott; 1985.
72. Holt GA, Hollon JD, Hughes SE, Coyle R. OTC labels: can consumers read and understand them? Am Pharm. 1990;NS30(11):51–4.
73. Davis TC, Mayeaux EJ, Fredrickson D, Bocchini Jr JA, Jackson RH, Murphy PW. Reading ability of parents compared with reading level of pediatric patient education materials. Pediatrics. 1994;93(3):460–8.
74. Petterson T. How readable are the hospital information leaflets available to elderly patients? Age Ageing. 1994;23(1):14–6.
75. Morgan PP. Illiteracy can have major impact on patients' understanding of health care information. CMAJ. 1993;148(7):1196–7.
76. Feldman SR, Quinlivan A, Williford P, Bahnson JL, Fleischer Jr AB. Illiteracy and the readability of patient education materials. A look at Health Watch. N C Med J. 1994;55(7):290–2.
77. Jubelirer SJ, Linton JC, Magnetti SM. Reading versus comprehension: implications for patient education and consent in an outpatient oncology clinic. J Cancer Educ. 1994;9(1):26–9.
78. Reid JC, Klachko DM, Kardash CA, Roinson RD, Scholes R, Howard D. Why people don't learn from diabetes literature: influence of text and reader characteristics. Patient Educ Couns. 1995;25(1):31–8.
79. Berner ES, Webster GD, Shugerman AA, Jackson JR, Algina J, Baker AL, Ball EV, Cobbs CG, Dennis VW, Frenkel EP, et al. Performance of four computer-based diagnostic systems. N Engl J Med. 1994;330(25):1792–6.

Chapter 11
Diagnostic Decision Support Systems

Randolph A. Miller

Abstract Since primeval times, mankind has attempted to explain natural phenomena using models. For the past five decades, a new kind of modeler, the healthcare informatician, has developed and proliferated a new kind of model, the clinical Diagnostic Decision Support System (DDSS). This chapter presents a definition of clinical diagnosis and of DDSS; a discussion of how humans accomplish diagnosis; a survey of previous attempts to develop computer-based clinical diagnostic tools; a discussion of the problems encountered in developing, implementing, evaluating, and maintaining clinical diagnostic decision support systems; and a discussion of current and future systems.

Keywords Diagnostic decision support • Diagnosis • Human reasoning • Evaluation • Decision support system development

Since primeval times, mankind has attempted to explain natural phenomena using models. For the past five decades, a new kind of modeler, the healthcare informatician, has developed and proliferated a new kind of model, the clinical Diagnostic Decision Support System (DDSS). Modeling was historically, and still remains, an inexact science. Ptolemy, in the Almagest, placed the earth at the center of the universe and still could explain why the sun would rise in the east each morning. Newton's nonrelativistic formulation of the laws of mechanics works well for earth-bound engineering applications. Yet mankind, using imperfect models, has built machines that fly, and has cured many diseases. Past and present DDSS incorporate

Portions of this chapter have been taken verbatim, with permission of the American Medical Informatics Association (AMIA), which owns the copyrights, from: Miller RA, Medical Diagnostic Decision Support Systems—Past, Present, and Future: A Threaded Bibliography and Commentary. J Am Med Inform Assoc 1994;1:8–27; and from Miller RA, Evaluating Evaluations of Medical Diagnostic Systems, J Am Medical Inform Assoc 1996;3:429–431. Dr. Miller acknowledges the earlier contributions of Antoine Geissbuhler, MD, of the Hospital of the University of Geneva, Switzerland, who co-authored a previous version of this chapter. The author thanks Joyce Green for her assistance with copy editing.

R.A. Miller, M.D. (✉)
Department of Biomedical Informatics, Vanderbilt University Medical Center, 2525 West End Avenue, Ste 1475, Nashville, TN 37203, USA
e-mail: randolph.a.miller@vanderbilt.edu

E.S. Berner (ed.), *Clinical Decision Support Systems*, Health Informatics,
DOI 10.1007/978-3-319-31913-1_11

inexact models of the incompletely understood and exceptionally complex process of clinical diagnosis. Because DDSS augment the natural capabilities of human diagnosticians, they have the potential to be employed productively [1].

This chapter presents a definition of clinical diagnosis and of DDSS; a discussion of how humans accomplish diagnosis; a survey of previous attempts to develop computer-based clinical diagnostic tools; a discussion of the problems encountered in developing, implementing, evaluating, and maintaining clinical diagnostic decision support systems; and a discussion of current and future systems.

11.1 Definitions of Diagnosis

To understand the history of clinical diagnostic decision support systems and envision their future roles, one must first define clinical diagnosis and computer-assisted clinical diagnosis. A simple definition of diagnosis is: [2]

> *the placing of an interpretive, higher level label on a set of raw, more primitive observations* [Definition 1].

By this definition one form of diagnosis might consist of labeling as "abnormal" any laboratory test results falling outside 1.5 times the 95 % confidence intervals for the "normal" values seen in the general population as measured by that laboratory. Another level of diagnosis under the same definition might consist of labeling the combination of a low serum bicarbonate level, a high serum chloride level, and an arterial blood pH of 7.3 as "metabolic acidosis." A more involved definition of diagnosis, specific for clinical diagnosis, is: [2]

> *a mapping from a patient's data (normal and abnormal history, physical examination, and laboratory data) to a nosology of disease states* [Definition 2].

Both of these definitions treat diagnosis improperly as a single event, rather than as a process. A more accurate definition appeared in the Random House Collegiate Dictionary: [3]

> *the process of determining by examination the nature and circumstances of a diseased condition* [Definition 3].

Skilled diagnosticians develop an understanding of what the patient's life situation was like before the illness began, how the illness has manifested itself, and how it has affected the life situation [2]. The clinician must also determine the patient's understanding of, and response to, an illness. The process of diagnosis entails a sequence of interdependent, often highly individualized tasks: evoking the patient's initial history and physical examination findings; integration of the data into plausible scenarios regarding known disease processes; evaluating and refining diagnostic hypotheses through selective elicitation of additional patient information, such as laboratory tests or serial examinations; initiating therapy at appropriate points in time (including before a diagnosis is established); and evaluating the effect of both the illness and the therapy, on the patient, over time [2].

Diagnosis is a process composed of individual steps. These steps go from a point of origin (a question and a set of "presenting findings" and "previously established diagnoses"), to a point of destination (an answer, usually consisting of a set of "new established diagnoses" and/or "unresolved differential diagnoses"). While the beginning and end points may be identical, the steps one diagnostician follows may be very different from those taken by another diagnostician, and the same diagnostician may take different steps in two nearly identical cases. Because expertise varies among clinicians, different individuals will encounter different diagnostic problems in evaluating the same patient. For instance, they may experience dissimilar difficulties at disparate steps in the diagnostic process, even if they follow exactly the same steps.

Studies of clinicians' information needs help us to understand the variability in diagnostic problem solving among clinicians. Osheroff and colleagues [4, 5] used participant observation, a standard anthropological technique, to identify and classify information needs during the practice of medicine in an academic health center. They identified three components of "comprehensive information needs:" (1) currently satisfied information needs (information recognized as relevant to a question and already known to the clinician); (2) consciously recognized information needs (information recognized by the clinician as important to know to solve the problem, but which is not known by the clinician); and (3) unrecognized information needs (information that is important for the clinician to know to solve a problem at hand, but is not recognized as being important by the clinician). Failure to detect a diagnostic problem at all would fall into the latter category. Different clinicians will experience different diagnostic problems within the same patient case, based on each clinician's varying knowledge of the patient and unique personal store of general medical knowledge. Osheroff et al. noted the difficulty people and machines have in tailoring general medical knowledge to specific clinical cases. There may be a wealth of information in a patient's inpatient and outpatient records, and also a large medical literature describing causes of the patient's problems. The challenge is to quickly and efficiently reconcile one body of information with the other [1, 4].

A DDSS can potentially facilitate that reconciliation. A DDSS can be defined as:

> *a computer-based algorithm that assists a clinician with one or more component steps of the diagnostic process* [Definition 4].

While individual clinicians attach different meanings to "diagnosis", users of DDSS are often slow to recognize that each system functionally defines diagnosis as the set of tasks that the DDSS can perform. Experienced users employ DDSS as tools to supplement, rather than replace, their own diagnostic capabilities. Naive users view diagnosis on their own terms, based on their own experiences, and expect DDSS to behave in accordance with their assumptions. Untrained DDSS users' unrealistic, preconceived expectations can engender subsequent frustrations. For example, a DDSS cannot solve a vague problem with minimal input; nor is a DDSS likely to help in understanding how an illness has affected a patient's lifestyle. Conversely, system developers sometimes create useful diagnostic tools that provide capabilities outside the experience of everyday clinical practice. For example, the relationships function of R-QMR[1] (a DDSS), takes, as input, up to ten findings that the clinician-user would like to explain as the key or "pivotal" findings from a diagnostically challenging case, and produces, as output, a rank-ordered list of "disease complexes" that each explain all of the input findings [7]. Each disease complex is made up of from one to four interrelated disorders (e.g., disease A predisposing to disease B and causing disease C). Because busy clinicians can spare little free time for extraneous activities, user training for DDSS utilization is extremely critical and must address the potential cognitive mismatch between user expectations and system capabilities.

That the problem to be solved originates in the mind of the clinician-user is conceptually critical for DDSS development, implementation, and evaluation. The diagnostic problem cannot be defined in an absolute sense, for example, by presenting an arbitrary set of input findings selected from a case—i.e., if clinical findings are extracted from a patient case in the absence of a query from a clinician caring for the patient, do those findings comprise a diagnostic problem to be solved? In only one situation can the findings of a case, in isolation, define a diagnostic problem: when the diagnostic problem is the global one. In the global problem, the DDSS, through its own initiative, takes all the steps in the diagnostic process required to explain all patient findings, by "concluding" new diagnoses (or listing unresolved differential diagnoses if no solution exists). Practicing clinicians rarely encounter the "global" diagnostic problem. Healthcare providers usually complete a portion of the diagnostic evaluation process before they encounter difficulty in making a diagnosis, and, correspondingly, once they overcome the difficulty (e.g., by consulting a colleague), they are usually capable of completing the evaluation without further assistance. While early DDSS developers often assumed the only problem worth solving was the global diagnostic problem, emphasis over the last decades has shifted to helping clinicians with problems they encounter during individual steps in the diagnostic process. This has led to the demise of the "Greek Oracle" model, wherein the DDSS was expected to take all of the patient's findings and come up with "the answer"[8]. Current DDSS models assume that the user will interact with the DDSS in an iterative fashion, selectively entering patient information and using the DDSS output to assist with the problems that the user has encountered in the diagnostic process [9].

To interact optimally with a DDSS, users must understand assumptions built into the system. Each DDSS functionally defines diagnosis as the tasks it can perform (or assist users in performing). The subtle nature of underlying assumptions incorporated into DDSS can be deceptive. As an example, one of the most well-known diagnostic systems is the Bayesian program for diagnosis of acute abdomi-

[1] In this chapter, R-QMR refers to the noncommercial, research version of QMR, the DDSS developed by Miller et al. [6]. The commercial version of QMR, previously marketed by First DataBank, while initially identical to R-QMR in 1990, was developed independently of R-QMR after that time. The commercial version of QMR is no longer marketed. Since 2014 Miller and colleagues at Vanderbilt have been developing a third-generation non-commercial successor system, "AskVanderbilt".

nal pain developed by de Dombal and colleagues [10, 11]. The system's original goal, not stated explicitly, was to discriminate among surgical and nonsurgical causes of acute abdominal pain in an emergency room (or similar) setting. The system supported a limited number of explicit diagnoses; all except "nonspecific abdominal pain," were potentially surgical conditions (such as acute appendicitis, acute pancreatitis, and acute diverticulitis). The performance of the system was evaluated in multicenter studies [11] and shown to be exemplary with respect to the circumstances for which it was designed. Nevertheless, de Dombal's system would most likely disappoint naive users relying on it to diagnose patients presenting with acute abdominal pain in more general settings. The system could not properly diagnose patients presenting with acute intermittent porphyria, lead poisoning, early T10 dermatome herpes zoster, or familial Mediterranean fever. The system would correctly label those conditions as "nonspecific abdominal pain," even though some are potentially life threatening and treatable. Clinical users of DDSS in general should recognize the potential for errors when using DDSS. This mandates that clinicians supplement DDSS-based suggestions with their own expert knowledge.

The utility of making specific diagnoses lies in the selection of effective therapies, making accurate prognoses, and providing detailed explanations [1]. In some situations, it is not necessary to arrive at an exact diagnosis in order to fulfill one or more of these objectives. Treatment is often initiated before an exact diagnosis is made (e.g., patients in the emergency room receive oxygen for shortness of breath, before the etiology is known). Furthermore, the utility of making certain diagnoses is debatable, especially if there is a small probability of effective treatment.

The cost of eliciting all possible patient data is potentially staggering—temporally, economically, and ethically—since there are real risks of morbidity and/or mortality associated with many diagnostic procedures such as liver biopsy or cardiac catheterization. Given the impossibility and impracticality of gathering every conceivable piece of diagnostic information with respect to each patient, the "art" of diagnosis lies in the ability of the diagnostician to carefully evoke enough relevant information to justify all important and ultimately correct diagnoses in each case, as well as to initiate therapies at appropriate points during the evaluation [2].

The knowledge of how to "work up" the patient depends critically on the ability to evoke history, symptoms, and physical examination findings, concurrently with the ability to generate diagnostic hypotheses that suggest how to further refine or pursue the findings already elicited, or to pursue completely different additional findings. In addition, this must be done in a compassionate and cost-effective manner [2].

11.2 Human Diagnostic Reasoning

Diagnostic reasoning involves diverse cognitive activities, including information gathering, pattern recognition, problem solving, decision-making, judgment under uncertainty, and empathy. Large amounts of highly organized knowledge are necessary to function in this relatively unstructured cognitive domain. Our knowledge of human diagnostic reasoning is based on generic psychological experiments about reasoning and on direct studies of the diagnostic process itself. Relevant principles of human problem-solving behavior have been unveiled through focused studies examining constrained problem spaces such as chess-playing and cryptarithmetic [12]. Such studies have documented that experts recognize patterns of activity within a domain at an integrated, higher level ("chunking") than novices. Additional psychological experiments about judgments made under uncertainty [13] have provided insights into individuals' imperfect semi-quantitative reasoning skills.

To investigate the complex intellectual task of clinical diagnosis, many researchers [14, 15] have used behavioral methods that combine protocol analysis with introspection. Researchers record clinicians as they think aloud while performing specified cognitive tasks related to diagnosis (including normal clinical activities). Post facto, the clinicians themselves, or others, are asked to interpret the motives, knowledge, diagnostic hypotheses, and strategies involved in the recorded sessions. However, there is no proof that the stories constructed by experts to explain their diagnostic reasoning correspond to the actual reasoning methods they use subconsciously.

Most models of diagnostic reasoning include the following elements: the activation of working hypotheses; the testing of these hypotheses; the acquisition and interpretation of additional information; and confirming, rejecting, or adding of new hypotheses as information is gathered over time. Working hypotheses are generated early in the process of information gathering, at a time when only few facts are known about the patient [14, 15]. Only a limited number of these hypotheses, rarely more than five, are entertained simultaneously, probably due to the limited capacity of human short term memory [16]. Early hypothesis generation is accomplished through some form of pattern recognition, with experts more capable of applying compiled knowledge and experiences than novices. Comparing clinical reasoning in novices and experts, Evans and Patel [17] showed that experts rarely rely directly on causal reasoning and knowledge of basic sciences, except when reasoning outside their domain of expertise.

As noted by Pople and others [8], clinical diagnosis fits Nobel Laureate Herbert Simon's criteria for being an ill-structured problem [18]. Simon gave as an example of an ill-structured problem, the task an architect faces in creatively designing a new house "from scratch"—the realm of possible solutions encompasses a great variety of applicable methods and a broad set of alternative outcomes. As noted by Pople, Simon observed that one can solve ill-structured problems by splitting the problems into smaller, well defined subtasks that are each more easily accomplished [8].

In clinical diagnosis, early hypothesis generation helps to constrain reasoning to "high yield" areas, and permits the use of heuristic methods to further elucidate a solution [19]. Studies have shown that most clinicians employ the hypothetico-deductive method after early hypothesis generation [14, 15]. Data are collected with a view to their usefulness in refining, rejecting, or substituting for the original set of hypotheses. In the setting of clinicopathological exercises, Eddy and Clanton [20] showed that identification of a pivotal finding is often used to simplify the diagnostic problem and to narrow the focus to a limited set of hypotheses. Kassirer and Gorry [15] described the "process of case building," where hypotheses are evaluated against the model of a disease entity using techniques that can be emulated in computers using Bayes' rule, Boolean algebra, or template matching (see Chap. 2 for an explanation of these terms). They also recognized that heuristic methods are commonly used to confirm, eliminate, discriminate between, or explore hypotheses. Weed [21] and later Hurst and Walker [22] suggested that clinical problem solving can be approached by splitting complex, composite problems into relatively independent, discrete "problem areas." With respect to diagnosis, Pople (like Gorry earlier) observed that separating complex differential diagnoses into problem areas allows diagnosticians to apply additional powerful reasoning heuristics. They can assume that the differential diagnosis list within a problem area that contains mutually exclusive hypotheses and that the list can be made to be exhaustive (i.e., complete), so that it is assured that the correct diagnosis is on the list for the problem area, and that only one diagnosis on the list is the correct one [8].

Kassirer identified three abstract categories of human diagnostic reasoning: probabilistic, causal, and deterministic [23]. Formal models for each type of reasoning have been developed—at times independently of observational studies on how actual reasoning occurs. Approaches such as Brunswik's lens model [24], Bayesian algorithms [25, 26], and decision analysis [27, 28] define statistical associations between clinical variables and use formal mathematical models to derive "optimal" decisions. While diagnosticians clearly consider prevalence and other likelihood-related concepts during their reasoning [14, 15], observational and experimental studies show that clinicians do not calculate probabilities subconsciously during their own diagnostic reasoning [13, 29]. Human problem solvers tend to rely on judgmental heuristics. Experiments document that humans improperly evaluate subjective probabilities, misuse prior probabilities, and fail to recognize important phenomena, such as the regression towards the mean.

Evidence indicates that humans have more difficulty reasoning with probabilities than they do understanding the concepts that underlie them [30]. Humans also fall prey to reasoning errors such as reluctance to revise opinions when new data do not fit with working hypotheses, even when the data's diagnostic significance is properly understood [13, 29].

Models of causal (pathophysiological) reasoning, such as those developed by Feinstein [31, 32] in the 1970s, establish cause-and-effect relations between clinical variables within anatomic, physiologic, cellular, molecular, and biochemical representations of the reality. Although causal inferences (deductive reasoning from causes to consequences) can be viewed as the inverse of diagnostic inferences (abductive reasoning from consequences to causes), studies have shown that when making judgments under uncertainty, humans assign greater impact to causal relationships over other forms of diagnostic data of equal informative weight. Subjects commonly make overconfident predictions when dealing with highly uncertain models [13]. Causal (pathophysiological) reasoning uses shared, global, patient-independent knowledge [32] and provides an efficient means of verifying and explaining diagnostic hypotheses. Nevertheless, how much causal reasoning is actually used in early hypothesis generation and other stages of non-verbalized diagnostic reasoning is unclear; simple pattern recognition is far more prevalent. Previous studies indicate that experts tend to employ causal, pathophysiological reasoning only when: (a) faced with problems outside the realm of their expertise; (b) solving highly atypical problems, or (c) when they are asked to explain their reasoning to others [5].

In deterministic models, production rules, i.e., specifying appropriate actions in response to certain conditions, are used to represent the basic building blocks of human problem-solving. Such if—then rules representing compiled knowledge can also be expressed in the form of branching-logic flowcharts and clinical algorithms for non-experts to follow. However, production rules do not deal effectively with uncertainty [33], which is a disadvantage in clinical practice, where uncertainty is a common feature.

The late M. Scott Blois, a great philosopher-informatician-clinician, used a funnel to illustrate the spectrum of clinical judgment [34]. Consideration of patients' ill-structured problems, including undifferentiated concerns and vague complaints, occurs at the wide end of the funnel. Focused decisions in response to specific clinical questions (e.g., choosing an antibiotic to treat the exact bacterial species isolated as the cause of a pneumonia) were represented at the narrow end. This model is consistent with Simon's view of how humans solve ill-structured problems [18].

Blois noted that decision support systems were best applied toward the narrow end of the funnel, since circumscribed, well-structured problems are encountered there. Those problems are more amenable to solution through application of computational models of cognitive skills, requiring only focused and specific knowledge. On the other hand, at the open end of the funnel, one has to deal with common-sense knowledge and the general scope of ordinary human judgment in order to make meaningful progress, and few computer-based systems (other than those for record-keeping) are applicable.

11.3 Historical Survey of Diagnostic Decision Support Systems

The literature prior to 1976 described a majority of the important concepts still relevant to current DDSS development. In a comprehensive 1979 review of reasoning strategies employed by early DDSS, Shortliffe, Buchanan, and Feigenbaum identified the following classes of DDSS: clinical algorithms, clinical databanks that include analytical functions, mathematical pathophysiological models, pattern recognition systems, Bayesian statistical systems, decision-analytical systems, and symbolic reasoning (sometimes called "expert" systems) [35]. This section, without being comprehensive, will describe how some of the early pioneering efforts led to many classes of systems present today.

The many types of DDSS result from the large number of clinical domains to which diagnostic reasoning can be applied, from the multiple steps of diagnostic reasoning described above, and from the variety of difficulties that diagnosticians may encounter at each step. Health care informaticians encountering the term "clinical diagnostic decision-support systems" think primarily of general-purpose, broad-spectrum consultation systems [1].

A useful dichotomy separates DDSS into systems for general diagnosis (no matter how broad or narrow their application domains), and systems for diagnosis in specialized domains such as interpretation of ECG tracings [36]. The general notion of DDSS conveyed in the biomedical literature sometimes overlooks specialized, focused, yet highly successful medical device-associated diagnostic systems. Some simple DDSS help to interpret blood gas results, or assist in categorizing diagnostic possibilities based on the output of serum protein electrophoresis devices, or aid in the interpretation of standardized pulmonary function tests. DDSS for cytological recognition and classification have found successful application in devices such as automated differential blood count analyzers and systems to analyze Papanicolaou smears [1]. Small, focused DDSS are the most widely used form of diagnostic decision support programs, and their use will grow as they are coupled with other automated medical devices [1].

In their classic 1959 Science paper, Ledley and Lusted [25] observed that physicians have an imperfect knowledge of how they solve diagnostic problems. Ledley and Lusted stated that both logic (as embodied in set theory and Boolean algebra) and probabilistic reasoning (as embodied in Bayes' rule) were essential components of medical reasoning. They mentioned the importance of protocol analysis in understanding human diagnostic reasoning. They stated that they had examined how physicians solve New England Journal of Medicine CPC (clinicopathological conference) cases as the foundation for their work on diagnostic computer systems. Their insights provided the basis for work on Bayesian and decision-analytic diagnostic systems carried out over subsequent decades. Both for practical reasons and for philosophical reasons, much work on DDSS has focused on the differences between logical deductive systems and probabilistic systems. Chapter 2 describes these approaches in more detail. What follows is a description of how DDSS have embodied varied reasoning principles.

Logical systems, based on "discriminating questions" to distinguish among mutually exclusive alternatives, have played an important role since the pioneering work by Bleich and his colleagues [37] on acid base and electrolyte disorders. To this day, such systems are applicable to narrow domains, especially those where it is fairly certain that only one disorder is present. When users of a branching logic system incorrectly answer one of the questions posed by the system, they may find themselves "out on a limb" with no way to recover except by starting over from the beginning; the likelihood of such problems increases when multiple independent disease processes interact in the patient. Thus, ideal application areas are those where detailed knowledge of pathophysiology or extensive epidemiological data make it possible to identify parameters useful for dividing diagnostic sets into non-intersecting subsets, based on specific characteristics.

Bayes' rule is applicable to many clinical domains. Following Ledley and Lusted's 1959 publication [25], Warner and colleagues developed one of the first medical application systems based on Bayes' rule. In a 1961 JAMA paper [26], Warner et al. described a Bayesian DDSS for the diagnosis of congenital heart diseases. It utilized probabilities obtained from literature review, from their own series of over 1,000 cases, and from experts' estimates based on self-knowledge of pathophysiology. They emphasized that straightforward application of Bayes' theorem requires independence among the diagnoses and among the findings encompassed in the DDSS. They proposed a method for eliminating the influence of redundant findings. Warner et al. observed how diagnostic systems can easily fail due to false positive case findings and due to errors in the system's database. In their evaluation of their system's performance, they pointed out the need for an independent "gold standard" against which evaluators can judge the performance of the system. For that purpose, they used cardiac catheterization data and/or anatomical (postmortem) data excluded from the inputted case descriptions to confirm the actual patient diagnoses. Warner et al. continued to develop and refine models for Bayesian diagnosis over the years [1]. In 1968, Gorry and Barnett developed a model for sequential Bayesian diagnosis that extended Warner's earlier approach [38].

Many regard the system for the diagnosis of acute abdominal pain developed by de Dombal and colleagues at the University of Leeds as the first practical Bayesian system. It was utilized at widespread clinical sites [1, 10]. A large number of groups have subsequently developed, implemented, and refined Bayesian methods for diagnostic decision making. Ongoing enthusiasm surrounds current work on use of the more general Bayesian belief network approach for clinical diagnosis [1]. Probabilistic systems have played, and will continue to play, an important role in DDSS development.

An additional DDSS alternative exists to categorical (predicate calculus) [39] and probabilistic reasoning that combines features of both but retains a fundamental difference. That alternative is heuristic reasoning, reasoning based on empirical rules of thumb. The HEME program for diagnosis of hematological disorders was one of the earliest systems to employ heuristics and also one of the first systems to use, in effect, criteria tables for diagnosis of disease states. Lipkin, Hardy, Engle, and their colleagues developed HEME in the late 1950s [1, 40–42]. Programs that heuristically match terminology from stored descriptions of disease states to lexical descriptions of patient cases are similar conceptually to HEME. The CONSIDER program developed by Lindberg et al. [43] and the RECONSIDER program developed by Blois and his colleagues [44] used heuristic lexical matching techniques to identify diseases detailed in the Current Medical Information and Terminology (CMIT), a manual of diseases previously compiled and maintained by the American Medical Association. The EXPERT system shell, developed by Weiss and Kulikowski [45], has been used extensively in developing systems that utilize criteria tables, including AI/Rheum [46, 47], for diagnosis of rheumatic disorders, as well as other systems.

G. Anthony Gorry was an enlightened pioneer in the development of heuristic diagnostic systems that employ symbolic reasoning (artificial intelligence, or expert systems). In a classic paper published in 1968, Gorry [48] outlined the general principles underlying expert system approaches to medical diagnosis that have been incorporated into subsequent systems from the 1970s through the present time. Gorry proposed a formal definition of the diagnostic problem. In a visionary manner, he analyzed the relationships among a generic inference function (used to generate diagnoses from observed findings), a generic test-selection function that dynamically selects the best test to order (in terms of cost and information content), and a pattern-sorting function that is capable of determining if competing diagnoses are members of the same "problem area" (i.e., whether diagnostic hypotheses should be considered together because they are related to pathology in the same organ system). He pointed out the difference between the information value, the economic cost, and the morbidity or mortality risk of performing tests; discussed the cost of misdiagnosis of serious, life-threatening or disabling disorders; noted the potential influence of "red herring" findings on diagnostic systems; described the "multiple diagnosis" problem faced by systems when patients have more than one disease; and suggested that the knowledge bases underlying diagnostic systems could be used to generate simulated cases to test the diagnostic systems.

Gorry's schemata represent the intellectual ancestors of a diverse group of medical diagnostic systems, including, among others: PIP (the Present Illness Program), developed by Pauker et al.; MEDITEL for adult illnesses, which was developed by Waxman and Worley from an earlier pediatric version; INTERNIST-1, developed by Pople, Myers, and Miller; QMR, developed by Miller, Masarie, and Myers; DXplain, developed by Barnett and colleagues; Iliad, developed by Warner and colleagues; the commercial system ISABEL; and a large number of other systems [1, 49–61].

Shortliffe introduced the clinical application of rule-based expert systems for diagnosis and therapy through his development of MYCIN [1, 62] in 1973–1976. MYCIN used backward chaining through its rule base to collect information to identify the organism(s) causing bacteremia or meningitis in patients (see discussion of backward and forward chaining in Chap. 2). A large number of rule-based DDSS have been developed over the years, but most rule-based DDSS have been devoted to narrow application areas due to the extreme complexity of maintaining rule-based systems with more than a few thousand rules [1].

With the advent of the microcomputer came a change in philosophy in regard to the development of DDSS. For example, the global style of diagnostic consultation in the original 1974 INTERNIST-1 program treated the physician-user as unable to solve a diagnostic case [61]. The model assumed that the physician would transfer all historical information, physical examination findings, and laboratory and imaging data to the INTERNIST-1 expert diagnostic consultant program. The physician's subsequent role was that of a passive observer, answering yes or no to questions generated by INTERNIST-1. Ultimately, the omniscient "Greek Oracle" (consultant program) was expected to provide the correct diagnosis and explain its reasoning.

By the late 1980s and early 1990s, DDSS developers abandoned this Greek Oracle mode [9] of diagnostic decision support. For example, the critiquing model developed by Perry Miller [1, 63] and his colleagues, embodied the goal of creating a combined system that could take advantage of the strengths of both the user's knowledge and the system's abilities.

Several innovative models for computer-assisted medical diagnosis were developed in the 1980s and 1990s. These embodied more formal models that add mathematical rigor to the successful, but more arbitrary, heuristic explorations of the 1970s and early 1980s. However, such models engender tradeoffs, often related to less than perfect underlying data quality, that in many ways make them heuristic as well [64]. Systems based on fuzzy set theory and Bayesian belief networks were developed to overcome limitations of heuristic and simple Bayesian models [1]. Reggia et al. [1, 65] developed set covering models as a formalization of ad hoc problem-area formation (partitioning) schemes, originally described by Gorry in 1968, and later embodied in systems such as Pople's diagnostic algorithms for INTERNIST-1 [66].

Neural networks presented an entirely new approach to medical diagnosis, although the weights learned by simple one-layer networks were analogous or identical to Bayesian probabilities [1]. While neural networks have found applicability in narrow, focused application domains, problems limited their applicability to general diagnosis in broad clinical fields. The difficulties involved selecting the best topology, preventing overtraining and undertraining, and determining what cases to use for training. The more complex a neural network is (number of input and output nodes, number of hidden layers), the greater the need for a large number of appropriate training cases. Often, one cannot obtain large epidemiologically representative data sets that have rigorously determined diagnostic labels. Some developers resort to simulation techniques to generate training cases, but use of artificial cases to train neural networks may lead to suboptimal performance on real cases. Chapters 2 and 3 provide additional detail on the models mentioned above.

11.4 Developing, Implementing, Evaluating, and Maintaining Diagnostic Decision Support Systems

Any successful DDSS must complete a series of developmental stages [2, 67]. First, a new DDSS should meet well-studied and well-documented information needs [4, 5, 68]. Developers must perform a clinical needs assessment to determine the utility of the proposed system and the frequency with which it might be used in various real-world settings. Clinical systems should not be developed simply because a scientist wants to test an exciting new computational algorithm. The rule, "if it's not broke, don't fix it" applies to the development of DDSS, as well as other aspects of technology. Developers must carefully define the scope and nature of the process to be automated. They must also understand the process to be automated well enough to reduce it to an algorithm. All systems, especially DDSS, have boundaries (both in domain coverage and algorithm robustness) beyond which the systems often fail. Developers must understand these limits and make users aware of them—during

DDSS use, if possible. Developers must study DDSS algorithms to determine the ways in which they might fail, both due to inherent limitations and to flaws that might occur during the processes of implementation and use [2].

Evaluation must first occur carefully, initially "in vitro" (outside of the patient care arena, with no risks to patients), and, once warranted, in vivo (prospectively, on the front lines of actual patient care delivery) in order to determine if the DDSS improves or promotes important outcomes that are not possible with the pre-existing manual system [69]. Finally, developers and users must demonstrate the practical utility of the system by showing that clinicians can adopt it for productive daily use [2]. A potentially great system that is not used cannot have a beneficial impact on clinical outcomes. Unfortunately, few existing DDSS have yet fulfilled these criteria.

A number of problems have limited the ultimate success of DDSS to date. These include: difficulties with domain selection and knowledge base construction and maintenance; problems with the diagnostic algorithms and user interfaces; the problem of system evolution, including evaluation, testing, and quality control; issues related to machine interfaces and clinical vocabularies; and legal and ethical issues. These issues are discussed below.

11.4.1 Clinical Domain Selection

DDSS domain selection can pose problems. Substantial clinical domains require construction of corresponding, high-quality DDSS knowledge bases. Their construction and maintenance can consume dozens of person-years of effort in broad domains such as general internal medicine. To date, most large DDSS knowledge bases have at least initially been created in the academic environment. Many projects do not have adequate funding to sustain such activity over time [70]. Availability of adequate domain expertise is also a problem. Clinical collaborators generally earn their wages through patient care or clinical research, and sustaining high-level input from individuals with adequate clinical expertise can be difficult in the face of real-world demands. Commercial vendors must hire an adequate and well qualified staff of physicians in order to maintain medical knowledge bases. The number of users willing to purchase a DDSS program and its updates, as well as the price they are willing to pay, limit the income generated through the sale of the DDSS. Obtaining a critical volume of sales to support ongoing developments and updates is difficult.

Different types of problems afflict DDSS that target narrow domains. One problem is garnering an adequate audience. The CASNET system was an exemplary prototypic system for reasoning pathophysiologically about the diagnosis and therapy of glaucoma [71]. It typifies a problem that can occur with successful focal experimental expert systems with limited scope—the persons most likely to require such a specialized system's use in clinical medicine are the domain experts whose knowledge was used to develop the system. The persons who routinely diagnose and treat glaucoma are ophthalmologists, who are by definition board-certified specialists in the domain of ophthalmology. Programs like CASNET, in effect, run the risk of preaching to the choir. It is more difficult for an automated system to provide useful expertise in a given narrow specialty; human subspecialists in that area may rightly or wrongly believe they need not use it. Conversely, generalists are also unlikely to use a system with very narrow range of function. Specialty-specific, focused DDSS programs like the CASNET system must be extremely robust and provide more than one kind of service (e.g., by providing integrated record management and other functions in addition to DDSS functionality) in order to find use in clinical practice.

11.4.2 Knowledge Base Construction and Maintenance

Knowledge base maintenance is critical to the clinical validity of a DDSS [1]. Yet it is hard to determine when new clinical information becomes established as "fact." First reports of new clinical discoveries in highly regarded medical journals must await confirmation by other groups over time before their content can be added to a medical knowledge base. The nosological labels used in diagnosis reflect the current level of scientific understanding of pathophysiology and disease. They may change over time without the patient or the patient's illness, per se, changing [1]. For example, changes occur in how a label is applied when the "gold standard" for making a diagnosis shifts from a pathological biopsy result to an abnormal serological or genetic test—patients with earlier, previously unrecognized forms of the illness may be labeled as having the disease. Corresponding changes must be made to keep a DDSS knowledge base up to date.

Knowledge base construction must become a scientifically reproducible process that qualified individuals can successfully undertake at any site [72]. Knowledge base construction should be clinically grounded, based on objective, peer-reviewed information (e.g., literature-based) whenever possible. Attempts to "tune" a DDSS knowledge base to improve DDSS performance on a given case or group of cases should be strongly discouraged. A general system tuned in that manner lacks lasting calibration across all cases—changes improving performance for one specific case may degrade performance on other previously diagnosable cases. Any updates should have an objective basis, such as information culled from the medical literature.

If the process of knowledge base construction is highly dependent on a single individual, or can only be carried out at a single institution, then the survival of that system over time is in jeopardy. While much of the glamour of computer- based diagnostic systems lies in the computer algorithms and interfaces, the long-term value and viability of a system depends on the quality, accuracy, and timeliness of its knowledge base [1].

Even initially successful DDSS cannot survive unless the medical knowledge bases supporting them are kept current. This can require Herculean efforts. Shortliffe's MYCIN program [62] was developed as a research project to demonstrate the applicability of rule-based expert systems to clinical medicine. MYCIN was a brilliant, pioneering effort in this regard. The evaluation of MYCIN in the late 1970s by Yu and colleagues demonstrated that the program could perform at the expert level on challenging cases [73]. But MYCIN was never put into routine clinical use, nor was an effort made to update its knowledge base over time. After 1980, lack of maintenance led its antibiotic therapy knowledge base to become out of date.

11.4.3 Diagnostic Algorithms and User Interfaces

Just as computer-based implementation of many complex algorithms involves making trade-offs between space (memory) and time (CPU cycles), development of real-world diagnostic systems involves a constant balancing of theory (model complexity) and practicality (ability to construct and maintain adequate medical databases or knowledge bases, and ability to create systems which respond to users' needs in an acceptably short time interval) [64]. We may understand, in theory, how to develop systems that take into account gradations of symptoms, the degree of uncertainty in the patient and/or physician-user regarding a finding, the severity of each illness under consideration, the pathophysiological mechanisms of disease, and/or the time course of illnesses. Such complexities may ultimately be required to make actual systems work reliably. Nevertheless, it is not yet practical to build such complex, broad-based systems for patient care. The effort required to build and maintain superficial knowledge bases is measured in dozens of person-years of effort, and more complex knowledge bases are likely to require an order of magnitude greater effort [1]. The evidence to support many fine-grained diagnostic knowledge representation schemes may not yet exist in objective repositories such as the peer-reviewed literature.

Although some have posited that DDSS will eventually replace physicians as primary diagnosticians [74], that position seems untenable. A clinician cannot easily convey his or her complete understanding of a complex patient case to a computer program. One should never assume that a computer program "knows" all that needs to be known about a patient case, no matter how much time and effort is spent on data input. As a result, the clinician-user who directly evaluated the patient must be considered to be the definitive source of information about the patient during the entire course of any computer-based consultation [2]. In addition, the highly skilled health care practitioner—who understands the patient as a person—possesses the most important intellect to be employed during a consultation. That user should control the intellectual process of computer-based consultation, determining the sequence of steps to take place, which questions to pose, and whether those questions have been addressed. Systems must provide flexible environments that adapt to the user's needs and problems, rather than providing an interface that is inflexible and which penalizes the user for deviating from the normal order of system operation.

11.4.4 Testing, Evaluation, and Quality Control

System evaluation in biomedical informatics should take place as an ongoing, strategically planned process, not as a single event or small number of episodes [67, 69]. Complex software systems and accepted medical practices both evolve rapidly, so evaluators and readers of evaluations face moving targets. As previously noted, systems are of value only when they help users to solve users' problems. Users, not systems, characterize and solve clinical diagnostic problems. In keeping with that observation—that the DDSS user defines the problem to be solved—the ultimate unit of evaluation should be whether the user plus the system is better than the unaided user with respect to a specified task or problem (usually one generated by the user) [2, 69, 75].

Extremely important during system development are lessons learned (and modifications) based on informal formative evaluations. Developers of DDSS should analyze new DDSS cases on a regular (e.g., weekly) basis. After each failure of the DDSS to make a "correct" diagnosis, careful analysis of both the system's knowledge base and diagnostic algorithms must be carried out. Both the information in the knowledge base on the "correct" diagnosis, and the information on any diagnoses offered in error, must be reviewed and potentially updated. Updates should be evidence-based, not just arbitrary "tuning" of the system for a specific problematic case. In addition, periodic rerunning of all previous test cases, done on an annual (or similar) basis, can verify that no significant "drift" in either the knowledge base or the diagnostic programs have occurred.

Formal evaluations of DDSS should take into account the following four perspectives: (1) appropriate evaluation design; (2) specification of criteria for determining DDSS efficacy in the evaluation; (3) evaluation of the boundaries or limitations of the DDSS; and (4) identification of potential reasons for "lack of system effect" [69]. Each of these issues is discussed below.

Appropriate Evaluation Design

Evaluation plans should be appropriate for the information needs being addressed, the level of system maturity, and users' intended form of DDSS usage (or specific system function evaluated) [67, 69]. The same DDSS may serve as an electronic textbook for one user, a diagnostic checklist generator for another user, a consultant to determine the next useful step in a specific patient's evaluation for a third user, and a tool to critique/reinforce the users' own pre-existing hypotheses for a fourth user. Each system function would require a different form of evaluation whenever anticipated user benefits depend on which system function is used. Evaluations should clearly state which user objective is being studied and which of the available system functions are relevant to that objective.

In 1994, Berner and colleagues evaluated the ability of several systems to generate first-pass differential diagnoses from a fixed set of input findings [76]. These findings were not generated by everyday clinical users, but from written case summaries of real patient data. That approach was dictated by the desire to standardize system inputs and outputs for purposes of multisystem use. The primary goal of Berner et al. was to develop methods and metrics that would characterize aspects of system performance in a manner useful for rationally comparing different systems and their functions. All of the systems in that study were capable of generating questions to further refine the initial differential diagnoses, which is the intended mode of clinical use for such systems. Because that study was not intended to produce a definitive rating or comparison of the systems themselves, the involved systems were not placed in the hands of end users, nor were the systems used in a manner to address common end-user needs. Even though the evaluation did not examine this capability, the methods used by Berner were sound. Generating a first-pass differential diagnosis is a good initial step, but subsequent evidence gathering, reflection, and refinement are required.

There are important questions that must be answered in the evaluation. Are the problems ones that clinical users generate during clinical practice, or artificial problems generated by the study design team? Is the case material accurately based on actual patient cases? Note that there can be no truly verifiable diagnosis when artificial, manually constructed or computer-generated cases are used. Are the evaluation subjects clinical users whose participation occurs in the clinical context of caring for the patients used as "test cases?" Are clinical users evaluating abstracts of cases they have never seen, or are nonclinical personnel evaluating abstracted clinical cases using computer systems? Are users free to use all system components in whatever manner they choose, or is it likely that the study design will constrain users to exercise only limited components of the system? The answers to these questions will determine the generalizability of the results of the evaluation.

Specification of Criteria for Determining Efficacy in the Evaluation

Evaluations must identify criteria for "successful" system performance similar to what clinical practitioners would use during actual practice. Diagnosis, or more properly, "diagnostic benefit," must be defined in such contexts. Similarly, what it means to establish a diagnosis must be carefully defined. For example, it is not adequate to accept hospital discharge diagnoses at face value as a "gold standard" since discharge diagnoses are not of uniform quality—they have been documented to be influenced by physician competency, coding errors, and economic pressures. Furthermore, some discharge diagnoses may be "active" (undiagnosed at admission and related to the patient's reason for hospitalization), while others may be relevant but inactive. Criteria for the establishment of a "gold standard" diagnosis should be stated prospectively, before beginning data collection.

Evaluation of the Boundaries or Limitations

A system may fail when presented with cases outside its knowledge base domain, but if an evaluation uses only cases from within that domain, this failure may never be identified. The limits of a system's knowledge base are a concern because patients do not accurately triage themselves to present to the most appropriate specialists. For instance, as discussed earlier, de Dombal's abdominal pain system performed very well when used by surgeons to determine if patients presenting with abdominal pain required surgery [10]. However, a patient with atypical appendicitis may present to an internist, and a patient with abdominal pain due to lead poisoning may first see a surgeon.

Identification of Potential Reasons for "Lack of System Effect"

DDSS operate within a system that not only includes the DDSS itself, but also the user and the healthcare environment in which the user practices. A model of all of the possible influences on the evaluation outcomes would include DDSS-related factors (knowledge base inadequacies, inadequate synonyms within vocabularies, faulty algorithms, etc.), user-related factors (lack of training or experience with the system, failure to use or understand certain system functions, lack of medical knowledge or clinical expertise, etc.) and external variables (lack of available gold standards, failure of patients or clinicians to follow-up during study period). It is important to recognize that studies that focus on one aspect of system function may have to make compromises with respect to other system or user-related factors in order to have an interpretable result. Additionally, in any DDSS evaluation, the user's ability to generate meaningful input into the system, and the system's ability to respond to variable quality of input from different users, is an important concern.

Evaluations of DDSS must each take a standard objective (which may be only one component of system function) and measure how effectively the system enhances users' performances, using a study design that incorporates the most appropriate and rigorous methodology relative to the stage of system development. The ultimate clinical end user of a given DDSS must determine if published evaluation studies examine the system's function in the manner that the user intends to use it. This is analogous to a practitioner determining if a given clinical trial (of an intervention) is relevant to a specific patient by matching the given patient's characteristics to the study's inclusion and exclusion criteria, population demographics, and the patient's tolerance for the proposed forms of therapy as compared to alternatives. The reporting of an individual "negative study" of system performance should not, as it often does now, carry the implication that the system is globally suboptimal. A negative result for one system function does not mean that, for the same system, some users cannot derive significant benefits for other system functions. Similarly, complete evaluation of a system over time should examine basic components (e.g., the knowledge base, ability to generate reasonable differential diagnoses, ability to critique diagnoses, and so on), as well as clinical functionality (e.g., can novice users, after standard training, successfully employ the system to solve problems that they might not otherwise solve as efficiently or completely?). The field of DDSS evaluation will become mature only when clinical system users regularly derive the same benefit from published DDSS evaluations as they do from evaluations of standard clinical interventions.

11.4.5 Interface and Vocabulary Issues

A critical issue for the success of large-scale, generic DDSS is their environment. Small, limited, "niche" systems may be adopted and used by the focused community for which they are intended, while physicians in general medical practice, for whom the large-scale systems are intended, may not perceive the need for diagnostic assistance on a frequent enough basis to justify purchase of one or more such systems. Therefore, it is common wisdom that DDSS are most likely to succeed if they can be integrated into a clinical environment so that patient data capture is already performed by automated laboratory and/or hospital information systems. In such an environment, the physician will not have to manually enter all of a patient's data in order to obtain a diagnostic consultation. However, automated transfer of all the information about a patient from a hospital information system to a diagnostic consultation system is nontrivial. If 100 hematocrits were measured during a patient's admission, which one(s) should be transferred to the consultation system—the mean, the extremes, or the value typical for a given time in a patient's illness? Should all findings be transferred to the consultation system, or only those findings relevant to the patient's current illness? These questions must be resolved by careful study before one can expect to obtain patient consultations routinely and automatically within the context of a hospital information system. Another reason for providing an integrated environment is that users will not use a system unless it is sufficiently convenient to do so. By integrating DDSS into healthcare provider results reporting and order entry systems, the usual computer-free workflow processes of the clinician can be replaced with an environment conducive to accomplishing a number of computer-assisted clinical tasks, making it more likely that a DDSS will be used.

Interfaces between automated systems are, at times, as important as the man-machine interface [77, 78]. Fundamental questions, such as the definition of diseases and of findings, limit our ability to combine data from the literature, from clinical databanks, from hospital information systems, and from individual experts' experiences in order to create DDSS. Similar problems exist when trying to match the records from a given case with a computer-based diagnostic system. A diagnostic system may embody different definitions for patient descriptors than those of the physician who evaluated the patient, even though the words used by each may be identical.

In order to facilitate data exchange among local and remote programs, it is mandatory to have a lexicon or interlingua which facilitates accurate and reliable transfer of information among systems that have different internal vocabularies (data dictionaries). The United States National Library of Medicine Unified Medical Language System (UMLS) project, which started in 1987 and continues through the present time, represents one such effort [79].

11.4.6 Legal and Ethical Issues

Proposals have suggested that governmental agencies, such as the United States Food and Drug Administration (FDA), which oversees medical devices, regulate use of clinical software programs such as DDSS. These proposals include a variety of recommendations that manufacturers of such systems would be required to perform to guarantee that the systems would function per specifications.

There is debate about whether these consultation systems are actually devices in the same sense as other regulatable devices. In the past, governmental regulation has not been considered necessary when a licensed practitioner is the user of a DDSS [80]. It would be both costly and difficult for the government to regulate DDSS more directly, even if a decision were made to do so. For general DDSS programs like Iliad, QMR, Meditel and DXplain, with hundreds to thousands of possible diagnoses represented in their knowledge bases [76], conducting prospective clinical trials, to demonstrate that the system worked for all ranges of diagnostic difficulty for a variety of patients with each diagnosis, would require enrollment of huge numbers of patients and would cost millions of dollars.

Other approaches, such as a "software quality audit" to determine, prospectively, if a given software product has flaws would also be clinically impractical. The clinician seeking help may have any of several dozen kinds of diagnostic problems in any given case. Unless it is known, for a given case, which kind of problem the practitioner will have, performing a software quality audit could not predict if the system would be useful.

Consider the dilemma the FDA or other responsible regulatory agency would face if it agreed to review situations when a user files a complaint. First, one must note that few patients undergo definitive enough diagnostic evaluations to make it possible to have a "gold standard" (certain) diagnosis. So if the doctor claims the program was wrong, a major question would be how governmental auditors would know what the actual "right" diagnosis was. Second, the reviewers would need to know all of the information that was knowable about the patient at the time the disputed diagnosis was offered. This could potentially violate patient confidentiality if the records were sent to outsiders for review. All sources of information about the patient would have to be audited, and this could become as difficult as evidence gathering in a malpractice trial. To complete the sort of audit described, the governmental agency would have to determine if the user had been appropriately trained and if the user used the program correctly. Unless the program had an internally stored complete audit trail of each session (down to the level of saving each keystroke the user typed), the auditors might never be able to recreate the session in question. Also, the auditors would have to study whether the program's knowledge base was appropriate. Initial development of the R-QMR knowledge base at the University of Pittsburgh required an average of three person-weeks of a clinician's time, which went into literature review of 50–150 primary articles about each disease, with additional time for synthesis and testing against cases of real patients with the disease. For an auditor to hire the required expertise to review this process for hundreds to thousands of diseases for each of the programs that it would have to review and subsequently monitor would be costly and cumbersome. The ultimate question, very difficult to answer, would be whether the original user in the case in question used the system in the best way possible for the given case. Making such a determination would require the governmental agency to become expert in the use of each DDSS program. This could take up to several months of training and practice for a single auditor to become facile in the use of a single system. It would be difficult for a governmental agency to muster the necessary resources for even a small number of such complaints, let alone nationwide for multiple products with thousands of users. The complexity of these issues makes it very difficult to formulate appropriate regulatory policy. In addition to legal issues concerning regulation, there are other legal and ethical issues relating to use of DDSS that are discussed in Chap. 8.

11.5 Diagnostic Decision Support Systems Circa 2015

Recent emphasis on preventable errors in clinical practice originated in the 1980s with published studies on adverse drug effects, and peaked with the Institute of Medicine's more comprehensive report, To Err Is Human [81]. Many researchers neglected or downplayed the frequency and importance of diagnostic errors, especially in the outpatient setting, because little was known at the time. Recently, increased interest has focused on diagnostic errors and their prevention [82–92]. The Society to Improve Diagnosis In Medicine (SIDM) grew out of the momentum generated by post-2000 annual conferences on diagnostic errors. In 2014, SIDM began publishing a journal, Diagnosis [92]. In 2015, the Agency for Healthcare Research and Quality (AHRQ) emphasized the importance of diagnosis by issuing new RFAs for methods to reduce diagnostic errors in the outpatient setting. The Institute of Medicine (National Academy of Medicine) of the National Academy of Sciences published its summary of a multi-year study of diagnostic errors [93]. The potential for implementation of DDSS in clinical practice, and the ability to study their impact has never been greater.

Three general, non-focal DDSS available in 2015 merit mention as exemplars: VisualDx® [94–99], DXplain [54, 56, 57, 100], and ISABEL [60, 101–105]. VisualDx® and ISABEL are marketed commercially; DXplain is available via institutional licenses for an annual fee. The web-based DXplain DDSS represents the current evolution of a system initially developed in 1984 by G. Octo Barnett and colleagues at the Massachusetts General Hospital [100]. Dr. Barnett, the primary developer of DXplain, often stated that the inspiration for the system grew out of his respect for INTERNIST-1 [58, 59]. According to the 2015 DXplain web site, "the current DXplain knowledge base (KB) includes over 2400 diseases and over 5000 clinical findings (symptoms, signs, epidemiologic data and laboratory, endoscopic and radiologic findings)" [100]. The ISABEL DDSS was developed as a commercial application from the outset. It originally covered Pediatric diagnosis [101–104] and its knowledge base has grown to now include adult disorders. In 2003, the developers of ISABEL published an evaluation of ISABEL, proposing that previous rigorous standards for DDSS evaluation might be unnecessary [105]. Berner discussed the implications of evaluating DDSS using less than absolute gold standards, as was proposed by the ISABEL team, in a well-balanced perspective covering "correctness" of diagnosis, "appropriateness" of management suggestions, end-user acceptance and satisfaction, degree of adoption and use of a DDSS, and issues related to human-computer system interfaces [106]. Like many heuristic systems before them, DXplain and ISABEL behaviorally follow Gorry's 1968 DDSS template.

A current DDSS that satisfies many of the previously discussed desiderata for a creating, maintaining, and distributing a successful system is VisualDx, developed by Dr. Art Papier and colleagues [94–99]. Dr. Papier is an academically-based dermatologist who has developed an extensive consortium of collaborating institutions to construct and maintain the VisualDx knowledge base, consisting of dermatological images, a standardized lexicon of text descriptions for each of the images, and summary characterizations of the disorders associated with each image and with each text description. The web site "visualdx.com" [94] states the following: "VisualDx is a diagnostic clinical decision support and reference tool that combines high-quality, peer-reviewed medical images and expert information to support today's internists and infectious disease physicians in the accurate recognition and management of disease ...over 1500 hospitals and large clinics ... recognize VisualDx as a ... quality and safety system."

11.6 The Future of Diagnostic Decision Support Systems

It is relatively safe to predict that specialized, focused DDSS will proliferate, and a sizable number of them will find widespread application [1]. As new medical devices are developed and older devices automated, DDSS software that enhances the performance of the device, or helps users to interpret the output of the device, will become essential.

Computerized electrocardiogram (ECG) analysis, automated arterial blood gas interpretation, automated protein electrophoresis reports, and automated differential blood cell counters, are but a few examples of such success at the present time. Since Miller's 1994 article summarizing past DDSS developmental activities [1], the great majority of new articles on "diagnosis, computer-assisted" indexed in

MEDLINE have described focused systems for the interpretation of images (radiological studies and pathology cytology/sections/slides), signals (ECGs, electroencephalograms (EEGs), and so on), and diagnosis of very narrowly defined clinical conditions. One by-product of the success of these systems is that users may be less vigilant in questioning system accuracy. In a 2003 article, Tsai and colleagues pointed out the potential clinical dangers of overreliance of inexpert clinicians on computer systems for advice—they tend to follow the advice even when it is wrong [107].

For the foreseeable future, machine-learning approaches to DDSS will find success in the realm of specialized, focused systems. There, adequate training exemplars can be found, and the number of categories to discriminate is relatively small (typically dozens). A somewhat related example, IBM's Watson™ analytic engine [108], is also more likely to find success in DDSS applications in focal domains rather than general diagnosis for medicine or pediatrics. Watson uses natural language processing to draw statistical relationships among terms extracted from textual documents [108], such as the biomedical literature or patients' charts. In reviewing the literature for the INTERNIST-1 and QMR projects, project members noticed that human expertise at a high level must resolve among conflicting reports as to whether a given disorder causes a given finding. Furthermore, in a given case summary appearing in either the literature or an EMR, patients often have multiple conditions that can cause or, in combination, exacerbate a given finding—e.g., a patient with shortness of breath who has both emphysema and heart failure. Purely automated systems would likely experience more difficulty than an expert clinician in sorting out which disorder caused the finding on an algorithmic basis. Furthermore, for extremely rare disorders, such as primary sarcoma of the heart, a sufficient number of case reports may not exist for algorithmic extraction of findings with certainty. The whole field of meta-analysis, which attempts to determine from published randomized controlled trials the quality of evidence supporting various therapeutic approaches to a given disorder, indicates the complexity of decision-making involved in collating evidence. Machine learning and Watson-like attempts to summarize the literature on diagnosis, which lacks the rigor of randomized controlled trials, will also encounter extreme difficulty when attempting to derive evidence bases to support DDSS in broad fields such as medicine or pediatrics.

So manual, or quasi-manual approaches to DDSS knowledge base curation by qualified clinical experts will remain the best method to construct and maintain DDSS knowledge bases in the near-term future. Watson-like systems may, however, provide useful assistance to humans or heuristic DDSS in general clinical domains by, upon request, searching for evidence supporting (or refuting) a given specific diagnosis within a single patient's voluminous EMR record.

The future of large-scale, "generic" diagnostic systems is hopeful, although less certain. As discussed in this and other chapters, a small number of large-scale, generic DDSS are in limited use in clinical practice. Systems like VisualDx provide hope that a model for ongoing maintenance and distribution for DDSS can be feasible. Nevertheless, it is well established that DDSS can play a valuable role in medical education [1]. The process of knowledge base construction, utilization of such knowledge bases for medical education in the form of patient case simulations, and the use of DDSS have all been shown to be of educational value in a variety of institutional settings.

In summary, the future of DDSS appears to be promising. The number of researchers in the field is growing. The diversity of DDSS is increasing. The number of commercial enterprises interested in DDSS is expanding. Rapid improvements in computer technology continue to be made. A growing demand for cost-effective clinical information management, and the desire for better health care, is sweeping the United States [109]. Evidence-based medicine is now in vogue. All these factors will insure that new and productive DDSS applications will be developed, evaluated, and used.

References

1. Miller RA. Medical diagnostic decision support systems—past, present, and future: a threaded bibliography and commentary. J Am Med Inform Assoc. 1994;1:8–27.
2. Miller RA. Why the standard view is standard: people, not machines, understand patients' problems. J Med Philos. 1990;15:581–91.
3. Flexner SB, Stein J, editors. The Random House college dictionary. Revised ed. New York: Random House; 1988. p. 366.
4. Osheroff JA, Forsythe DE, Buchanan BG, Bankowitz RA, Blumenfeld BH, Miller RA. Physicians' information needs: an analysis of questions posed during clinical teaching in internal medicine. Ann Intern Med. 1991;114:576–81.
5. Forsythe DE, Buchanan BG, Osheroff JA, Miller RA. Expanding the concept of medical information: an observational study of physicians' information needs. Comput Biomed Res. 1992;25:181–200.
6. Miller R, Masarie FE, Myers J. Quick Medical Reference (QMR) for diagnostic assistance. MD Comput. 1986;3:34–8.
7. Miller RA, Masarie FE Jr. The quick medical reference (QMR) relationships function: description and evaluation of a simple, efficient "multiple diagnoses" algorithm. Medinfo. 1992;512–18.
8. Pople Jr HE. Heuristic methods for imposing structure on ill-structured problems: the structuring of medical diagnostics. In: Szolovits P, editor. Artificial intelligence in medicine, AAAS symposium series. Boulder: Westview Press; 1982. p. 119–90.
9. Miller RA, Masarie Jr FE. The demise of the "Greek Oracle" model for medical diagnosis systems. Methods Inf Med. 1990;29:1–2.
10. de Dombal FT, Leaper DJ, Horrocks JC, Staniland JR, McCann AP. Human and computer-aided diagnosis of abdominal pain: further report with emphasis on performance of clinicians. Br Med J. 1974;1:376–80.
11. Adams ID, Chan M, Clifford PC, et al. Computer aided diagnosis of acute abdominal pain: a multicentre study. Br Med J (Clin Res Ed). 1986;293:800–4.
12. Newell A, Simon HA. Human problem solving. Englewood Cliffs: Prentice Hall; 1972.
13. Kahneman D, Slovic P, Tversky A, editors. Judgment under uncertainty: heuristics and biases. Cambridge, UK: Cambridge University Press; 1982.
14. Elstein AS, Shulman LS, Sprafka SA. Medical problem solving: an analysis of clinical reasoning. Cambridge, MA: Harvard University Press; 1978.
15. Kassirer JP, Gorry GA. Clinical problem-solving—a behavioral analysis. Ann Intern Med. 1978;89:245–55.

16. Miller GA. The magical number seven, plus or minus two: some limits on our capacity for processing information. Psychol Rev. 1956;63:81–97.
17. Evans DA, Patel VL, editors. Cognitive science in medicine. Cambridge, MA: MIT Press; 1989.
18. Simon HA. The structure of ill-structured problems. Artif Intell. 1973;4:181–201.
19. Miller RA, Pople Jr HE, Myers J. INTERNIST-1, an experimental computer-based diagnostic consultant for general internal medicine. N Engl J Med. 1982;307:468–76.
20. Eddy DM, Clanton CH. The art of diagnosis: solving the clinicopathological conference. N Engl J Med. 1982;306:1263–9.
21. Weed LL. Medical records that guide and teach. N Engl J Med. 1968;278:593–600. 652–657.
22. Hurst JW, Walker HK, editors. The problem-oriented system. New York: Medcom Learning Systems; 1972.
23. Kassirer JP. Diagnostic reasoning. Ann Intern Med. 1989;110:893–900.
24. Brunswik E. Representative design and probabilistic theory in a functional psychology. Psychol Rev. 1955;62:193–217.
25. Ledley RS, Lusted LB. Reasoning foundations of medical diagnosis; symbolic logic, probability, and value theory aid our understanding of how physicians reason. Science. 1959;130:9–21.
26. Warner HR, Toronto AF, Veasey LG, Stephenson R. Mathematical approach to medical diagnosis. JAMA. 1961;177:75–81.
27. Raiffa H. Decision analysis. Reading: Addison-Wesley; 1970.
28. Pauker SG, Kassirer JP. Decision analysis. N Engl J Med. 1987;316:250–8.
29. Dawes RM, Faust D, Meehl PE. Clinical versus actuarial judgment. Science. 1989;243:1668–74.
30. Gigerenzer G, Hoffrage U. How to improve Bayesian reasoning without instruction: frequency formats. Psychol Rev. 1995;102:684–704.
31. Feinstein AR. An analysis of diagnostic reasoning. I. The domains and disorders of clinical macrobiology. Yale J Biol Med. 1973;46:212–32.
32. Feinstein AR. An analysis of diagnostic reasoning. II. The strategy of intermediate decisions. Yale J Biol Med. 1973;46:264–83.
33. Horvitz EJ, Heckerman DE. The inconsistent use of measures of certainty in artificial intelligence research. In: Kanal LN, Lemmer JF, editors. Uncertainty in artificial intelligence, vol. 1. Amsterdam: Elsevier Science; 1986. p. 137–51.
34. Blois MS. Clinical judgment and computers. N Engl J Med. 1980;303:192–7.
35. Shortliffe EH, Buchanan BG, Feigenbaum EA. Knowledge engineering for medical decision-making: a review of computer-based clinical decision aids. Proc IEEE. 1979;67:1207–24.
36. Willems JL, Abreu-Lima C, Arnaud P, et al. The diagnostic performance of computer programs for the interpretation of electrocardiograms. N Engl J Med. 1991;325:1767–73.
37. Bleich HL. Computer evaluation of acid-base disorders. J Clin Invest. 1969;48:1689–96.
38. Gorry GA, Barnett GO. Experience with a model of sequential diagnosis. Comput Biomed Res. 1968;1:490–507.
39. Szolovits P, Pauker SG. Categorical and probabilistic reasoning in medical diagnosis. Artif Intell. 1978;11:114–44.
40. Lipkin M, Hardy JD. Differential diagnosis of hematological diseases aided by mechanical correlation of data. Science. 1957;125:551–2.
41. Lipkin M, Hardy JD. Mechanical correlation of data in differential diagnosis of hematological diseases. JAMA. 1958;166:113–23.
42. Lipkin M, Engle Jr RL, Davis BJ, Zworykin VK, Ebald R, Sendrow M. Digital computer as aid to differential diagnosis. Arch Intern Med. 1961;108:56–72.
43. Lindberg DAB, Rowland LR, Buch CR Jr, Morse WF, Morse SS. Consider: a computer program for medical instruction. In: Proceedings of the ninth IBM medical symposium. White

Plains: IBM, 1968. Conference dates: 9th IBM Medical Symposium, Burlington, Vermont, October 24–26, 1969.
44. Nelson SJ, Blois MS, Tuttle MS, et al. Evaluating RECONSIDER: a computer program for diagnostic prompting. J Med Syst. 1985;9:379–88.
45. Weiss S, Kulikowski CA. EXPERT: a system for developing consultation models. In: Proceedings of the sixth international joint conference on artificial intelligence. Tokyo; 1979.
46. Lindberg DAB, Sharp GC, Kingsland III LC, et al. Computer-based rheumatology consultant. In: Linberg DAB, Kaihara S, editors. Proceedings of MEDINFO 80 Tokyo, third world conference on medical informatics. Amsterdam: North Holland Publishing Company; 1980. p. 1311–5.
47. Moens HJ, van der Korst JK. Development and validation of a computer program using Bayes' theorem to support diagnosis of rheumatic disorders. Ann Rheum Dis. 1992;51:266–71.
48. Gorry A. Strategies for computer-aided diagnosis. Math Biosci. 1968;2:293–318.
49. Pauker SG, Gorry GA, Kassirer JP, Schwartz WB. Towards the simulation of clinical cognition. Taking a present illness by computer. Am J Med. 1976;60:981–96.
50. Waxman HS, Worley WE. Computer-assisted adult medical diagnosis: subject review and evaluation of a new microcomputer-based system. Medicine. 1990;69:125–36.
51. Pople HE, Myers JD, Miller RA. DIALOG: a model of diagnostic logic for internal medicine. In: Proceedings of the fourth international joint conference on artificial intelligence. Tiblisi; 1975. p. 848–55.
52. First MB, Soffer LJ, Miller RA. QUICK (Quick Index to Caduceus Knowledge): using the INTERNIST-1/Caduceus knowledge base as an electronic textbook of medicine. Comput Biomed Res. 1985;18:137–65.
53. Miller RA, McNeil MA, Challinor S, Masarie Jr FE, Myers JD. Status report: the Internist-1/ Quick Medical Reference project. West J Med. 1986;145:816–22.
54. Hupp JA, Cimino JJ, Hoffer EF, Lowe HJ, Barnett GO. DXplain—a computer- based diagnostic knowledge base. In: Proceedings of the fifth world conference on medical informatics (MEDINFO 86). Amsterdam. p. 117–21.
55. Warner HR, Haug P, Bouhaddou O, Lincoln M. ILIAD as an expert consultant to teach differential diagnosis. In: Greenes RA, editor. Proceedings of the twelfth annual symposium on computer applications in medical care. Los Angeles: IEEE Computer Society; 1988. p. 371–6.
56. Barnett GO, Cimino JJ, Hupp JA, Hoffer EP. DXplain. An evolving diagnostic decision-support system. JAMA. 1987;258:67–74.
57. Elkin PL, Liebow M, Bauer BA, Chaliki S, Wahner-Roedler D, Bundrick J, Lee M, Brown SH, Froehling D, Bailey K, Famiglietti K, Kim R, Hoffer E, Feldman M, Barnett GO. The introduction of a diagnostic decision support system (DXplain™) into the workflow of a teaching hospital service can decrease the cost of service for diagnostically challenging Diagnostic Related Groups (DRGs). Int J Med Inform. 2010;79(11):772–7.
58. Barnett GO. The computer and clinical judgment. N Engl J Med. 1982;307(8):493–4.
59. Barnett GO. Personal communications to RA Miller, 1988–2002.
60. Graber ML, Mathew A. Performance of a web-based clinical diagnosis support system for internists. J Gen Intern Med. 2008;23 Suppl 1:37–40.
61. Miller RA. A history of the INTERNIST-1 and Quick Medical Reference (QMR) computer-assisted diagnosis projects, with lessons learned. Yearb Med Inform. 2010;121–136.
62. Shortliffe EH. Computer-based medical consultations: MYCIN. New York: Elsevier; 1976.
63. Miller PL. A critiquing approach to expert computer advice: ATTENDING. Boston: Pittman; 1984.
64. Aliferis CF, Miller RA. On the heuristic nature of medical decision support systems. Methods Inf Med. 1995;34:5–14.
65. Reggia JA, Nau DS, Wang PY. Diagnostic expert systems based on a set covering model. Int J Man Mach Stud. 1983;19:437–60.

66. Berman L, Miller RA. Problem area formation as an element of computer aided diagnosis: a comparison of two strategies within quick medical reference (QMR). Methods Inf Med. 1991;30:90–5.
67. Stead WW, Haynes RB, Fuller S, et al. Designing medical informatics research and library-resource projects to increase what is learned. J Am Med Inform Assoc. 1994;1:28–33.
68. Covell DG, Uman GC, Manning PR. Information needs in office practice: are they being met? Ann Intern Med. 1985;103:596–9.
69. Miller RA. Evaluating evaluations of medical diagnostic systems. J Am Med Inform Assoc. 1996;3:429–31.
70. Yu VL. Conceptual obstacles in computerized medical diagnosis. J Med Philos. 1983;8:67–75.
71. Weiss S, Kulikowski CA, Safir A. Glaucoma consultation by computer. Comput Biol Med. 1978;8:24–40.
72. Giuse NB, Giuse DA, Miller RA, et al. Evaluating consensus among physicians in medical knowledge base construction. Methods Inf Med. 1993;32:137–45.
73. Yu VL, Fagan LM, Wraith SM, et al. Antimicrobial selection by computer: a blinded evaluation by infectious disease experts. JAMA. 1979;242:1279–82.
74. Mazoue JG. Diagnosis without doctors. J Med Philos. 1990;15:559–79.
75. Friedman CP. A "fundamental theorem" of biomedical informatics. J Am Med Inform Assoc. 2009;16(2):169–70.
76. Berner ES, Webster GD, Shugerman AA, et al. Performance of four computer-based diagnostic systems. N Engl J Med. 1994;330:1792–6.
77. Rosenbloom ST, Miller RA, Johnson KB, Elkin PL, Brown SH. Interface terminologies: facilitating direct entry of clinical data into electronic health record systems. J Am Med Inform Assoc. 2006;13(3):277–88.
78. Rosenbloom ST, Miller RA, Johnson KB, Elkin PL, Brown SH. A model for evaluating interface terminologies. J Am Med Inform Assoc. 2008;15(1):65–76.
79. Lindberg DA, Humphreys BL, McCray AT. The unified medical language system. Methods Inf Med. 1993;32:281–91.
80. Young FE. Validation of medical software: present policy of the Food and Drug Administration. Ann Intern Med. 1987;106:628–9.
81. Kohn LT, Corrigan JM, Donaldson MS, editors. To err is human: building a safer health system. Washington, DC: National Academy Press; 2000.
82. Friedman CP, Gatti GG, Franz TM, et al. Do physicians know when their diagnoses are correct? Implications for decision support and error reduction. J Gen Intern Med. 2005;20:334–9.
83. Shojania KG, Burton EC, McDonald KM, et al. Changes in rates of autopsy-detected diagnostic errors over time: a systematic review. JAMA. 2003;289:2849–56.
84. Studdert DM, Mello MM, Gawande AA, et al. Claims, errors, and compensation payments in medical malpractice litigation. N Engl J Med. 2006;354:2024–33.
85. Gandhi TK, Kachalia A, Thomas EJ, et al. Missed and delayed diagnoses in the ambulatory setting: a study of closed malpractice claims. Ann Intern Med. 2006;145:488–96.
86. Berner ES, Graber ML. Overconfidence as a cause of diagnostic error in medicine. Am J Med. 2008;121:S2–23.
87. Newman-Toker D, Pronovost P. Diagnostic errors—the next frontier for patient safety. JAMA. 2009;301:1062.
88. Zwaan L, De Bruijne MC, Wagner C, et al. A record review on the incidence, consequences and causes of diagnostic adverse events. Arch Intern Med. 2010;170:1015–21.
89. Schiff G, Bates D. Can electronic clinical documentation help prevent diagnostic errors? N Engl J Med. 2010;362:1066–9.
90. Singh H, Giardina T, Meyer A, et al. Types and origins of diagnostic errors in primary care settings. JAMA Int Med. 2013;173:418–25.
91. McDonald K, Matesic B, Contopoulos-Ioannidis D, et al. Patient safety strategies targeted at diagnostic errors- a systematic review. Ann Intern Med. 2013;158:381–90.

92. Society to Improve Diagnosis in Medicine. http://www.improvediagnosis.org. Accessed 26 Jul 2015.
93. National Academies of Sciences, Engineering, and Medicine. Improving diagnosis in health care. Washington, DC: The National Academies Press; 2015.
94. Visualdx. http://www.visualdx.com. Accessed 27 Jul 2015.
95. Papier A. Decision support in dermatology and medicine: history and recent developments. Semin Cutan Med Surg. 2012;31(3):153–9.
96. Goldsmith LA, Papier A. Fighting Babel with precise definitions of knowledge. J Invest Dermatol. 2010;130(11):2527–30.
97. Tleyjeh IM, Nada H, Baddour LM. VisualDx: decision-support software for the diagnosis and management of dermatologic disorders. Clin Infect Dis. 2006;43(9):1177–84.
98. Papier A, Chalmers RJ, Byrnes JA, Goldsmith LA, Dermatology Lexicon Project. Framework for improved communication: the Dermatology Lexicon Project. J Am Acad Dermatol. 2004;50(4):630–4.
99. Papier A, Peres MR, Bobrow M, Bhatia A. The digital imaging system and dermatology. Int J Dermatol. 2000;39(8):561–75.
100. Dxplain. http://www.mghlcs.org/projects/dxplain. Accessed 27 Jul 2015.
101. Greenough A. Help from ISABEL for paediatric diagnoses. Lancet. 2002;360:1259.
102. McKenna C. New online diagnostic tool launched to help doctors. BMJ. 2002;324:1478.
103. Thomas NJ. ISABEL. Crit Care. 2003;7:99–100.
104. Ramnarayan P, Tomlinson A, Rao A, Coren M, Winrow A, Britto J. ISABEL: a web-based differential diagnostic aid for paediatrics: results from an initial performance evaluation. Arch Dis Child. 2003;88:408–13.
105. Ramnarayan P, Kapoor RR, Coren M, et al. Measuring the impact of diagnostic decision support on the quality of decision-making: development of a reliable and valid composite score. J Am Med Inform Assoc. 2003;10:563–72.
106. Berner E. Diagnostic decision support systems: how to determine the gold standard? J Am Med Inform Assoc. 2003;10:608–10.
107. Tsai TL, Fridsma DB, Gatti G. Computer decision support as a source of interpretation error: the case of electrocardiograms. J Am Med Inform Assoc. 2003;10:478–83.
108. Kohn MS, Sun J, Knoop S, Carmeli B, Sow D, Syed-Mahmood T, Rapp W. IBM's health analytics and clinical decision support. IMIA Yearb Med Inform. 2014;9:154–62.
109. Blumenthal D. Stimulating the adoption of health information technology. N Engl J Med. 2009;360(15):1477–149.

Chapter 12
Use of Clinical Decision Support to Tailor Drug Therapy Based on Genomics

Joshua C. Denny, Laura K. Wiley, and Josh F. Peterson

Abstract Clinical decision support (CDS) has been an effective tool to improve prescribing to prevent errors, avoid adverse events, and optimize dosing. The imminent adoption of inexpensive panel assays to generate dense molecular data offers new opportunities to improve prescribing. Yet realizing the potential of such data to improve care faces many challenges to clinical informatics. These 'omic' data are large, are frequently stored and presented within non-computable narrative reports, require maintenance of an updated interpretation, and lack widespread representation standards for interoperability. In this chapter, we focus on using genomic data to guide drug therapy as a prototypic class of omic data with the greatest evidence base to support its clinical use in routine clinical care. We provide an overview of the challenges and opportunities of using genomic information within CDSS, the evidence for clinical utility, the emergence of genomic data standards, and examples of systems of pharmacogenomic prescribing. We conclude that the opportunities for genomic-guided therapy will likely increase over time. Clinical informatics development will be required to meet rapidly evolving needs, toward an outcome of improved patient care with the right drug at the right dose the first time, decreasing "idiopathic" adverse events.

Keywords Clinical decision support • Genomics • Pharmacogenomics • Electronic health records • Adverse drug events • Health level 7 • Pharmacology

---

J.C. Denny, M.D., M.S. (✉) • J.F. Peterson, M.D., M.P.H.
Biomedical Informatics and Medicine, Vanderbilt University Medical Center, 2525 West End Ave, Suite 1475, Nashville, TN 37203, USA
e-mail: josh.denny@vanderbilt.edu; josh.peterson@vanderbilt.edu

L.K. Wiley, M.S., Ph.D.
Department of Biomedical Informatics, Vanderbilt University Medical Center, 2525 West End Ave, Suite 1050, Nashville, TN 37215, USA
e-mail: laura.k.wiley@vanderbilt.edu

E.S. Berner (ed.), *Clinical Decision Support Systems*, Health Informatics,
DOI 10.1007/978-3-319-31913-1_12

One of the visions from the Human Genome Project was the ability to use genetic information to tailor therapeutic decisions for individuals. The scientific validity of this potential has been validated as numerous cases of common and rare genomic variations have been found to influence drug effects. Many prototypical rare "idiopathic" adverse drug events have been shown to have genetic influences, such as Stevens Johnson Syndrome with the antiepileptic carbamazepine [1] and drug induced liver injury with flucloxacillin [2]. The efficacy of other drugs has been shown to be influenced by genetic variation [3]. Other types of medications that are influenced by genetic variation are oncology medications [4]. Two types of genetic variation, termed germline and somatic, have been recognized as contributing to drug response. Germline variants are present since conception essentially in all cells and can affect an enzyme's activity, a receptor to which a drug binds, or alter the probability of an immune reaction to a drug. Somatic variations are mutations that have arisen after birth in a subpopulation of cells; typically they refer to neoplastic cells and allow a provider to target chemotherapy medications based on the specific genetic makeup of an individual's cancer. Accordingly, the US Food and Drug Administration (FDA) now includes genetic biomarker data (germline or somatic) in drug labels for 167 medications [4], some of which have acquired "Black Box" status.

Genomic data are just one type of high dimensionality data that could potentially be incorporated into clinical care for purposes of drug prescribing. Other types of 'omic' data being pursued in research settings include the proteome, transcriptome, microbiome, or even clinical phenome that could be considered; however, none of these have yet reached the necessary level of evidence to incorporate into actionable clinical testing. Genomic data also present many of the same challenges that are seen with using other forms of -omic testing (such as large scale and naming schema that may not make the actionability clear) were they to become clinically actionable. For these reasons, we focus this chapter on the use of genomic information in building Clinical decision support systems (CDSS), primarily in the context of drug prescribing.

Growth in available genomic testing and knowledge combined with reductions in costs have led to increasing availability of genetic testing and the possibility of integration of genomic information within the EHR. Indeed, during an interview in 2009, Dr. Francis Collins, current Director of the National Institutes of Health (NIH), remarked on the potential of the inevitability of pharmacogenomic-based prescribing with genomic information embedded in the EHR [5]. However, translating the basic science knowledge of genetic variation's influence on drug response into clinical action is not trivial. The nomenclature of genomic variants can be confusing, the data are high dimensional, and the knowledge base changes frequently. Thus, it is an ideal application for clinical decision support (CDS). In this chapter, we will review the evidence for incorporating genomic information into drug prescribing and some of the challenges and successes in doing so.

12.1 Opportunities for Integration of -Omic Technologies into CDSS

Until recently, use of genetic and genomic information to guide care has largely been relegated to esoteric situations driven by experts in the field. These include specialized genetic tests, often by clinical geneticists, to aid in diagnosis of suspected conditions or prenatal screening. Arguably, because genetics experts usually interpret the results, CDSS may not be needed for diagnostic support (e.g., does the patient have cystic fibrosis) or prenatal screening. The types of interpretation and patient education needed require experts to interpret and relay the information, and the breadth of possible results and integration with clinical knowledge would go beyond the capabilities of most CDSS for many genetic disorders.

One of the earliest uses of genetics to guide drug therapy involves testing of thiopurine methyltransferase (TPMT) activity during thoipurine (e.g., azathioprine) therapy for cancers and autoimmune therapies. Since this medication is ordered by a select few types of physicians, there has arguably been less of a need for CDS to guide what to do for individuals with altered TPMT activity. However, it is interesting to note that while this is a fairly widely-known pharmacogenomics trait and taught routinely in medical schools, TPMT activity or genotype testing is not always ordered routinely before prescribing azathioprine, which suggests a potential need for CDS to remind clinicians to order the appropriate tests.

Knowledge about genomic biomarkers affecting drug efficacy or influencing drug response has increased dramatically in the last decade. Specific evidence is discussed more in the next section.

12.2 How Is Genomic Decision Support Different from Other Types of CDS?

Use of genomic information has a number of unique challenges compared to typical use cases for CDS, such as for drug-drug interactions, dose or drug adjustment based on biologic factors such as body surface area, concomitant medications, or kidney function. One of the most common forms of variants is single nucleotide polymorphisms, or SNPs, which indicate variation (inserted, deletion, or variation) at a single base pair. SNPs are typically identified by their "rsID" (e.g., rs2359612). The National Center for Biotechnology Information's dbSNP lists nearly 150 million human SNPs in build 144, points in which variation has been detected amongst the three billion base pairs in the human genome [6]. Other variations include copy number variants (CNVs), larger insertions or deletions, and translocations. The latter are arguably less commonly studied and less comprehensively understood.

Table 12.2 Summary of drug-gene guideline sources

Resource	Number of guidelines
Food and Drug Association http://www.fda.gov/drugs/scienceresearch/researchareas/pharmacogenetics/ucm083378.htm	158 Drug-variant pairs (105 germline, 42 somatic)
Clinical Pharmacogenetics Consortium (CPIC) https://www.pharmgkb.org/page/cpic	34 Drug-variant pairs (16 guidelines, 5 updates)
Evaluation of Genomic Applications in Practice and Prevention (EGAPP) http://www.egappreviews.org/	1 Drug class-gene pair

The FDA issues pharmacogenomic guidance through affected drug product labels. The locations of these alerts indicate the type, severity of the interaction, and level of recommendation. The pharmacogenomic biomarkers in drug labeling cover genomic biomarkers that describe: (1) drug exposure and clinical response variability, (2) risk for adverse events, (3) genotype-specific dosing, (4) mechanisms of drug action, and/or (5) polymorphic drug targets and disposition genes. Importantly, FDA pharmacogenomic guidance includes both germline and somatic variation. The most serious warnings are presented as "black box" warnings where: (1) the adverse reaction is so severe that the genetic variant must be considered to properly assess the risk or benefit of the drug, (2) a serious adverse reaction can be reduced in frequency or severity based on use of the genetic variation, or (3) FDA approved the drug based on the pharmacogenomic restriction to ensure safe use. A recent study of the FDA Table of Pharmacogenomic Biomarkers reviewed the 158 drug-gene pairs present in the table as of June 2014. Of the 108 germline drug-gene pairs listed at that time, 6 were subject to black box warnings [10]. The study interpreted the FDA guidance as requiring genetic testing for nine germline drug-gene pairs and recommending genetic testing for a further four pairs. As of September 2015, the count had risen to a total of 167 drug-gene pairs, 111 of which included germline variants. Of these germline variants, eight had black box warnings.

Established in 2009 to address the lack of clear, curated guidelines for germline pharmacogenomic interventions, CPIC developed procedures to evaluate the levels of evidence needed to implement pharmacogenomic interventions [11]. Importantly, CPIC guidelines are based on the assumption that genetic test results are already available to the physician and the guidelines only provide guidance on how to interpret those results to improve drug therapy. Thus, unlike certain FDA recommendations, guidelines produced by CPIC do not address whether a patient should be tested for the gene-drug interaction. Drug-gene interactions are chosen by CPIC for guideline development based on surveys of CPIC members, availability of clinical testing for the indicated genotype, the potential for alternate treatments, and/or the severity of consequences of ignoring the interaction. Once written, drug-gene interaction recommendations are subject to ongoing updates (typically every 2 years) consisting of literature review of newly published data as well as possible guideline modifications. Guidelines and their updates have been published in the journal *ClinicalPharmacologyand Therapeutics*, and are posted to the NIH Genetic Testing

Registry, the AHRQ National Guideline Clearinghouse and the Pharmacogenomic Knowledge Base (PharmGKB) website (www.pharmgkb.org). In addition to these human readable guidelines, there are efforts to translate all recommendations into computer readable formats for easier integration into clinical systems.

12.4 Who, What, and When to Test

Clinical use of these markers can be considered in two broad contexts. The first is "reactive" – genotyping for specific variants is undertaken in individual subjects at the point of care, and then acted on when the results become available. This is the most common type of testing pursued in medicine, including not just genomic interrogation but any testing done in response to an individual's changing clinical status (presentation of a new symptom, family member diagnosed with a new disease, etc.). In the case of genetic testing for drug response, the reactive approach is to test an individual when they are about to be prescribed a drug with a pharmacogenomic variant known to affect a drug's effect, so a provider tests for the variant before or concomitant with prescribing the medication. Ideally the first therapy prescribed would be the correct one, taking into account the results of genetic testing. However, this is not feasible in the case of medications needed acutely, such as following a myocardial infarction or anticoagulation for a thromboembolic event, given that genetic information generally takes at least a few days to return. Thus, in reactive testing, providers have three options: (1) wait to prescribe the medication until genetic test results are available, delaying therapy; (2) prescribe a standard of care therapy (exposing some fraction of the population to increased risk of harm) and then revise as necessary once genetic test results are returned; or (3) avoid the therapy requiring genetic guidance and start with an alternate therapy that does not need genetic testing. While option 3 may seem ideal in many circumstances, it is important to remember that the initial therapy was chosen for a reason – it may be cheaper, have better efficacy, be better tolerated, or be generally more trusted by the provider or in the marketplace. In fact, as shown in Hong Kong, option 3 has been observed in practice, with negative outcomes. After requiring HLA testing to prevent Stevens Johnson Syndrome, or SJS, before prescribing carbamazepine for epilepsy, the prescription rates of alternative antiepileptic drugs increased. However, since the adverse reactions to the alternative medications could not be averted via genetic testing, the overall population rate of SJS did not decrease despite eliminating SJS from carbamazepine, as cases of SJS from other antiepileptic drugs increased significantly [12].

An alternative testing strategy is preemptive, in which dense genotypic information is routinely stored in advanced electronic health record (EHR) systems, allowing genotype-based advice to be delivered to providers prior to or during prescribing. Preemptive genotyping is analogous to a screening test. Screening tests in medicine are performed for a wide variety of conditions in medicine that have high morbidity or mortality in the absence of early treatment. These conditions are effectively intervenable if diagnosed. When diagnostic screening tests perform well, they are cost-efficient and cause little harm. Examples of screening tests commonly performed in medicine include mammography for breast cancer, colonoscopy for colon cancer, and glucose testing for diabetes. These screening procedures have broadly established evidence bases and cost-effectiveness studies, unlike prospective pharmacogenomic testing. However, it can be argued that pharmacogenomic testing has little toxicity, costs relatively little [several hundred dollars for Clinical Laboratory Improvement Act (CLIA)-compliant testing], and may need to be performed only once for an individual, unlike many other screening tests.

An advantage of preemptive genetic testing is that the genetic information can be embedded in the individual's chart or EHR before such information is needed, so that the genotype-guided care can be the first therapy initiated, theoretically leading to better outcomes. This approach is dependent on the fact that one's genotype does not (generally) change over one's lifetime, such that once genotyped, that information can be used for many years. A disadvantage is that that genotypes needed for testing vary based on the drug one is to be prescribed. Fortunately, some pharmacogenomic variants influence multiple drugs, most commonly driven by cytochrome P450 and Human Leukocyte Antigen (HLA) variants. Thus, testing for a limited set of variants can cover many of the important variants determined by CPIC.

Another disadvantage of preemptive testing is the cost of testing. Schildcrout et al. studied 52,942 "medical home" patients (≥3 outpatient visits at Vanderbilt within 2 years) and found that 64.8 % were exposed to at least 1 of 57 medications with FDA pharmacogenomic guidance within 5 years, including 14 % having exposure to more than 4 of these medications over 5 years. Assuming reduction of risk of adverse events to baseline with alternative therapies, they estimated that, in this population over a 5-year period, implementation of pharmacogenomic testing could avert 383 serious adverse events such as myocardial infarction, warfarin-related bleeds, and myelosuppression [13].

12.5 Types of CDS Useful for Genomic Medicine

The three major types of CDS implementation methods include active, passive, and surveillance methods.

12.5.1 Passive Decision Support

Passive decision support amounts to providing education for providers and patients. Such efforts involve creation of human-readable documents and straightforward action steps for providers to follow when they prescribe medications where the patients' response is influenced by genetic factors. This process can be very effective for medications prescribed by a select group of providers knowledgeable about the drug-genome interactions, such as the TMPT/thiopurine example above, or for genetic tests done for diagnostic support. Chemotherapeutics for cancer are another example, in which often a provider (or team of providers) orders a complex battery of tests, which increasingly includes somatic variants in the cancer, before deciding on a therapy plan. A human-readable interpretation (e.g., as a static, non-computable document) of genetic testing can effectively guide therapy for such cases.

12.5.2 Active Decision Support

Active decision support is a process that monitors provider activity and then actively advises the provider toward a path based on actionable information. It can be either synchronous or asynchronous. Synchronous CDS describes a workflow in which a clinician order, such as prescribing a medication, is monitored in real-time by rules embedded within the EHR, and clinician behavior is influenced when the rule is triggered. The most widely recognized approach is an alert window warning the user of a potentially risky order, such as an allergy or severe drug-drug interaction. Active decision support modules can contain both interpretation and advice (as would passive CDS) but active decision support has the added value of happening during the workflow and linking to actionable decisions, such as suggesting alternative therapies or doses. For genetic examples, this would involve taking into account the drug being prescribed, the genetic variants, and applying a rule to yield a recommendation. Since most examples in pharmacogenetics known to date involve genetic variants present in a minority of the population yielding increased risk of an ADE, most individuals would not need altering from typical therapies based on genetics. Thus, in many cases, active synchronous CDS may be invisible to the provider during the ordering process, and would only intervene on those individuals with the genetic variant.

Active CDS can also be deployed asynchronously, though this is less common. An example could be a system that evaluates for possible drug-drug interactions or gene-drug interactions in batch (e.g., once nightly) and delivers a clinical communication to a provider of a possible interaction. It can also suggest alternatives and would have the potential to provide a direct, actionable alternative suggestion. This model, however, may be desirable for lab results that are delivered after the medication is prescribed. Such decision support has been successfully applied when a medication that should take into account renal function has been prescribed. The CDS may suggest dosing changes when the lab results documenting an individual's kidney function are returned [14].

12.5.3 Surveillance Decision Support Mechanisms

In contrast to active decision support mechanisms, surveillance systems are designed to provide centrally-monitored "dashboards" for monitoring and managing something intervenable, such as drug dosing. One example of surveillance systems commonly used includes the anticoagulant warfarin, which can be implemented via a combination of human, workflow, and electronic means. In this chapter, we focus on electronic means for centralized decision support and surveillance of targeted drug-outcomes.

Surveillance systems have been used for germline genomic decision support at Vanderbilt University Medical Center [15]. Individuals with high-risk genotypes can be viewed as panels and their most recent medication lists searched for target medications to see if these individuals were still on these medications. These potential drug-genome interactions are reviewed by pharmacists, who contact each patient's provider for possible change in drug therapy according to genomic guidance. This type of CDS is important for individuals whose results are returned after an interacting medication is prescribed, especially so for tests ordered during acute events by non-primary providers (e.g., hospitalization for acute myocardial infarction for which *CYP2C19* testing was ordered to tailor antiplatelet therapy).

12.6 Standardized Representation of Genetic Variation

For genomic data to be actionable as inputs into a CDSS, they must be represented in computable forms in the EHR. Genotyping patients on a multiplexed panel generates a large set of potentially actionable genomic results that have persistent relevance over a patient's lifetime. Currently, systems that are using genomic CDS have typically represented their genomic results in the EHR in a variety of locally-developed, locally-computable formats [16–19]. Creating a portable version of results that can be shared across electronic medical records is a high priority for implementation of genomic medicine or any health analytics task that relies on uniform specification of genomic variation across EHRs. Standard representation of genetic results will also be important for broader adoption of genomic CDSS and to allow interaction of genomic data with a variety of systems.

Health Level Seven (HL7) has created a specification for genomic variation that leverages existing nomenclature standards for variant identification such as the HUGO Gene Nomenclature Committee (HGNC; http://www.genenames.org), Human Genome Variation Society (HGVS; http://www.hgvs.org), and the RefSeq ID (http://www.ncbi.nlm.nih.gov/refseq/). Additionally, it allows stipulation of brief coded interpretative phenotype text such as "poor metabolizer" using a controlled set of descriptors from the Logical Observation Identifiers Names and Codes (LOINC) vocabulary. The standard is focused on coding genetic test results from genotyping technologies where variants from a reference standard are defined as opposed to raw sequence data. HL7 has released an implementation guide to generate messages on version 2.5.1 of the parent HL7 messaging standard. The clinical genomics standard is sufficiently robust to support interpretations at the allele (e.g., *CYP2C19**2) and gene (e.g., *CYP2C19*) level, and can describe in a single message a phenotype based on the combined impact of multiple gene effects. Such is the case with warfarin sensitivity, which is based on both *CYP2C9* and *VKORC1* variation. However, some common pharmacogene interpretation terms are not currently present in LOINC, such as the phenotypes of variants in *SLCO1B1*, which affect hepatic uptake of most statins and are known to be associated with simvastatin toxicity [20]. Additionally, momentum is building for newer standards to feature standard representations of genetic variation, such as the Fast Healthcare Interoperability Resource (FHIR) [21].

Direct support of clinical genomics standards from laboratory information systems and EHR vendors would accelerate the communication and interoperable use of interpreted genotype and sequencing results. Similar standards could be applied to family history and pedigree data as well. Currently, there are a number of systems that will structure family history/pedigree data in computable formats. The MyTree system, which is the focus of one of the grants in the Implementing Genomics in Practice (IGNITE) Network, [22] has been developed to be a consumer of FHIR information to receive EHR data in a standard format, though structured return of family history/pedigree data into the EHR has not yet been standardized.

12.7 CDS Knowledge Bases

Traditionally, clinical decision support content is developed by institutions or knowledge vendors and delivered by EHR vendors after undergoing extensive local customization. The scale and complexity of genomic medicine highlights the difficulty of recreating the rule set for every health system looking to implement across an enterprise. Several prior efforts within clinical decision support have aimed to publically standardize rule sets encouraging dissemination. A recent effort by two genomic medicine consortia, Electronic Medical Records and Genomics (eMERGE) and IGNITE, aims to collect local versions of genomic CDS and the design documents that were created during the course of implementation. The implementation 'artifacts' generated by consortia members have traditionally not been published or shared and include algorithms or logic, genotype to phenotype maps, optimizations of clinical workflow, design of clinician and physician facing user interfaces, and design or presentation of patient and provider communications.

A working version of the Clinical Decision Support Knowledge Base (CDS-KB, hosted at http://cdskb.org) has gathered a preliminary set of knowledge artifacts from academic medical centers and integrated health systems that have piloted genomic medicine programs. The site is supported through grants given by the National Human Genome Research Institute (NHGRI). The artifacts on the site are stored, indexed, and disseminated by the site. In addition, the site facilitates exchanges and discussions between implementers across institutions and features a monthly educational webinar. While the majority of artifacts currently hosted represent a pharmacogenomics scenario given the accumulated years of experience within this domain, a few examples of CDS created for germline variation predicting disease state are included as well (such as *BRCA1* mutations and breast cancer or *APOL1* variants and kidney disease). The site is part of a larger effort being pursued by IGNITE and eMERGE to develop tools to help implement genomic medicine.

12.8 Examples of Genomic CDS in Practice

Pharmacogenomic testing to guide drug prescribing, often through use of complex CDS interfaces, has increased dramatically over the last 5 years. Sarkar identified genomic medicine clinical implementation efforts as one of the major recent informatics developments in his 2012 International Medical Informatics Association Yearbook Survey [23]. He noted only two clinical pharmacogenomics programs at that time: the Vanderbilt Pharmacogenomic Resource for Enhanced Decisions in Care & Treatment (PREDICT) [17] and a similar effort targeted for the pediatric cancer population at St. Jude Children's Research Hospital [16]. Figure 12.1 shows

Drug-Genome Advisor
Intermediate Metabolizer - clopidogrel (Plavix) - Rare Risk Allele
Substitution recommended due to increased cardiovascular risks

If not otherwise contraindicated:

☐ Prescribe prasugrel (Effient) 10 mg daily

Prasugrel should not be given to patients:
- history of stroke or transient ischemic attack
- >= 75 years of age [Current patient age: 51]
- with body weight < 60 kg [Current patient weight: 59.0 kg as of 10/12/2012]

☐ Prescribe ticagrelor (Brilinta) 90 mg twice daily

Ticagrelor should not be given to patients:
- history of severe hepatic impairment
- intracranial bleed

☑ Continue with clopidogrel (Plavix) prescription

Primary override reason:

☐ Contraindicated for prasugrel or ticagrelor
☐ Potential side effects
☐ Provider/Patient opts for clopidogrel
☐ Cost

Evidence Link

This patient has been tested for CYP2C19 variants which has identified the presence of one copy of a rare risk allele which is associated with intermediate metabolism of clopidogrel. Intermediate metabolizers treated with clopidogrel at normal doses are associated with higher rates of stent thrombosis and other cardiovascular events. The Vanderbilt P&T Committee recommends that prasugrel or ticagelor replace clopidogrel for poor metabolizers unless contraindicated. If not feasible, maintain standard dose of clopidogrel. The guidelines above were developed based on the outcome studies of patients who received a drug-eluting stent into a coronary artery. However, there is not a national consensus on drug/dose guidance particularly associated with the population possessing extremely rare genetic variants.

Continue Cancel

Fig. 12.1 Decision support for clopidogrel guidance as part of the Vanderbilt PREDICT program

a screenshot of a PREDICT CDS alert. Both of these efforts employed multiplexed genotyping assays to evaluate common pharmacokinetic and pharmacodynamic variants for germline variants affecting commonly prescribed drugs. To do so, both placed interpreted genetic results within the EHR in a structured format. A number of academic programs using genetic testing to guide care have since gotten underway. The University of Chicago is enrolling about 1,200 patients from 12 preselected physicians for prospective genetic testing [24]. Information on genetic variants is provided through a custom web interface that displays summarized phenotype information. The University of Florida/Shands Hospital's Personalized Medicine Program is testing individuals undergoing cardiac catheterization to genetically-guide clopidogrel prescribing [18]. They have since expanded to include other drug-genome interactions.

Each of the eMERGE Network sites developed systems to integrate genomic information within their EHR to guide prescribing. Specifically, the eMERGE-PGx project involved testing patients at pediatric and adult sites using a custom sequencing platform that investigated 84 pharmacogenes, with clinical validation and EHR implementation of select actionable variants. eMERGE sites have pursued a variety of genomic CDS implementation projects by leveraging either communicating with the EHR, infobutton technologies, or custom EHR solutions [25, 26]. In each of these solutions, a common theme of those with dense genomic information is a separate repository linked to the EHR, with actionable genomic information inserted into the EHR is computable formats (Fig. 12.2) [27, 28].

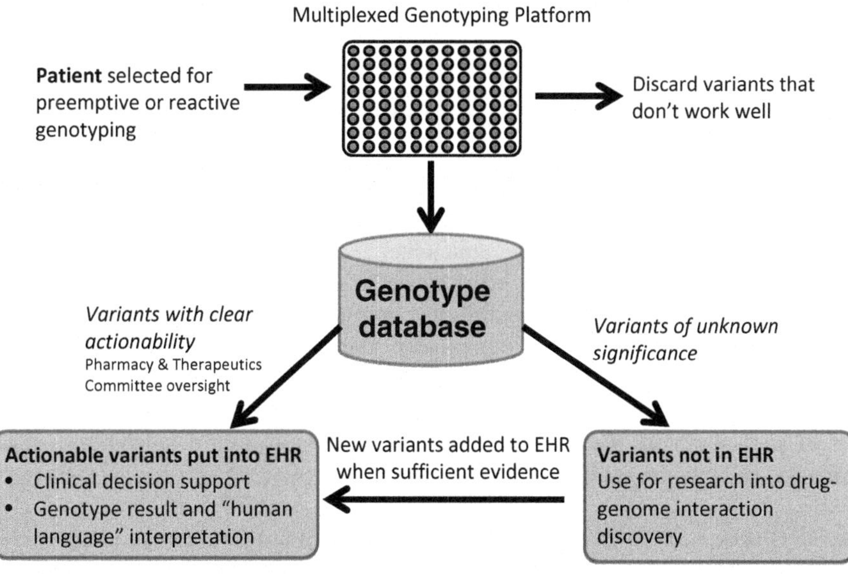

Fig. 12.2 Schematic for testing and storage of genetic variants in multiplexed testing (Adapted from Denny [27])

Although the use cases for somatic variation driving precision cancer care are becoming increasingly common, fewer systems have integrated somatic variant testing into CDSS. Typically, cancer genetic testing is performed by reference labs, which return results as documents containing non-computable information. One such example of computable variant information returned into the EHR is the Personalized Cancer Medicine Initiative [29] project, which includes structured somatic mutation testing with links to the MyCancerGenome website. The website serves as a central repository of cancer genetic variants, their interpretation, and relevant clinical trials. Thus, a provider looking at a given patient's cancer testing results can quickly discover the relevance of their genetic variants and can find out if there were open clinical trials for which the patient might be eligible. This report structure is a type of passive CDS. The authors are not aware of active CDSS that have been implemented based on somatic mutations.

In 2012, NHGRI funded the IGNITE network to integrate genomic information into EHRs and develop genomic clinical decision support at sites beyond large academic hospitals [22]. IGNITE consists of six member projects. Three of these projects are pursing pharmacogenomics, two others genome-based disease care, and another a computable family history module. Many of these sites are implementing genomic medicine across many sites. Duke University's Family History project is implementing within 28 primary care clinics across 5 different health systems. The Integrated, Individualized, and Intelligent Prescribing (I^{3}P) Network will be implementing germline and somatic pharmacogenomics in five different health systems. The Sanford Health System in the Dakotas, part of IGNITE, represents a large non-academic health system that has implemented genomic CDSS for a variety of medications (Fig. 12.3) [30].

12.9 Direct-to-Consumer Genetic Testing

Direct-to-consumer (DTC) genetic testing provides an avenue for patients to pursue genetic testing without requiring a doctor's order. Although initially there were several companies offering DTC genomic testing, 23andMe (Mountain View, CA) is the only major company still offering dense genomic testing to the public without requiring physician orders. 23andMe has currently tested more than one million individuals, and provides information to consumers on a consumer-friendly website that allows individuals to explore traits and ancestry information based on their genetic testing, which is performed on a high-density genotyping array performed in a CLIA laboratory. These personalized results initially also included health information, such as the individual's genetic risk for a number of diseases and some advice on pharmacogenomics, including warfarin sensitivity and clopidogrel efficacy. However, in November of 2013, the Food and Drug Administration ordered 23andMe to stop providing clinical guidance for genetic test results, citing "potential health consequences that could result from false positive or false negative assessments" [31]. As a result, 23andMe stopped providing disease risk and drug

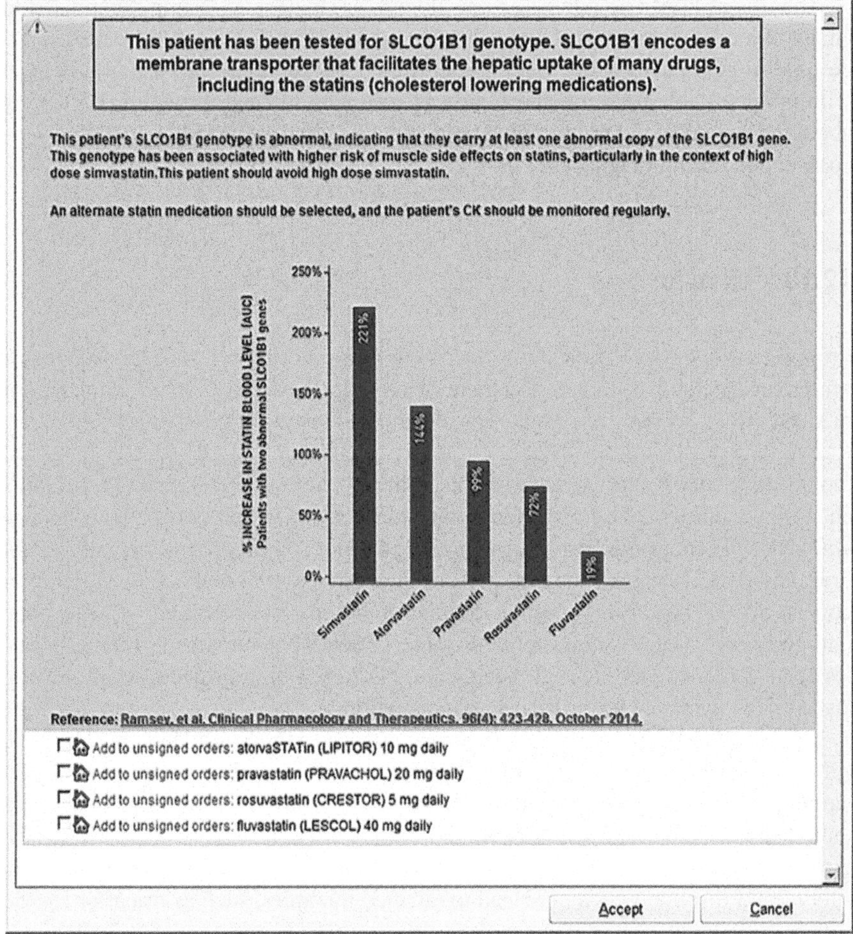

Fig. 12.3 Automated statin advisor implementing in an Epic environment. (Reprinted from Larson and Wilke [30], Copyright 2015, with permission from Elsevier)

response information to new enrollees, though such information remains available to prior enrollees at the time of this writing. In February 2015, 23andMe obtained FDA approval to release clinical information on Bloom syndrome carrier status, a rare Mendelian disease, as a first return to providing clinical data back to patients [32]. In addition, 23andMe offers the ability for customers to download, in bulk, their genome-wide genetic data, which include hundreds of thousands of variants. Thus, a particular savvy consumer (regardless of timing with respect to the FDA ruling) could go to 23andMe and download their genetic data and find and use the genetic data relevant to particular drugs (e.g., specific alleles at rs9923231 and warfarin sensitivity).

There is at least one published anecdote of DTC genetic testing being used to change care. Tenenbaum et al. described a model for how DTC genetic testing could be used to guide care with clinical input [33]. They reported the case of a woman with unremarkable personal and family history who learned through DTC testing about the presence of a prothrombin gene mutation, and as a result, underwent anticoagulation during pregnancy.

12.10 Conclusions

From the early days of clinical informatics to support order entry, CDS has been an important mechanism to effect change in provider behavior toward avoidance of medical errors, adherence to standards of care, and faster adoption of best practices. Researchers have leveraged CDS to not only enhance provider prescribing and monitoring, but also to engage multidisciplinary teams and to monitor a patient's changing conditions. Use of genomic information in CDS provides a new, but not altogether different, modality to enhance a provider's ability to prescribe the right drug at the right dose, at the first prescription. An exciting realization of pharmacogenomics is the shrinking of the domain of "idiopathic" reactions as some once unpredictable reactions become predictable. Much work remains to realize seamless genomic medicine through healthcare, but initial pilot projects are promising and provide guidance for broader implementation.

On January 20, 2015, President Obama announced a Precision Medicine Initiative (PMI), which has two major arms: precision cancer therapy and the creation of a natural, longitudinal cohort of more than one million individuals who will share their health data and biospecimens for research. One of the envisioned use cases for the PMI cohort initiative is study of pharmacogenomics and genetically-defined subtypes of disease, which may lead to targeted therapies, such as ivacaftor for the subset of cystic fibrosis patients with a particular CFTR mutation [34]. Individuals in the PMI cohort will receive genetic testing over time, which will include biomarkers of disease response (including but not limited to dense genomic investigation). A goal of the resource is that individuals will have access to their own data, and if they have genetic testing on relevant biomarkers, participants in the initiative could become advocates for use of their genomic data in prescribing. Similarly, the precision cancer therapy initiative will seek new knowledge for genomically-driven (as opposed to histologically-driven) cancer therapy. Both of these initiatives foreshadow a future with potential for dramatic growth in the opportunities for genomically-tailored care. Patients may catalyze the growth in use of these new classes of information, such as genetics, to guide their care. In order to achieve these goals, we will need adoption of EHRs capable of genomic decision support, agreed-upon standards for genomic representation, processes to maintain and update knowledge bases and CDSS, and report interpretations that are easily understood by both providers and patients.

References

1. McCormack M, et al. HLA-A*3101 and carbamazepine-induced hypersensitivity reactions in Europeans. N Engl J Med. 2011;364:1134–43.
2. Daly AK, et al. HLA-B*5701 genotype is a major determinant of drug-induced liver injury due to flucloxacillin. Nat Genet. 2009;41:816–9.
3. Shuldiner AR, et al. Association of cytochrome P450 2C19 genotype with the antiplatelet effect and clinical efficacy of clopidogrel therapy. JAMA. 2009;302:849–57.
4. Pharmacogenomic biomarkers in drug labels. At <http://www.fda.gov/Drugs/ScienceResearch/ResearchAreas/Pharmacogenetics/ucm083378.htm>.
5. Collins F. Opportunities and challenges for the NIH – an interview with Francis Collins. Interview by Robert Steinbrook. N Engl J Med. 2009;361:1321–3.
6. dbSNP Summary. At <http://www.ncbi.nlm.nih.gov/SNP/snp_summary.cgi?view+summary=view+summary&build_id=144>.
7. DNA Sequencing Costs. At http://www.genome.gov/sequencingcosts/.
8. Ramirez AH, et al. Predicting warfarin dosage in European-Americans and African-Americans using DNA samples linked to an electronic health record. Pharmacogenomics. 2012;13:407–18.
9. Relling MV, Klein TE. CPIC: Clinical pharmacogenetics implementation consortium of the pharmacogenomics research network. Clin Pharmacol Ther. 2011;89:464–7.
10. Vivot A, Boutron I, Ravaud P, Porcher R. Guidance for pharmacogenomic biomarker testing in labels of FDA-approved drugs. Genet Med Off J Am Coll Med Genet. 2015;17:733–8.
11. Caudle KE, et al. Incorporation of pharmacogenomics into routine clinical practice: the Clinical Pharmacogenetics Implementation Consortium (CPIC) guideline development process. Curr Drug Metab. 2014;15:209–17.
12. Chen Z, Liew D, Kwan P. Effects of a HLA-B*15:02 screening policy on antiepileptic drug use and severe skin reactions. Neurology. 2014;83:2077–84.
13. Schildcrout JS, et al. Optimizing drug outcomes through pharmacogenetics: a case for preemptive genotyping. Clin Pharmacol Ther. 2012;92:235–42.
14. McCoy AB, et al. A computerized provider order entry intervention for medication safety during acute kidney injury: a quality improvement report. Am J Kidney Dis Off J Natl Kidney Found. 2010;56:832–41.
15. Peterson JF, et al. Electronic health record design and implementation for pharmacogenomics: a local perspective. Genet Med Off J Am Coll Med Genet. 2013;15:833–41.
16. Hicks JK, et al. A clinician-driven automated system for integration of pharmacogenetic interpretations into an electronic medical record. Clin Pharmacol Ther. 2012;92:563–6.
17. Pulley JM, et al. Operational implementation of prospective genotyping for personalized medicine: the design of the Vanderbilt PREDICT project. Clin Pharmacol Ther. 2012;92:87–95.
18. Johnson JA, et al. Institutional profile: University of Florida and Shands Hospital Personalized Medicine Program: clinical implementation of pharmacogenetics. Pharmacogenomics. 2013;14:723–6.
19. Rasmussen-Torvik LJ, et al. Design and anticipated outcomes of the eMERGE-PGx project: a multicenter pilot for preemptive pharmacogenomics in electronic health record systems. Clin Pharmacol Ther. 2014. doi:10.1038/clpt.2014.137.
20. Link E, et al. SLCO1B1 variants and statin-induced myopathy – a genomewide study. N Engl J Med. 2008;359:789–99.
21. Alterovitz G, et al. SMART on FHIR Genomics: facilitating standardized clinico-genomic apps. J Am Med Inf Assoc. 2015;22(6):1173–8. doi:10.1093/jamia/ocv045. ocv045.
22. Implementing Genomics in Practice (IGNITE). At http://www.genome.gov/27554264.
23. Sarkar IN. Bringing genome tests into clinical practice. Yearb Med Inform. 2013;8:172–4.
24. O'Donnell PH, et al. The 1200 patients project: creating a new medical model system for clinical implementation of pharmacogenomics. Clin Pharmacol Ther. 2012;92:446–9.

25. Gottesman O, et al. The CLIPMERGE PGx Program: clinical implementation of personalized medicine through electronic health records and genomics-pharmacogenomics. Clin Pharmacol Ther. 2013;94:214–7.
26. Overby CL, et al. A template for authoring and adapting genomic medicine content in the eMERGE Infobutton project. AMIA Annu Symp Proc AMIA Symp. 2014;2014:944–53.
27. Denny JC. Surveying recent themes in translational bioinformatics: big data in EHRs, omics for drugs, and personal genomics. Yearb Med Inform. 2014;9:199–205.
28. Starren J, Williams MS, Bottinger EP. Crossing the omic chasm: a time for omic ancillary systems. JAMA. 2013;309:1237–8.
29. Lovly CM, et al. Routine multiplex mutational profiling of melanomas enables enrollment in genotype-driven therapeutic trials. PLoS One. 2012;7:e35309.
30. Larson EA, Wilke RA. Integration of genomics in primary care. Am J Med. 2015. At http://www.sciencedirect.com/science/article/pii/S0002934315004520.
31. 2013 – 23andMe, Inc. 11/22/13. At http://www.fda.gov/ICECI/EnforcementActions/WarningLetters/2013/ucm376296.htm.
32. Press Announcements > FDA permits marketing of first direct-to-consumer genetic carrier test for Bloom syndrome. At http://www.fda.gov/NewsEvents/Newsroom/PressAnnouncements/UCM435003.
33. Tenenbaum J, James A, Paulyson-Nuñez K. An altered treatment plan based on Direct to Consumer (DTC) genetic testing: personalized medicine from the patient/pin-cushion perspective. J Pers Med. 2012;2:192–200.
34. Solomon GM, Marshall SG, Ramsey BW, Rowe SM. Breakthrough therapies: cystic fibrosis (CF) potentiators and correctors. Pediatr Pulmonol. 2015. doi:10.1002/ppul.23240.

Chapter 13
Clinical Decision Support: The Experience at Brigham and Women's Hospital/Partners HealthCare

Paul Varghese, Adam Wright, Jan Marie Andersen, Eileen I. Yoshida, and David W. Bates

Abstract In this chapter, we review clinical decision support systems (CDSS) at Brigham and Women's Hospital (BWH), including design, implementation, and evaluation. BWH has over 40 years active experience in the development of clinical information systems. Here we focus specifically on BWH's work in assessing the impact of CDSS in critical areas of patient safety, quality, and cost outcomes, and offer generalizable lessons for current and future applications of CDSS. CDSS examined include both inpatient and outpatient systems, medication related, laboratory and radiology decision support as well as documentation-related CDSS, clinical reminders, and patient-centric applications. Also included are descriptions of studies on the impact on the user and cost-effectiveness of CDSS.

Keywords Clinical decision support • Brigham and Women's Hospital • Partners healthcare • Clinical reminders • Patient-centric • Cost-effectiveness

---

P. Varghese, M.D. • A. Wright, M.S., Ph.D. (✉) • D.W. Bates, M.D., M.Sc.
Clinical and Quality Analysis, Information Systems, Partners HealthCare System, Inc., 93 Worcester Street, Suite 201, Wellesley, MA 02481, USA

Division of General Internal Medicine and Primary Care, Brigham and Women's Hospital, 1620 Tremont Street - OBC-3, Boston, MA 02120, USA

Department of Medicine, Harvard Medical School, 75 Francis Street, Boston, MA 02115, USA
e-mail: paul_varghese@hms.harvard.edu; awright@bwh.harvard.edu; dbates@partners.org

J.M. Andersen, M.A.
Clinical and Quality Analysis, Information Systems, Partners HealthCare System, Inc., 93 Worcester Street, Suite 201, Wellesley, MA 02481, USA

Division of General Internal Medicine and Primary Care, Brigham and Women's Hospital, 1620 Tremont Street - OBC-3, Boston, MA 02120, USA
e-mail: jmandersen@partners.org

E.I. Yoshida, B.Sc.Phm., M.B.A.
Partners eCare, Partners Healthcare System Inc., 93 Worcester Street, Wellesley, MA 02481, USA
e-mail: eyoshida1@partners.org

E.S. Berner (ed.), *Clinical Decision Support Systems*, Health Informatics, DOI 10.1007/978-3-319-31913-1_13

13.1 Background

Located in Boston, MA and with origins dating to 1832, BWH is a non-profit 793-bed facility, providing clinical practice ranging from primary care to tertiary/quaternary care. In 2014, BWH had approximately 46,000 inpatient admissions, over 4.2 million patient visits and 59,000 emergency department visits. In 1994, BWH joined with the Massachusetts General Hospital (MGH) to found Partners HealthCare System, which in 20 years has grown to include nine hospitals and five community health centers as well as a managed care organization and physician network [1].

A major teaching hospital for Harvard Medical School, BWH has done leading research in clinical medicine, population health, and health services research and this has directly shaped its approach in implementing and evaluating health information technology (HIT), particularly with clinical information systems for computerized provider order entry (CPOE) and Clinical Decision Support (CDS).

The key systems developed and deployed are the *Brigham Integrated Computing System* (*BICS*) and the *Longitudinal Medical Record* (*LMR*), both of which have been in use at BWH for close to 20 years. In this chapter, we review clinical decision support systems (CDSS) at BWH, including design, implementation, and evaluation.

13.1.1 Brigham Integrated Computing System (BICS)

In 1984, BWH initiated development of its clinical information system, the Brigham Integrated Computing System (BICS). Richard Nesson, MD, CEO of BWH at the time, had previously been instrumental in one of the first implementations of an automated medical record system (COSTAR) to support patient care, quality assurance and billing at Harvard Community Health Plan [2]. With this formative influence, BWH leadership moved to build upon technology developed at neighboring Boston hospitals to further improve quality of care and patient safety.

The predecessor to BICS began in 1976 as a direct port of the clinical information system created by Howard Bleich, MD and Warner Slack, MD, at the then Beth Israel Hospital in Boston [3]. Based upon a MUMPS database (a development of the Laboratory of Computer Science at MGH) and utilizing client-server architecture, BICS initially provided review access to clinical reports including lab values, imaging and pathology reports. However, the central vision of BICS was well-established from its inception: transition information systems from being a passive repository of clinical data to playing an active role contributing to improved quality of care and reduction of both adverse events and cost [1].

To fulfill this objective, BICS was expanded to include sophisticated order entry, under the leadership of John Glaser, PhD, BWH's chief information officer and Jonathan Teich, MD, PhD, the system's lead architect. The BICS design philosophy emphasized: (1) *broad content* using coded/structured information (building the root data for alerts and recommendations); (2) *workflow support*, where screens display relevant contextual data useful to a particular clinical scenario; (3) *clinical decision support*, providing appropriate interventions to modify current processes of care; (4) *efficient communication*, to bring to disparate care team members urgent data reflected in real-time display; (5) *education*, so clinicians have context for CDS recommended interventions; and (6) *added value*, where advanced services provide users with greater efficiency and satisfaction [1].

Later expansion of features included: alerts for panic-value labs (1991); automatic email notifications of a patient's emergency department visits to a primary care provider (1992); and a clinical reference system ("Handbook") (1992). To improve transitions of care, BICS incorporated both cross-coverage lists (continuously tracking relationship between provider coverage and patients) and automatically generating sign-out communications (1993) [1].

In 1993–1994, two significant developments set the foundation for the long-term success of BICS: the introduction of CPOE within BICS, providing a substrate to influence treatment plans at the time of creation through decision support; and deployment of a flexible, configurable rule-based Event Engine, which provided a platform for monitoring data in real time and notifying physicians [1].

CPOE used a text-mode interface with structured windows. Screens were designed specifically for each type of order, and were often enhanced with relevant clinical information. For example, a digoxin order screen presented the physician with the latest renal function values, serum potassium value and digoxin level; blood product orders displayed transfusion restrictions and results of last cross-match. In 1995, order sets, starting with chemotherapy, were deployed [1].

The Event Engine system was created for the purpose of detecting important events, testing them for importance to the patient, and rapidly conveying enough information to the caregiver that swift action could be taken in response. This was made possible by the combination of a logic-triggering system which detected new clinical data which might trigger a rule, a dispatcher which directed the data to the proper logic, an inference engine which evaluates logic states defined using a collection of standard logic primitives, a notification system to quickly contact clinicians (by text page or alert), and an action-item processor which made taking action on alerts straightforward [1].

With these functions in place, BICS had the essential elements as a platform for successful CDSS, allowing for the steady expansion of functionality and remaining in continuous use for over 20 years, with transitions from Visual Basic front end to a full Windows environment. BICS received Office of the National Coordinator-Authorized Certification Body (ONC-ACB) certification in 2014.

Of note, BICS was designed for use in both the inpatient and ambulatory settings, with BICS ambulatory record module ("MiniAmb") implemented in 1990. MiniAmb contained problem lists, medications, allergies, vital signs and progress notes (free text entry or transcription from dictation), along with a health maintenance section which organized key data, including cholesterol values and Pap smear results to support management [1].

With the creation of Partners HealthCare, the founding hospitals of BWH and MGH confronted the challenge of unifying different clinical information systems.

Each hospital would continue with its own inpatient information systems, but would adopt a common ambulatory medical record, built upon the success of MiniAmb and called the Longitudinal Medical Record (LMR).

13.1.2 Longitudinal Medical Record (LMR)

The Longitudinal Medical Record (LMR) was implemented in 1997 as a full-featured electronic health record (EHR) in all Partners HealthCare ambulatory settings. The LMR includes notes for primary care and subspecialties, coded and uncoded problem lists, medication lists, coded allergies and results from laboratory tests and radiographic studies (drawn from a Partners-wide clinical data repository). The LMR provides facilities for e-prescribing and radiology ordering; however direct laboratory order entry is not supported. As described by Linder et al. the LMR implements a wide range of CDS, including "reminders for preventive services and chronic care management; medication monitoring; medication dosing alerts and medication alerts for drug-drug, drug-lab, and drug-condition and drug-allergy interactions" [4]. The LMR also has a registry and quality management function, which provides panel management tools which draw from a data warehouse [4].

The LMR, now web-based, was first certified by the Certification Commission for Healthcare Information Technology (CCHIT) as a complete ambulatory EHR in 2007, with subsequent ONC-ACB certifications in 2014 (see Fig. 13.1 for a screenshot from the LMR).

Since the initial implementation of BICS and the LMR, BWH has been motivated by the belief that CDSS via EHRs are the means to improved performance in a wide range of patient care domains: clinical outcomes, utilization and performance measures, and in particular, patient safety. What follows next are the salient observations from a series of studies evaluating CDSS impact in these areas, focused in the inpatient and ambulatory settings.

13.2 Clinical Decision Support: Inpatient Applications and Assessment

13.2.1 Medication-Related Decision Support

General Applications

BICS supports medication ordering and was designed to reduce errors and encourage appropriate and cost-effective ordering. Interventions at appropriate points during the ordering process display warnings, reminders, and/or suggested alternatives related to the ordered medication [5].

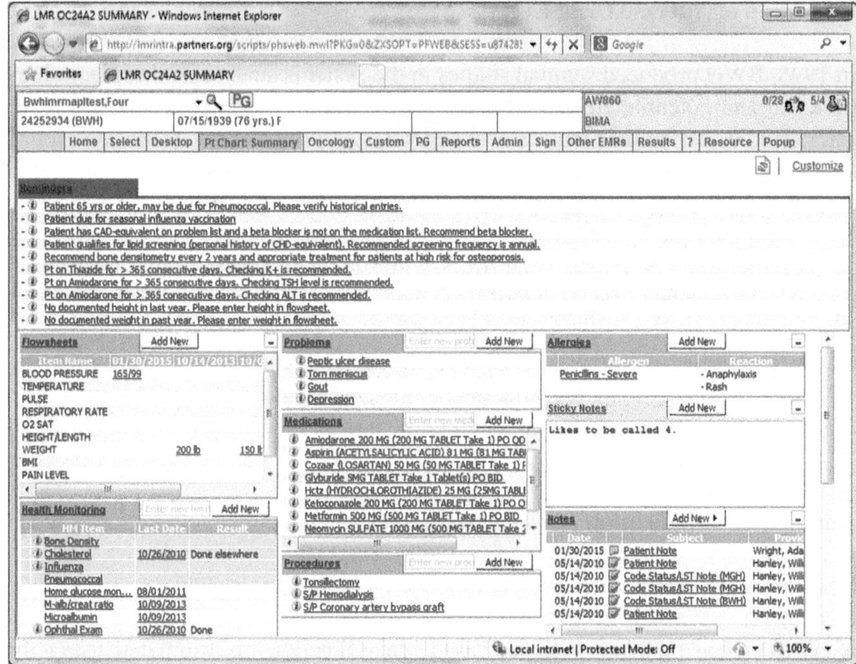

Fig. 13.1 Screenshot of LMR

When ordering a medication for a patient, the system suggests a patient-specific dose and frequency of medication to the prescriber. In addition, common CDS features such as drug-allergy, drug-drug interactions, duplicate medications, and possible alternative medications for the given clinical situation are also presented. All of these CDS tools have been developed using a process of iterative refinement [5].

After an initial order, consequent order recommendations are triggered which alert the physician to possible additional orders that should follow. For example, after a patient is placed on bed rest, BICS checks for preexisting heparin orders and, if none are found, BICS will suggest that an order be placed for subcutaneous heparin to prevent deep vein thrombosis [5].

Evaluation of medication-related interventions showed positive impact on medication selection (improvement in the use of lower-cost histamine$_2$-blocking agents); dosage guidance (reduction in dosages exceeding highest recommended dose for all medications); frequency recommendations (increase in ondansetron TID vs. QID dosing); and consequent orders (a doubling of heparin orders placed in conjunction with bed rest orders) [5].

Reduction of Adverse Drug Events

In 1995, BWH produced seminal studies in the systems analysis and epidemiology of actual and potential adverse drug events (ADEs) in hospitalized patients [6,7]. These studies determined that 42 % of serious or life-threatening ADEs were found to be preventable, with 52 % of these occurring at the ordering stage. A consequence of these results was a sharp focus on using and evaluating BICS as a means of reducing the frequency of ADEs.

An initial study established that BICS, with simple medication-ordering decision support (drug names from standard lists, default drug dosages, and limited checks for drug-allergy, drug-drug and drug-laboratory interactions), reduced serious ADEs by 55 % [8]. A follow-up study, which was performed after iterative improvement of drug-allergy and drug-drug interaction checking, showed an 88 % reduction of serious ADEs and an 81 % reduction in the overall medication error rate [9].

Anticipatory Medication Decision Support

In 1996, BWH implemented a CDS module (Nephros) to provide dosing recommendations for a subset of drugs which are renally cleared or nephrotoxic. In Nephros, when patients with decreased renal function (as estimated using the Cockcroft-Gault equation), are prescribed these potentially dangerous medications, a recommendation of a modified dose list (dose and frequency) is triggered and/or a recommendation of an alternative medication. When studied in a controlled trial, this functionality was found to increase the rate of appropriate prescriptions (59 % vs. 35 %) in patients with impaired renal function, and to decrease a patient's length of stay (4.3 vs. 4.5 days) [10].

Subsequently, a companion CDS module (Gerios) was developed to deliver evidence-based prescribing recommendations for psychotropic medications in hospitalized geriatric patients (age >65), with the goal of better drug selection and reduction in initial dosing where appropriate. For these medications, a modified dose list (dose and frequency) is presented and/or an alternative medication is recommended. In addition, in elderly patients with decreased renal function, who are prescribed a medication listed in both knowledge bases, the Nephros and Gerios CDSS work together and will only present one recommendation to the user.

In a controlled trial, orders written for patients in the cohort receiving the recommendations were (1) more likely to be at the recommended daily dose (29 % vs. 19 %), (2) less likely to have a tenfold misdose (2.8 % vs. 5.0 %), and (3) less likely to be for non-recommended drugs (7.6 % vs. 10.8 % of total orders). Additionally, patients in the cohort who got the CDS intervention had fewer falls in the hospital (0.28 vs. 0.64 falls per 100 patient-days). The recommendations were not found to have any effect on hospital length of stay or days of altered mental status [11]. Since the study, the knowledge base continues to be updated using the Beers criteria.

Medication-Specific Decision Support

BWH has evaluated the implementation of medication-specific recommendations as interventions. In a 1998 randomized control trial, vancomycin use guidelines based upon the Centers for Disease Control and Prevention's (CDC) recommendations were incorporated into BICS, to examine the effect on Vancomycin overuse. Physicians receiving the intervention placed 32 % fewer orders than physicians in the control group. Vancomycin orders were initiated or renewed for 28 % fewer patients in the intervention group. Compared with the control group, patients of the intervention physicians received courses of Vancomycin that were shorter by 36 % [12].

In another study focusing on the high utilization of the high-cost medication human growth hormone in the surgical intensive care unit, a targeted guideline requiring the indication and the tracking of the ordering provider was implemented. This seemingly small intervention reduced human growth hormone use by one-third [13].

13.2.2 Laboratory-Related Decision Support

BWH has evaluated the impact of CDS interventions to improve utilization and efficacy of clinical laboratory testing, with the studies showing a range of success.

Display of Charges at Test Ordering

In a randomized clinical trial, charges for 19 commonly ordered clinical laboratory tests and cumulative totals were displayed at the time the tests were ordered. This simple intervention had little or no impact on the number of tests ordered. Of note, although the results of the intervention were not statistically significant, they did show a trend toward fewer tests, in particular for more expensive tests. Given projected cost savings for this trend, the display of charges was continued after the conclusion of the trial [14].

Reduction in Redundant Testing

A 1998 utilization study at BWH identified that 9 % of ten common clinical laboratory tests were ordered in a redundant manner and potentially could be eliminated by CDSS, resulting in the projected reduction of $930,000 in charges [15].

A subsequent follow-up intervention to reduce redundant testing was evaluated in a 1999 randomized control trial. Tests targeted included a serum chemistry panel, therapeutic medication level monitoring for six medications, and three microbiology cultures. When a physician placed an order for a test that had previously been ordered within a given, test-specific interval, an alert was shown stating that the test had been performed recently – including the result, if available – or was pending. The default response after a reminder was delivered was cancellation of the redundant test order, but physicians could continue with the order if they so chose. With this intervention, the proportion of redundant tests that were performed was lowered from 51 % to 27 % [16].

However, the overall effect on costs was smaller than expected for three reasons: (1) over half (56 %) of the redundant tests did not have an associated computer order (the laboratory system at BWH was not directly integrated with the order entry system, so tests could be performed without orders), (2) not all tests were screened for redundancy; approximately half of computer-ordered tests were ordered using order sets, which were omitted from the algorithm, and (3) almost one third (31 %) of reminders were overridden, while the original estimate assumed 100 % of detected redundant orders would be canceled [16].

In a subsequent 2003 randomized clinical trial, BWH targeted potentially redundant therapeutic monitoring of anti-epileptic medication levels, primarily focused on reducing orders for test of serum drug levels which were placed before the medication level was expected to have reached a steady state. Additionally, the CDS intervention provided education aimed at increasing the appropriateness of non-redundant monitoring of drug levels. Following implementation of the CDSS, 13 % of all anti-epileptic drug tests ordered were cancelled and inappropriate repeat testing before steady state decreased from 54 % to 14.6 %. The total volume of anti-epileptic drug level testing decreased by 19.5 % [17].

Tests Pending at Discharge

Discharge from the hospital is a particularly dangerous time for communication failures and ambiguity about responsibility. In 2005, BWH research identified that 41 % of patients were discharged with tests pending at discharge (TPADs), but inpatient/primary care providers were aware of only 38 % of these pending tests [18]. To better manage TPADs, BWH developed an automated email system to notify the both the responsible inpatient-attending physician at discharge and the patient's primary care provider (PCP) of the final results of TPADs [19, 20].

The TPAD notification system was evaluated using a cluster-randomized controlled trial, investigating the impact on physician awareness of TPAD results and surveying physicians to assess overall satisfaction with the system. Attending physicians in the intervention group were significantly more aware of TPAD results than those in the control group: 76 % vs. 38 %. Intervention PCPs showed a slightly less dramatic though still significant increase in awareness of 57 % versus 33 % of control PCPs. Intervention attending physicians were more aware of actionable TPAD results, showing a level of awareness of these results of 59 % compared to 29 % in control attending physicians [21].

13.2.3 Radiology-Related Decision Support

Appropriateness of Ordered Studies

Effectiveness of CDSS interventions to improve utilization of radiology tests at BWH has progressed iteratively: as the CDSS has added more feedback information (e.g. pretest probabilities) to the providers, there has been greater impact on the appropriateness of test ordering.

In the initial implementation of BICS, the CDSS for radiology functioned in a critiquing mode. Providers were required to input coded patient condition information and test indications for radiology orders, which were used to provide feedback to providers on the appropriateness of the test ordered and suggested alternatives. An early study in 1997 showed limited acceptance of suggestions to cancel inappropriate abdominal radiographs (3–4 %). The addition of recommendations for alternative testing only resulted in 45 % compliance [22].

However, more recent evaluation of radiology CDSS interventions for CT orders has shown significant impact. By informing providers about the pretest probability of pulmonary embolism (PE) (based on clinical suspicion level and D-dimer status), orders for pulmonary angiograms by CT decreased 20 % for emergency department (ED) patients and by 12.3 % for hospitalized patients [23, 24]. Including guidelines for appropriate use of head CT in ED patients with minor traumatic brain injury led to a 56 % increase in guideline adherence [25].

Notification About Critical Radiology Results

In 2007, building on national patient safety initiatives to promote optimal communication of critical test results, BWH undertook a comprehensive effort to address timely delivery and assured receipt of critical radiology findings in the inpatient setting [26]. The process identified a need to develop an automated closed-loop notification system for critical results, leading to the creation of the Alert Notification of Critical Results (ANCR) tool, a web-based, open-source system which was integrated within the BICS environment in 2010.

ANCR allowed radiologists to communicate critical results through synchronous (e.g. paging) and asynchronous (e.g. secure HIPAA-compliant email) mechanisms with secure, auditable, web-enabled acknowledgement by ordering providers. A 4-year assessment of the ANCR system's impact on adherence to BWH critical results policy revealed adherence increased from 91.3 to 95 %, with a ninefold increase in critical results communicated via the system. Sixty percent of less urgent but still critical results were delivered and acknowledged via the ANCR system's non-interruptive communication (email) [27].

13.2.4 Transition of Care Support

Early in its implementation (1992–1993), BICS functionality was extended to support physician cross-coverage hand-offs of patient responsibilities, via Coverage List and Sign-out applications. CDS applications that detect significant clinical events can use the coverage list to route notifications to the responsible team member. The Sign-out application provides residents with abstracted patient lists that include medications, notable recent laboratory tests, and code status, which can be printed out. A case-controlled study demonstrated that Sign-out served to eliminate the previously identified sixfold increase in risk of adverse events associated with cross-coverage times [28, 29].

13.2.5 Assessment of CPOE Impact on Users

CPOE implementation at BWH was evaluated for impact on providers' satisfaction and time. A 1996 survey study of physicians and nurses (medical and surgical) showed good overall satisfaction with CPOE, including embedded CDS [30]. Formal assessment of CPOE's impact on productivity involved a prospective time-motion study. The study found that interns using CPOE spent 9.0 % of their time entering orders, compared to 2.1 % of their time before adoption. However, other features of CPOE yielded a 2 % time savings, making the net difference only 5 %. The interns' use of CPOE, however, saved time for other disciplines, including pharmacy and nursing [31].

13.3 Clinical Decision Support: Ambulatory Applications and Assessment

Many of the successful CDS interventions developed in the inpatient setting are also used in the outpatient systems at BWH.

13.3.1 Ambulatory Medication Decision Support

Medication-related CDSS in the LMR mirrors and extends the functionality of BICS in the inpatient setting. With iterative development, LMR offers alerts and recommendations for drug-allergy conflicts; drug-lab checks; drug-disease checks; drug-pregnancy checks; drug-drug interaction (DDI); drug and therapeutic duplication checks; and drug utilization costs. LMR also incorporates the Nephros (renal-based dosing) and Gerios (age-based dosing) systems previously described in this chapter.

BWH has evaluated the impact and utility of these types of alerts in the outpatient setting. To reduce alert fatigue, BWH developed highly targeted knowledge bases which contain only the most clinically relevant drug contraindications in the ambulatory setting. Alerts are divided into three tiers: "fatal or life-threatening interactions" (Level 1), "undesirable interactions with the potential for serious injury" (Level 2) and possible undesirable interactions where drug should be used with caution (Level 3) [32].

These tiers affect the presentation of DDI alerts in the system. Level 1 alerts are hard stops – clinicians cannot proceed without eliminating one of the interacting drugs. High severity alerts (Level 2) are interruptive, requiring clinicians to provide a reason before proceeding. The most common alerts, Level 3, are informational – a warning is shown on the ordering screen, but no reason for override is required, and no additional clicks are necessary [32].

A 6-month study of this tiered DDI system demonstrated that only 29 % were in the higher categories (Levels 1 and 2), with a 67 % acceptance rate (order either cancelled or modified) – a much higher acceptance rate than reported in other systems, suggesting that this high acceptance was due to limiting alert burden via selective knowledge base and minimizing workflow interruptions [33].

This particular BWH experience (developing selective knowledge bases for high-severity/interruptive DDI and non-interruptive DDI classifications) has subsequently served as the basis for consensus-based recommendations for standardized lists of DDI for incorporation in EHRs [34, 35].

Subsequent research to improve acceptance of alerts and reduce alert fatigue has better characterized the nature of outpatient alert overrides. A study of 157,483 CDS alerts in a 3-year period found providers overrode 52.6 % of alerts. Formulary substitutions had an 85.0 % override rate, followed by age-based recommendations with an override rate of 79.0 %, renal dosage recommendations showing a 78.0 % override rate, and allergies at 77.4 % of alerts overridden. Half of the total overrides were evaluated as clinically appropriate – drug-allergy alerts, drug duplication and therapeutic class duplication warnings and formulary-related alerts were particularly likely to be subject to appropriate overrides [36].

13.3.2 Laboratory-Related Decision Support

Although LMR does not support computerized laboratory ordering for ambulatory patients, a dedicated module within LMR, Results Manager (RM), provides CDS capabilities for laboratory result management. RM facilitates test result follow-up by collecting, organizing, and prioritizing these results. Functionality in RM includes sorting results by degree of abnormality, multi-lingual templates for sending letters to patients about lab results and guideline-based CDS about appropriate follow-up and management of abnormal results, along with reminders for repeat testing where indicated [37].

13.3.3 Radiology-Related Decision Support

Ambulatory radiology CPOE was first implemented at BWH in primary care offices in 2000, with the adoption of a web-enabled commercial product (Precipio) from Medicalis Corporation (San Francisco, CA) – the company was a joint venture between BWH and Harvard Medical School. The commercial product is fully integrated as a module within the LMR [38].

Orders are created from predetermined structured menus and controlled vocabularies to specify a requested imaging procedure and clinical indications. Clinicians are provided recommendations on diagnostic strategy based on the patient's clinical context and presentation data. For example, an order for an abdominal radiograph in a patient with suspected appendicitis triggers a "low-utility" message with a recommendation for a higher yield examination. Clinicians may choose to cancel the request or proceed with the order [38].

Targeted CDS interventions included alerting ordering providers to potentially redundant CT studies, resulting in 6 % cancellation of orders [39], and recommendations against ordering MRI imaging for patients with low back pain, resulting in 30 % reduction in orders [40].

13.3.4 Clinical Reminders

The LMR has a reminder system to alert clinicians to guideline-based screening, and preventive interventions. While these are well received by physicians, evaluation of the efficacy of reminders in improving care has demonstrated mixed results.

A 2005 randomized trial of LMR reminders for diabetic care (five total) and coronary artery disease care (four total) showed significant improvements in overall compliance with recommended care when physicians were shown reminders; however, the effect of individual reminders was variable [41].

A 2008 study provided suggestions for evidence-based laboratory monitoring for chronic medications, including testing for liver and kidney function and monitoring of drug levels. The study found no effect of the intervention, perhaps because the alerts were not actionable [42].

In 2011, a study investigated a set of actionable reminders for screening and monitoring, which also showed no effect. The limited effect of these reminders was thought to be strongly related to adoption of the reminders – notably, 79 % of responding physicians were either unaware of the functionality or almost never used it [43].

13.3.5 Documentation-Related Decision Support

Researchers at BWH led the development of the Smart Form, a clinical workflow tool integrating condition specific templates and knowledge-based orders to facilitate simultaneous clinical documentation, structured data capture, and actionable decision support [44]. Pilot studies showed modest improvement in the management and treatment of acute respiratory infection [45] and diabetes/coronary artery disease [46]; however, in both studies, overall physician use of the forms was low, and was likely impacted by the limited integration into LMR that required separate manual action by the users to initiate the form.

13.3.6 Problem-List Decision Support

Primary care providers at BWH do the majority of problem list maintenance (despite a policy of shared responsibility with specialists) [47]. To support them in this work, BWH developed a series of inference rules which identify potentially undocumented potential patient problems for 17 target conditions by evaluating a range of structured data, including laboratory results, medications, ICD-9 diagnosis codes and vital signs [48]. A randomized trial of an intervention implementing these inference rules as alerts suggesting problems resulted in a threefold increase in problem documentation for study conditions – in fact, in the intervention arm, 70.4 % of all study problems were added to the list via alerts [49].

13.3.7 Assessment of Ambulatory EHR Impact on Users

The incremental implementation of the LMR throughout the Partners HealthCare ambulatory clinics provided opportunity to assess impact on productivity. A formal time-motion study found that using the LMR did not require additional physician time to complete a primary care session compared to a clinic's existing paper-based system, nor were significant increases in administrative duties for physicians observed [50].

13.3.8 Patient-Centric Applications

In 2002, LMR incorporated a personal health record (PHR) called Patient Gateway (PG), which allowed patients web-based viewing of the contents of their medical record (medications, allergies, lab values) and on-line communication with their providers [51].

With the primary goal of improving patient experience and engagement, the PG was also intended to support quality of care improvements. A prospective, randomized trial of a PHR intervention including health screening questions, medication history documentation and diabetes management was carried out at BWH [52]. For the intervention arm, patients were given the opportunity to view/interact with components of their EHR and create "e-Journals" of information to be updated and/or addressed with their primary care doctors.

The study demonstrated the intervention group patients had increased rates of diabetes-related medication adjustment [53]. Providing direct-to-patient health maintenance reminders increased the rates of some types of preventive care (mammography and influenza vaccinations) [54]. Additionally, the intervention reduced potentially harmful medication discrepancies [55].

13.4 Clinical Decision Support: Cost-Effectiveness

Investigators at BWH have undertaken evaluation of the cost-effectiveness of implementing its EHR with CPOE/CDS, in both the inpatient and ambulatory settings. Between 1992 and 2003, BWH's total cost for developing, implementing and maintaining its inpatient CPOE system were $11.8 million, compared to savings of $28.5 million (largely due to reduction in harm from the renal dosing system, as well as increased efficiency for nurses and other drug-related CDS) [56].

Cost-effectiveness evaluation of the LMR also found significant financial benefit, estimated at $86,400 per provider over a 5 year period, driven largely by savings in drug costs, reduction in unnecessary imaging and better billing [57].

13.5 Overarching Lessons

In 2003, Bates et al. published "The Ten Commandments of Clinical Decision Support" and it remains a salient summary of the lessons learned during BWH experience with the implementation of CDSS [13]. The 'Ten Commandments' as identified in the paper are:

1. Speed Is Everything
2. Anticipate Needs and Deliver in Real Time
3. Fit into the User's Workflow
4. Little Things Can Make a Big Difference
5. Recognize that Physicians Will Strongly Resist Stopping
6. Changing Direction Is Easier than Stopping
7. Simple Interventions Work Best
8. Ask for Additional Information Only When You Really Need It
9. Monitor Impact, Get Feedback, and Respond
10. Manage and Maintain Your Knowledge-based Systems [13].

13.6 Future Directions

In 2013, BWH charted a new direction for CDSS and the EHR when Partners HealthCare made the transformative decision to move away from its long-standing model of self-developing clinical information systems in favor of a commercial EHR, selecting the Epic system. A key goal of this program, dubbed Partners eCare, is better integration across the large Partners HealthCare delivery network.

In May 2015, BWH was the first Partners site to go live on the Partners eCare Epic clinical system with a big-bang implementation in both inpatient and outpatient settings. Although not all the previously developed decision support could be deployed initially, the CDSS have all been inventoried, and with the strong commitment of BWH leadership, the intent is to implement additional CDSS as resources allow. Thus, BWH's years of experience in developing clinical information systems will now be applied to developing/implementing CDS features within this new environment. BWH researchers see new opportunities to innovate and to perform the rigorous systematic evaluation of CDS safety and efficacy they have practiced for the last 40 years.

References

1. Teich JM, Glaser JP, Beckley RF, Aranow M, Bates DW, Kuperman GJ, et al. The Brigham integrated computing system (BICS): advanced clinical systems in an academic hospital environment. Int J Med Inform. 1999;54(3):197–208.
2. Grossman JH, Barnett GO, Koepsell TD, Nesson HR, Dorsey JL, Phillips RR. An automated medical record system. JAMA. 1973;224(12):1616–21.
3. Bleich HL, Beckley RF, Horowitz GL, Jackson JD, Moody ES, Franklin C, et al. Clinical computing in a teaching hospital. N Engl J Med. 1985;312(12):756–64.
4. Linder JA, Schnipper JL, Middleton B. Method of electronic health record documentation and quality of primary care. J Am Med Inform Assoc: JAMIA. 2012;19(6):1019–24.
5. Teich JM, Merchia PR, Schmiz JL, Kuperman GJ, Spurr CD, Bates DW. Effects of computerized physician order entry on prescribing practices. Arch Intern Med. 2000;160(18):2741–7.
6. Leape LL, Bates DW, Cullen DJ, Cooper J, Demonaco HJ, Gallivan T, et al. Systems analysis of adverse drug events. ADE Prevention Study Group. JAMA. 1995;274(1):35–43.
7. Bates DW, Cullen DJ, Laird N, Petersen LA, Small SD, Servi D, et al. Incidence of adverse drug events and potential adverse drug events. Implications for prevention. ADE Prevention Study Group. JAMA. 1995;274(1):29–34.
8. Bates DW, Leape LL, Cullen DJ, Laird N, Petersen LA, Teich JM, et al. Effect of computerized physician order entry and a team intervention on prevention of serious medication errors. JAMA. 1998;280(15):1311–6.
9. Bates DW, Teich JM, Lee J, Seger D, Kuperman GJ, Ma'Luf N, et al. The impact of computerized physician order entry on medication error prevention. J Am Med Inform Assoc. 1999;6(4):313–21.
10. Chertow GM, Lee J, Kuperman GJ, Burdick E, Horsky J, Seger DL, et al. Guided medication dosing for inpatients with renal insufficiency. JAMA. 2001;286(22):2839–44.
11. Peterson JF, Kuperman GJ, Shek C, Patel M, Avorn J, Bates DW. Guided prescription of psychotropic medications for geriatric inpatients. Arch Intern Med. 2005;165(7):802–7.

12. Shojania KG, Yokoe D, Platt R, Fiskio J, Ma'luf N, Bates DW. Reducing vancomycin use utilizing a computer guideline: results of a randomized controlled trial. J Am Med Inform Assoc. 1998;5(6):554–62.
13. Bates DW, Kuperman GJ, Wang S, Gandhi T, Kittler A, Volk L, et al. Ten commandments for effective clinical decision support: making the practice of evidence-based medicine a reality. J Am Med Inform Assoc. 2003;10(6):523–30.
14. Bates DW. Does the computerized display of charges affect inpatient ancillary test utilization? Arch Intern Med. 1997;157(21):2501.
15. Bates DW, Boyle DL, Rittenberg E, Kuperman GJ, Ma'Luf N, Menkin V, et al. What proportion of common diagnostic tests appear redundant? Am J Med. 1998;104(4):361–8.
16. Bates DW, Kuperman GJ, Rittenberg E, Teich JM, Fiskio J, Ma'luf N, et al. A randomized trial of a computer-based intervention to reduce utilization of redundant laboratory tests. Am J Med. 1999;106(2):144–50.
17. Chen P, Tanasijevic MJ, Schoenenberger RA, Fiskio J, Kuperman GJ, Bates DW. A computer-based intervention for improving the appropriateness of antiepileptic drug level monitoring. Am J Clin Pathol. 2003;119(3):432–8.
18. Roy CL, Poon EG, Karson AS, Ladak-Merchant Z, Johnson RE, Maviglia SM, et al. Patient safety concerns arising from test results that return after hospital discharge. Ann Intern Med. 2005;143(2):121–8.
19. Dalal AK, Poon EG, Karson AS, Gandhi TK, Roy CL. Lessons learned from implementation of a computerized application for pending tests at hospital discharge. J Hosp Med. 2011;6(1):16–21.
20. Dalal AK, Schnipper JL, Poon EG, Williams DH, Rossi-Roh K, Macleay A, et al. Design and implementation of an automated email notification system for results of tests pending at discharge. J Am Med Inform Assoc: JAMIA. 2012;19(4):523–8.
21. Dalal AK, Roy CL, Poon EG, Williams DH, Nolido N, Yoon C, et al. Impact of an automated email notification system for results of tests pending at discharge: a cluster-randomized controlled trial. J Am Med Inform Assoc. 2014;21(3):473–80.
22. Harpole LH, Khorasani R, Fiskio J, Kuperman GJ, Bates DW. Automated evidence-based critiquing of orders for abdominal radiographs: impact on utilization and appropriateness. J Am Med Inform Assoc. 1997;4(6):511–21.
23. Raja AS, Ip IK, Prevedello LM, Sodickson AD, Farkas C, Zane RD, et al. Effect of computerized clinical decision support on the use and yield of CT pulmonary angiography in the emergency department. Radiology. 2012;262(2):468–74.
24. Dunne RM, Ip IK, Abbett S, Gershanik EF, Raja AS, Hunsaker A, et al. Effect of evidence-based clinical decision support on the use and yield of CT pulmonary angiographic imaging in hospitalized patients. Radiology. 2015;276(1):167–74.
25. Ip IK, Raja AS, Gupta A, Andruchow J, Sodickson A, Khorasani R. Impact of clinical decision support on head computed tomography use in patients with mild traumatic brain injury in the ED. Am J Emerg Med. 2015;33(3):320–5.
26. Anthony SG, Prevedello LM, Damiano MM, Gandhi TK, Doubilet PM, Seltzer SE, et al. Impact of a 4-year quality improvement initiative to improve communication of critical imaging test results. Radiology. 2011;259(3):802–7.
27. Lacson R, Prevedello LM, Andriole KP, O'Connor SD, Roy C, Gandhi T, et al. Four-year impact of an alert notification system on closed-loop communication of critical test results. AJR Am J Roentgenol. 2014;203(5):933–8.
28. Hiltz FL, Teich JM. Coverage list: a provider-patient database supporting advanced hospital information services. Proc Annu Symp Comput Appl Med Care. 1994;809–13.
29. Petersen LA, Orav EJ, Teich JM, O'Neil AC, Brennan TA. Using a computerized sign-out program to improve continuity of inpatient care and prevent adverse events. Jt Comm J Qual Improv. 1998;24(2):77–87.
30. Lee F, Teich JM, Spurr CD, Bates DW. Implementation of physician order entry: user satisfaction and self-reported usage patterns. J Am Med Inform Assoc. 1996;3(1):42–55.

31. Shu K, Boyle D, Spurr C, Horsky J, Heiman H, O'Connor P, et al. Comparison of time spent writing orders on paper with computerized physician order entry. Stud Health Technol Inform. 2001;84(Pt 2):1207–11.
32. Yu DT, Seger DL, Lasser KE, Karson AS, Fiskio JM, Seger AC, et al. Impact of implementing alerts about medication black-box warnings in electronic health records. Pharmacoepidemiol Drug Saf. 2011;20(2):192–202.
33. Shah NR, Seger AC, Seger DL, Fiskio JM, Kuperman GJ, Blumenfeld B, et al. Improving acceptance of computerized prescribing alerts in ambulatory care. J Am Med Inform Assoc. 2006;13(1):5–11.
34. Phansalkar S, Desai AA, Bell D, Yoshida E, Doole J, Czochanski M, et al. High-priority drug-drug interactions for use in electronic health records. J Am Med Inform Assoc. 2012;19(5):735–43.
35. Phansalkar S, van der Sijs H, Tucker AD, Desai AA, Bell DS, Teich JM, et al. Drug-drug interactions that should be non-interruptive in order to reduce alert fatigue in electronic health records. J Am Med Inform Assoc. 2013;20(3):489–93.
36. Nanji KC, Slight SP, Seger DL, Cho I, Fiskio JM, Redden LM, et al. Overrides of medication-related clinical decision support alerts in outpatients. J Am Med Inform Assoc. 2014;21(3):487–91.
37. Poon EG, Wang SJ, Gandhi TK, Bates DW, Kuperman GJ. Design and implementation of a comprehensive outpatient results manager. J Biomed Inform. 2003;36(1–2):80–91.
38. Ip IK, Schneider LI, Hanson R, Marchello D, Hultman P, Viera M, et al. Adoption and meaningful use of computerized physician order entry with an integrated clinical decision support system for radiology: ten-year analysis in an urban teaching hospital. J Am Coll Radiol. 2012;9(2):129–36.
39. Wasser EJ, Prevedello LM, Sodickson A, Mar W, Khorasani R. Impact of a real-time computerized duplicate alert system on the utilization of computed tomography. JAMA Int Med. 2013;173(11):1024–6.
40. Ip IK, Gershanik EF, Schneider LI, Raja AS, Mar W, Seltzer S, et al. Impact of IT-enabled intervention on MRI use for back pain. Am J Med. 2014;127(6):512–8. e1.
41. Sequist TD, Gandhi TK, Karson AS, Fiskio JM, Bugbee D, Sperling M, et al. A randomized trial of electronic clinical reminders to improve quality of care for diabetes and coronary artery disease. J Am Med Inform Assoc. 2005;12(4):431–7.
42. Matheny ME, Sequist TD, Seger AC, Fiskio JM, Sperling M, Bugbee D, et al. A randomized trial of electronic clinical reminders to improve medication laboratory monitoring. J Am Med Inform Assoc. 2008;15(4):424–9.
43. El-Kareh RE, Gandhi TK, Poon EG, Newmark LP, Ungar J, Orav EJ, et al. Actionable reminders did not improve performance over passive reminders for overdue tests in the primary care setting. J Am Med Inform Assoc. 2011;18(2):160–3.
44. Schnipper JL, Linder JA, Palchuk MB, Einbinder JS, Li Q, Postilnik A, et al. "Smart forms" in an electronic medical record: documentation-based clinical decision support to improve disease management. J Am Med Inform Assoc. 2008;15(4):513–23.
45. Linder JA, Schnipper JL, Tsurikova R, Yu T, Volk LA, Melnikas AJ, et al. Documentation-based clinical decision support to improve antibiotic prescribing for acute respiratory infections in primary care: a cluster randomised controlled trial. Inform Prim Care. 2009;17(4):231–40.
46. Schnipper JL, Linder JA, Palchuk MB, Yu DT, McColgan KE, Volk LA, et al. Effects of documentation-based decision support on chronic disease management. Am J Manag Care. 2010;16(12 Suppl HIT):SP72–81.
47. Wright A, Feblowitz J, Maloney FL, Henkin S, Bates DW. Use of an electronic problem list by primary care providers and specialists. J Gen Intern Med. 2012;27(8):968–73.
48. Wright A, Pang J, Feblowitz JC, Maloney FL, Wilcox AR, Ramelson HZ, et al. A method and knowledge base for automated inference of patient problems from structured data in an electronic medical record. J Am Med Inform Assoc. 2011;18(6):859–67.

49. Wright A, Pang J, Feblowitz JC, Maloney FL, Wilcox AR, McLoughlin KS, et al. Improving completeness of electronic problem lists through clinical decision support: a randomized, controlled trial. J Am Med Inform Assoc. 2012;19(4):555–61.
50. Pizziferri L, Kittler AF, Volk LA, Honour MM, Gupta S, Wang S, et al. Primary care physician time utilization before and after implementation of an electronic health record: a time-motion study. J Biomed Inform. 2005;38(3):176–88.
51. Wald JS, Middleton B, Bloom A, Walmsley D, Gleason M, Nelson E, et al. A patient-controlled journal for an electronic medical record: issues and challenges. Stud Health Technol Inform. 2004;107(Pt 2):1166–70.
52. Wald JS, Businger A, Gandhi TK, Grant RW, Poon EG, Schnipper JL, et al. Implementing practice-linked pre-visit electronic journals in primary care: patient and physician use and satisfaction. J Am Med Inform Assoc. 2010;17(5):502–6.
53. Grant RW, Wald JS, Schnipper JL, Gandhi TK, Poon EG, Orav EJ, et al. Practice-linked online personal health records for type 2 diabetes mellitus: a randomized controlled trial. Arch Intern Med. 2008;168(16):1776–82.
54. Wright A, Poon EG, Wald J, Feblowitz J, Pang JE, Schnipper JL, et al. Randomized controlled trial of health maintenance reminders provided directly to patients through an electronic PHR. J Gen Intern Med. 2012;27(1):85–92.
55. Schnipper JL, Gandhi TK, Wald JS, Grant RW, Poon EG, Volk LA, et al. Effects of an online personal health record on medication accuracy and safety: a cluster-randomized trial. J Am Med Inform Assoc. 2012;19(5):728–34.
56. Kaushal R, Jha AK, Franz C, Glaser J, Shetty KD, Jaggi T, et al. Return on investment for a computerized physician order entry system. J Am Med Inform Assoc. 2006;13(3):261–6.
57. Wang SJ, Middleton B, Prosser LA, Bardon CG, Spurr CD, Carchidi PJ, et al. A cost-benefit analysis of electronic medical records in primary care. Am J Med. 2003;114(5):397–403.

Chapter 14
Clinical Decision Support at Intermountain Healthcare

Peter J. Haug, Reed M. Gardner, R. Scott Evans, Beatriz H. Rocha, and Roberto A. Rocha

Abstract The medical community within the United States is adopting Electronic Health Records (EHRs) at an accelerating pace. These systems are designed to support medical documentation, communication, and billing practices and can bring the efficiencies of digital systems to these healthcare functions. However, one of the key advantages of an EHR is the availability of cognitive support provided during the care process in the form of embedded Clinical Decision Support Systems (CDSS). Historically, the initial exploration of CDS technologies occurred in a group of hospital-based EHRs. These pioneering institutions engaged in early experimentation with a variety of CDS interventions. In this chapter, we describe experience with a group of CDS applications developed and evaluated within the HELP Hospital Information System created and used by Intermountain Healthcare

P.J. Haug, M.D. (✉)
Department of Medical Informatics, Intermountain Healthcare,
5171 Cottonwood Street, Suite 220, Murray, UT 84107, USA
e-mail: Peter.Haug@imail.org

R.M. Gardner, Ph.D.
Department of Biomedical Informatics, University of Utah,
1745 Cornell Circle, Salt Lake City, UT 84108, USA
e-mail: reed.gardner@hsc.utah.edu

R.S. Evans, B.S., M.S., Ph.D.
Department of Medical Informatics, Intermountain Healthcare,
8th Ave & C Street, Salt Lake City, UT 84143, USA
e-mail: rscott.evans@imail.org

B.H. Rocha, M.D., Ph.D.
Division of General Internal Medicine and Primary Care, Department of Medicine, Brigham and Women's Hospital, Information Systems, Partners HealthCare System Inc., Harvard Medical School, 93 Worcester Street, Wellesley, MA 02481, USA
e-mail: b.h.rocha@icloud.com

R.A. Rocha, M.D., Ph.D.
Division of General Internal Medicine and Primary Care, Department of Medicine, Brigham and Women's Hospital, Partners eCare, Partners HealthCare System Inc., Harvard Medical School, 93 Worcester Street, Wellesley, MA 02481, USA
e-mail: r.rocha@computer.org

E.S. Berner (ed.), *Clinical Decision Support Systems*, Health Informatics,
DOI 10.1007/978-3-319-31913-1_14

of Utah. These CDS applications have employed several different approaches in their interactions with clinical users and their capture and processing of clinical data.

Keywords Intermountain Healthcare • HELP System • Antibiotic Assistant • Nosocomial infections • Ventilator management • Adverse drug events

As Electronic Health Records (EHRs) have become common components of the medical workplace, so have decision support technologies become increasingly available to medical practitioners. A variety of programs designed to assist with drug dosing, health maintenance, diagnosis, and other clinically relevant healthcare decisions have been developed to support medical decision making. A key driver of this change has been the growing dependency on computers to maintain part or all of the medical record. This has led to an expanded interest in and, in some cases, dependency on, automated medical decision making to support the delivery of economical, quality care.

The Electronic Health Record (EHR), itself, may be seen as a response to the increasing complexity and volume of both the clinical data available for the individual patient and the medical knowledge necessary to assimilate and respond to this data. Historical evidence emphasizes the cost of failures to properly integrate the patient's findings with the fruits of medical science. In 1999, the Institute of Medicine estimated that between 44,000 and 98,000 Americans die each year because of medical errors [1]. Computer-based systems have been proposed as a remedy for a large subset of these errors [2–5].

Clinical Decision Support systems (CDSS) are often described as a cure for these and other failings in traditional care delivery. A substantial part of the literature that has sparked this awareness comes from research done in early generations of medical information systems. These systems resided on large mainframe computing hardware. Many of them were designed to serve hospitals and have for decades supported the patient care given there [6, 7]. The applications and algorithms that were piloted in these systems provide the background for the modern decision support technologies which we see developing and evolving in client/server environments, on personal computers, on systems based in Internet technologies, and on personal devices.

Significant early contributions to the science of applying computer systems to clinical practice have been provided by the several sites where hospital-based, medical decision support has been implemented and studied. Among the leaders in these efforts have been groups at the Regenstrief Institute in Indianapolis[8], Columbia-Presbyterian Medical Center in New York [9], Beth Israel Hospital in Boston [10], Partners Healthcare in Boston, and the HELP System developed initially at the LDS Hospital in Salt Lake City and subsequently deployed across the 22 hospitals included in Intermountain Healthcare of Utah [11]. Efforts to incorporate decision support into order entry systems at the Brigham and Women's Hospital in Boston [12] and Vanderbilt University Medical Center in Nashville [13] have helped to provide further insight into this important healthcare computing function.

In this chapter, we will review the experience gained in 30 years of CDS delivered through Intermountain Healthcare's HELP System. We will present a set of examples of CDS that illustrate specific characteristics of decision support systems whose value has been confirmed through experience and comparative research.

At present, Intermountain Healthcare is in the midst of a conversion to a new healthcare computing platform. After decades of focus on systems developed exclusively for the use of Intermountain patients and clinicians, this integrated healthcare delivery system will install a commercially available EHR provided by Cerner Corporation (http://www.cerner.com/). This new system represents a fresh approach for Intermountain. Rather than depending exclusively on platforms engineered internally, we expect to take advantage of the extensive work on standardization and on compliance with national healthcare requirements supplied by Cerner and to use the computing infrastructure provided as a foundation for another generation of healthcare computing applications. The CDS experience presented in this chapter represents the foundation upon which we expect to apply the existing decision support capabilities found within our new healthcare computing environment and to develop a next generation of novel CDS applications consistent with the increased capabilities that modern information management technologies afford us.

Thus, in this chapter, we will focus on the experience of Intermountain Healthcare, a provider of integrated medical services in the Intermountain West, as an example of two phenomena readily recognized in a variety of healthcare organizations as they adopt or extend medical computing systems. These phenomena are the continuing value of decision support applications and the effort to project and expand the use of these technologies across the entire gamut of clinical care. Modern-day EHR developers are required to embrace both new and old CDS agendas and to apply them in both the inpatient and outpatient setting. Thus, the target for the next generation of clinical systems will be a comprehensive longitudinal patient record instrumented with the best available decision support technologies.

The history of the HELP system reaches back to 1972. As we illustrate lessons in decision support from this EHR, we will not restrict ourselves to the latest incarnation of CDS delivered by the system. Instead, we will describe a mixture of old and new. We will include a set of classic applications that evolved in the early HELP Hospital Information System (HIS) and the original research that proved their worth. In addition, we will discuss several current CDS examples that illustrate more recent uses of decision support technologies. As a part of these descriptions, we will discuss the data used and the mechanism through which suggested decisions are communicated to the user.

The applications described below were developed by teams from Intermountain Healthcare, the Department of Medical Informatics at the University of Utah, and commercial partners. They represent accumulated experience whose relevance is attested to by the continuing success of CDS solutions to comparable clinical problems.

14.1 The HELP System

The overall setting for the CDSS examples described here is the HELP Hospital Information System (HIS). This system is a culmination of more than 40 years of development and testing [11]. It currently operates on high availability hardware supplied by the Hewlett-Packard, NonStop Enterprise Division. Software components of the HELP system are provided to the 22 hospitals operated by Intermountain Healthcare over a proprietary wide area network from a single server located at the Lake Park Datacenter in Salt Lake City. The largest individual deployment is at the Intermountain Medical Center (IMC), which opened in 2007. IMC is Intermountain Healthcare's tertiary care facility, replacing the LDS Hospital in which much of the work described below was accomplished. At IMC the information system communicates with users and developers through more than 4000 terminals and approximately 450 printers. The system is interfaced with a variety of other computer systems, including a billing system, a laboratory system, a medical records system, a digital radiology system, and a collection of local area networks (LANs) used by a variety of departments forresearch and departmental management functions.

The HELP System itself consists of an integrated clinical database, a frame-based, medical decision support system, programs to support hospital and departmental clinical and administrative functions, and the software tools needed to maintain and expand these components. The integrated clinical database contains a variety of patient data (Table 14.1) kept online during the patient's stay to allow review by health-care professionals at terminals throughout each hospital. These terminals allow the entry of pertinent clinical data into the HELP system by personnel who are involved in patient care. In addition, automated systems capture clinical information directly from monitors and other instruments in the hospitals' ICUs.

Table 14.1 Clinical data captured by the HELP hospital information system (partial list)

Chemistry	Hematology
Medications	X-ray findings
Allergies	Dietary information
Blood gases	Surgical procedures
ED nursing assessment	ICU monitoring
Intake/output	Pulmonary function testing
Demographic information	Microbiology
Cardiac catheterization data	Respiratory therapy notes
Biopsy results	Nursing data
Select physical examination	Pathology department data
Admit/discharge information	History and physical exam reports
Consult reports	Intervenous fluid therapy
Ventilator management	Procedure reports

Use of the HELP System as a medical expert system has been a major focus of research since the system's inception. The result has been a set of embedded expert system development tools. The HELP System contains a decision support subsystem based on a modular representation of medical decision logic in frames [14]. These modules are used to: (1) identify the data used in making the target medical decision; and (2) encode the logic that converts the raw data into the proposed decision. Decisions encoded in these modules resemble small computer programs written in a Pascal-like language. They are each designed to represent a single simple decision capable of activation in a number of ways. The language supports either simple or multiple outputs from a frame. This flexibility can be used to create more complex modules capable of deriving several distinct decisions from the same data.

This form for computerized medical decisions represented an evolution from an earlier decision language whose focus was a more declarative representation designed to be developed using a simple authoring system. CDS examples from the 1970s are largely based on this older approach.

These sets of tools led to the successful development of expert systems in blood gas interpretation [15], intensive care settings [16], and medication monitoring [17], to name a few. The HELP System hardware and software environment has provided the setting for the implementation and testing of the decision support examples described below.

The history of decision support in the HELP System extends more than 40 years into the past. This classic hospital information system has been used to demonstrate two types of CDSS. The first type focuses on narrowly circumscribed medical conditions. The logic may be simple or complex and the data requirements are typically modest. The *computerized laboratory alerting, ventilator disconnect notification, early prediction of deterioration, blood ordering, and ventilator management systems* described below are examples of this type.

The second type of CDSS discussed here is less common. This type of tool attempts to discriminate among a group of important *diagnostic* entities using the raw medical data. Diagnostic systems often attempt the challenging task of managing large degrees of uncertainty using pattern matching algorithms. Several of these approaches have been tested in the HELP environment. Below, we will describe experience with four applications engaged in diagnostic behaviors. These are systems designed to diagnose *adverse drug events, nosocomial infections, pneumonia in the emergency department, and a variety of infectious diseases with a focus on the most relevant antibiotic regime to prescribe.*

We will also describe the behavior of two experimental applications that leverage diagnostic logic to drive other, *peri-diagnostic* behaviors. These are systems that use underlying diagnostic models to simulate knowledge-driven behaviors of clinicians. Two behaviors, the collection of relevant patient history and the critiquing of diagnostic x-ray interpretations, have been explored.

14.2 Categories of Decision Support Technologies

Independent of the environment in which they are used, two elements of medical decision support applications are critical to their success. These are:

(1) The mechanism by which the systems acquire the data used in their decision algorithms; and (2) the interface through which they interact with clinicians to report their results. These considerations have led us to focus here on different *categories* of decision support [18]. Although somewhat arbitrary, this categorization captures the idea that different models of computerized assistance may be needed for different types of clinical problems.

Four categories of CDSS have routinely been used to support medical decision makers who use the HELP system. These are:

1. Processes which respond to clinical data by issuing an *alert*;
2. Programs activated in response to recorded decisions (typically new orders) to alter care. These applications work by *critiquing* the decision and proposing alternative suggestions as appropriate;
3. Applications that respond to a request by the decision maker by *suggesting* a set of diagnostic or therapeutic maneuvers fitted to the patient's needs;
4. *Retrospective* quality assurance applications where clinical data are abstracted from multiple patient records and summary evaluations concerning the quality of care are derived and fed back to caregivers.

The first three types focus on individual patient decisions and center on a real-time CDS interaction with the clinical user while the fourth type provides global feedback reflecting healthcare decision-making for a clinical population. In this chapter, we will focus on the first three types.

14.3 Alerting Systems

Alerting processes are programs that operate by monitoring select clinical data as it is collected and stored in the patient's electronic record. They are designed to test specific types of data against predefined criteria. If the data meet the criteria, these systems alert medical personnel. The timing and character of the messages vary with the alerting goals.

14.3.1 Computerized Laboratory Alerting System

A typical example is a subsystem implemented within the HELP System that monitored common laboratory results and detected and alerted for potentially life-threatening abnormalities in the data acquired. This type of application is notable

Table 14.2 Alerts for which computerized alerting logic was created

Alerting condition	Criteria
Hyponatremia (NAL)	Na+ <120 mEq/l
Falling Sodium (NAF)	Na+ fallen 15+ mEq/l in 24 h and Na+ <130 mEq/l
Hypernatremia (NAH)	Na+ >155 mEq/l
Hypokalemia (KL)	K+ <2.7 mEq/l
Falling Potassium (KLF)	K+ fallen 1+ mEq/l in 24 h and K+ <3.2 mEq/l
Hypokalemia, patient on digoxin (KLD)	K+ <3.3 mEq/l and patient on digoxin
Hyperkalemia (KH)	K+ >6.0 mEq/l
Metabolic Acidosis (CO2L)	CO2 <15 and BUN <50 or CO2 <18 and BUN <50 or CO2 <18 (BUN unknown) or CO2 fallen 10+ in 24 h. and CO2 <25
Hypoglycemia (GL)	Glucose <45 mg%
Hyperglycemia (GH)	Glucose >500 mg%

for the simplicity of its decision logic as well as for the magnitude of its potential impact.

The HELP System captures results from the clinical laboratory through an interface to a dedicated laboratory information system (LIS). The results are collected and returned to the HELP System for storage in the clinical record as soon as they are collected and validated in the LIS.

Laboratory results are reviewed by personnel engaged in patient care both through terminals connected to the HELP System and through a variety of special and general-purpose printouts, such as rounds reports generated by the HELP System. The "times" when the data are reviewed have only a loose relationship to the "times" when these data become available. Instead, the principal determinants of the review times are typically the work schedules of the physicians and nurses involved with the patient. A physician, for instance, may round on inpatients twice a day and review patient data only during those times unless some aspect of the patient's condition prompts a more aggressive approach.

Under these circumstances, abnormalities in laboratory results, especially those that are unexpected, may not receive the prompt attention they deserve. In particular, unexpected laboratory abnormalities may go unseen for hours until a nurse or physician reviews them during their routine activities. Or, as some authors have noted, they may be missed entirely [19, 20].

As a response to this disparity, researchers at LDS Hospital have described an experiment with a Computerized Laboratory Alerting System (CLAS) designed to bring potentially life-threatening conditions to the attention of caregivers [21–24]. This system was constructed by reducing a set of 60 alerts developed during a previous pilot system [25] to the 10 most important (Table 14.2).

Six medical experts from the disciplines of surgery, cardiology, internal medicine, and critical care participated in the development of these alerts and the system used to deliver them. The alerts chosen were translated into computer logic and tested to determine that the logic functioned properly. Data from previously admitted patients were used to refine and test the logic.

Once the logic was deemed acceptable, an experiment was designed to evaluate the effect of the system on several intermediate outcome measures. Two approaches were tested for delivering the alerts. The first of these techniques was tested on a single nursing division to determine its acceptability. A flashing yellow light was installed in the division, and whenever an alert was generated for a patient in that division, the light was activated. It continued to flash until the alert was reviewed and acknowledged on a computer terminal.

Responses from clinicians rapidly convinced the researchers that this approach was too aggressive. In a number of cases, the flashing light was disabled within hours of initial implementation. A second approach was found less intrusive by the division staff. Whenever anyone accessed the program used to review a patient's laboratory results, any unacknowledged alerts for that patient were immediately displayed along with the data that had triggered them.

The results of this type of intervention were tested in three ways. First, appropriateness of treatment was evaluated. The alerting system was shown to result in a significant increase in appropriate therapy for conditions involving abnormalities of Na^+, K^+, and glucose (68.1–83.8 %). Second, time spent in the life-threatening condition with and without the alerting system was examined. Length of time spent in "life-threatening" conditions decreased significantly (30.4–15.7 h). Finally, the hospital length of stay was examined. A significant improvement in this parameter was also noted for the patients with abnormalities of Na^+, K^+, or glucose (350.6–211.9 h).

Alerting as a decision support intervention has become common as hospital information systems have evolved [26]. In the inpatient environment where the severity of illness is steadily increasing, the possibility of better alerting has the potential to improve the quality of patient care.

Interestingly, the original HELP system for alerting on critical laboratory values has been re-implemented since these initial studies. The Intermountain Healthcare laboratory that processes the inpatient laboratory values also serves a variety of locations into which the HELP System does not reach, notably a large number of outpatient clinics. Based upon the demonstrated value of this type of intervention, Intermountain's Laboratory Services has instituted the process of identifying laboratory abnormalities as the samples are processed and having personnel telephone ordering physicians or other caregivers whenever critical laboratory values are detected. Thus, the limitations of a model that was restricted to select inpatient locations have been circumvented.

14.3.2 Unit-Wide Notification of Ventilator Disconnections

Many of the most seriously ill patients in hospitals today require ventilatory assistance during some part of their admission. This assistance is delivered using mechanical ventilators that support a patient's breathing during periods when they cannot breathe for themselves. While mechanical ventilators are designed to detect disconnections, the alarms are only audible beeps that are often difficult to hear outside of the patient's room. Thus, some ventilator disconnection alarms go unnoticed for periods of time that result in permanent harm or death. This is a systems problem that is outside of the control of the ventilator and may be due to the physical layout of the ICU, staffing limitations, environmental acoustics and noise, or the patient being in isolation. Moreover, information concerning ventilator disconnections has been limited and was not included in our electronic medical record (EMR). Without this information, appropriate process changes to prevent future disconnections or improve patient safety were difficult to identify.

In response, Intermountain researchers determined to develop a method to notify medical personnel of critical ventilator events that was accurate, reliable, instantly recognizable, and would not report low-level ventilator alarms [27]. The ventilators used at LDS Hospital were connected to an external microcomputer that captures current alarm and ventilator settings every 5 s (Fig. 14.1). The microcomputer then

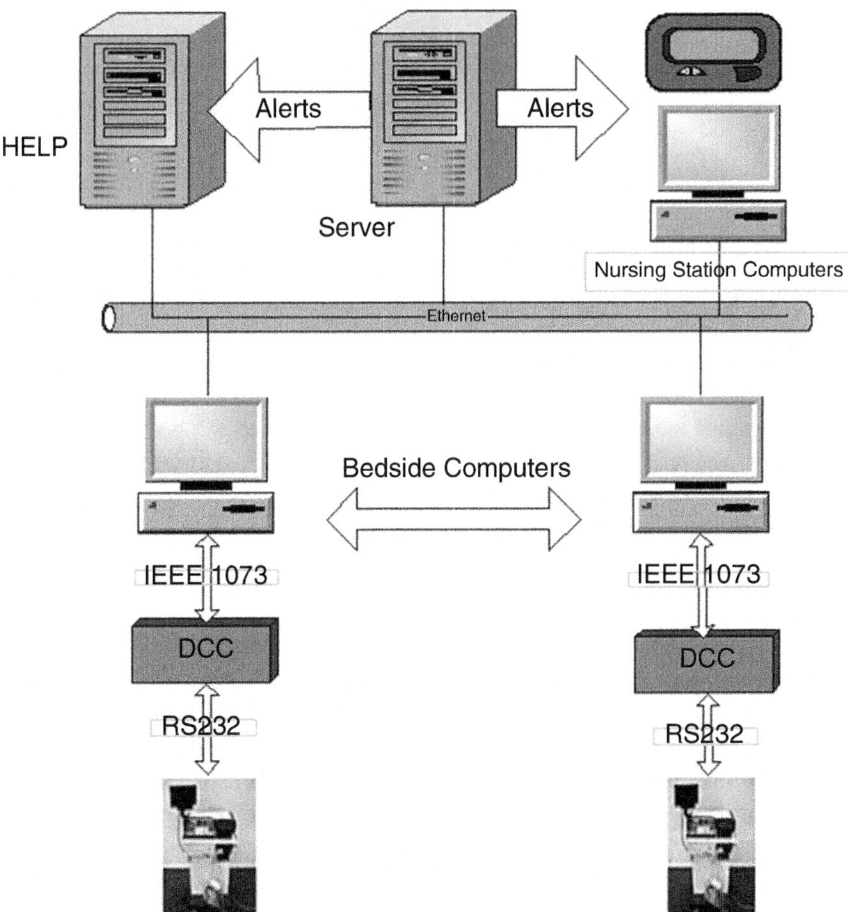

Fig. 14.1 Diagram of the enhanced ventilator event alerting system. (*DCC* = Device communications controller)

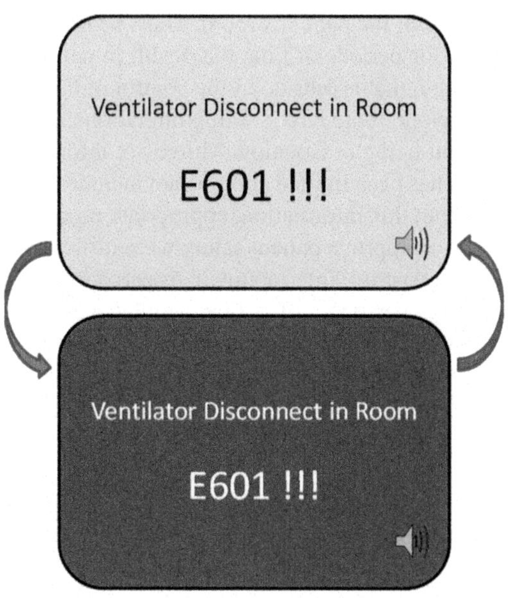

Fig. 14.2 Display found on every computer terminal in the same unit as the patient who generated the critical ventilator alarm. Screen color alternates between *red* and *black* every 3 s.

sends the ventilator information to the bedside computer. Each bedside computer then transmits this information to a server. When this server receives a disconnection alarm, it identifies all other computers in the same unit and runs a program loaded on those computers. This program takes control of each computer and begins managing the display. The result is that the background of each computers' screen alternates between red and black every three seconds and a message indicates that there is a ventilator disconnection and identifies the room (Fig. 14.2). An audio message containing the "submarine dive horn" is also sent to the non-bedside computers in the unit. The program then logs pertinent information concerning the alert. Once the alarm is corrected on the ventilator, all the computers are restored to the pre-alert status or application.

The respiratory therapy-charting program on the HELP System is also a part of this system. When they next sign-on, therapists are prompted to enter specific ventilator disconnection information to document the disconnect. That information is loaded into the enterprise data warehouse each night.

The new system was initially tested in the shock/trauma ICU for 6 months. The new audio/video alerts were easily distinguished from any other alarms and impossible to ignore. The approval of medical staff was so high that the alerting tool was requested to be installed in three other ICUs (medical/surgical, coronary care, thoracic). During a 4-month pilot study, 152 ventilator disconnections were identified in the four ICUs (2.5 per bed). Forty-two were for unintended disconnections, self-extubations or tube occlusions, all potential life threatening events. Other disconnections were due to ventilator asynchrony or occurred during patient procedures, which can result in patient discomfort and suggest a need for additional education on ventilator adjustment. Average disconnection time from the ventilator was 19.8 s. Ventilator disconnection information including the duration time is now stored in the patient's EMR and log files. Monthly and ad hoc reports now permit respiratory care management to identify each event and perform root cause analyses.

While the prevention of all ventilator disconnections is not possible, this alerting system improves patient safety through early notification of medical staff. We have reduced disconnection times to a level where patient harm does not occur. The system also facilitates root cause analyses and the development of new safety strategies.

14.3.3 Early Prediction of Deterioration (ePOD)

The average age of the US population is increasing as is the complexity of their medical care. As a result, up to 5 % of patients experience physiologic deterioration (PD) during their hospital stay resulting in admission to the intensive care unit (ICU) or death [28, 29]. Studies reveal that many of these adverse events are preceded by indicators of PD [30–38]. In many institutions, Medical emergency teams (MET) have been developed to prevent patient crises leading to a cardiopulmonary arrest [39]. However, delayed MET calls are common and patients who are attended to within 30–60 min of PD have significantly lower mortality rates [35, 40, 41]. Therefore, to be effective, MET must have an afferent limb (case detection and timely alerting) in addition to an efferent limb (medical response) [42].

We created a MET Risk committee comprised of critical care nurses from the MET and its nursing and medical directors, intensive care physicians, an infectious disease physician, and medical informaticists. A decision support tool was developed which monitored hospitalized patients every 5 min and used vital sign and neurologic data in our electronic medical record (EMR) to identify patients with early PD [43]. Once the positive predictive value (PPV) of our PD alert model was acceptable, we went live on a 33-bed medical and oncology floor (A) and a 33-bed non-ICU surgical trauma floor (B). During the intervention year, pager alerts of early PD were sent automatically to charge nurses along with access to a graphical point-of-care web page to help facilitate patient evaluation. Nurses were requested to fill out a form describing the validity of the PD alerts and their response to the alerts.

Patients on unit A were significantly older and had significantly more comorbidities than unit B. During the intervention year, unit A patients had a significant increase in length of stay and total hospital cost, a non-significant increase in ICU transfers (163 (5.1 %) of 3,189 compared to 146 (4.3 %) of 3,423 ($p=0.1163$)), and significantly more MET calls (60 vs 29, $p=0.0004$) while significantly fewer patients died (84 (2.6 %) vs 125 (3.7 %), $p=0.022$) compared to the pre-intervention year. No significant differences in outcome were found on unit B and no differences between pre-intervention and intervention patient populations were found in either unit. Nurses called a physician based on 51 % and 44 % of the PD alerts in units A and B and interventions were initiated based on 59 % and 52 % of the PD alerts.

The results of this 4 year effort to use the HELP EMR to develop, implement, and evaluate an automated case detection and alerting system for PD was designed to support nursing workflow and received nursing endorsement. Nurses on both study units reported an appreciated difference in their workflow based on the early identification of patients with PD.

In this study computerized alerting provided a way to constantly monitor patients and alert nursing of early PD. This resulted in a significant increase in appropriate MET calls and a significant decrease in mortality in the nursing unit containing older patients with multiple comorbidities. Moreover, with the patient trending information contained in the graphical alerts, nurses reported that they had the information they needed to evaluate the patient status, felt more confident about their assessment, and were more at ease about requesting additional help.

14.4 Critiquing Systems

In the alerting examples described above, the computer system responded to abnormalities in the data as they were captured by the EHR by prompting those caring for the patient to intervene. In contrast, critiquing processes begin functioning when an order for a medical intervention is entered into the information system. Such methods typically respond by evaluating the order and either pointing out disparities between the order and an internal definition of proper care or by proposing an alternative therapeutic approach. Below, we describe a computerized critiquing system that specifically targets orders for blood products.

14.4.1 Blood Product Order Critiquing

Over the years, it has become apparent that the transfusion of blood products is an important, often life-saving, therapy and that these same blood products must be ordered and administered with care. Not only are there significant reasons for anxiety concerning diseases that can be transmitted during transfusions, but also the limited supply and shelf life of blood products make them a scarce resource to be used sparingly. The system described here is an older system since supplanted by newer ordering procedures, but it effectively illustrates the place of detailed guidance in creating orders consistent with best practices.

In 1987, the Joint Commission [at that time, the Joint Commission for the Accreditation of Healthcare Organizations (JCAHO)] began to require healthcare institutions to develop criteria for the use of blood products and to carefully monitor compliance with these criteria. At the LDS Hospital, the response to these requirements was to develop a computer system designed specifically to manage the ordering of transfusions and to assist in ensuring compliance with criteria for proper use

Table 14.3 Simplified criteria for ordering red blood cells

Hemoglobin <12 g/dl or hematocrit <35 % if age ≥35 years Hemoglobin <10 g/dl or hematocrit <30 % if age <35 years Oxygen saturation (SaO2) <95 %
Active bleeding Blood loss >500 ml
Systolic blood pressure <100 mmHg or heart rate >100 bpm Adult respiratory distress syndrome (ARDS)

of blood products [44–46]. A central premise of the system design was that all orders would be entered into the computer and that physicians or nurses would be responsible for the entry of all blood orders.

Embedded in the blood-ordering program was a critiquing tool designed to ascertain the reason for every transfusion and to compare the reason against strict criteria. The approach used provides information specific to the type of transfusion planned. For instance, when an order was made for packed red blood cells, the criteria in Table 14.3 were used to critique the order.

The process for entering an order into this system included several points at which information bearing on the propriety of giving blood products is displayed. As a first step, the physician was shown the blood products ordered in the last 24 h. This was followed by a display of the applicable laboratory data. The user then chose the specific blood products required along with the number of units and the priority (stat, routine, etc.). At this point, the user was asked to document the reason for the order. A list of reasons, specific to the blood product chosen, was displayed, and the user chose the appropriate rationale for the intervention. The computer then applied the stored criteria and determined whether the order met the hospital's guidelines.

If the guidelines were met, the order was logged and the blood bank and nursing division were informed electronically and via computer printout. If the criteria were not met, the user was presented with a message stating the applicable criteria and relevant patient data. The physician or nurse could optionally decide to place or cancel the order. If the order was made, he or she was required to enter the reasons for the decision to override the system. The criteria used were the result of a consensus effort by the LDS Hospital medical staff. The criteria were developed using primarily published guidelines but with some adaptations for local conditions (altitude of 4,500 ft). The criteria underwent several modifications based on experience as well as new definitions of standards for these therapies.

One way of measuring the effectiveness of the system's various critiquing messages was to examine the frequency with which the process of ordering blood products was terminated as a result of the feedback. During one 6-month period, the ordering program was entered and then exited without an order 677 times. This was 12.9 % of the total uses. We estimate that one-half of these exits represent decisions not to order blood products based on feedback from the program.

The program relied heavily on the integrated clinical database in the HELP System. It accessed data from: (1) the admitting department; (2) the clinical laboratory; (3) surgical scheduling; (4) the blood bank; and (5) the orders entered by nurses and physicians.

The blood-ordering program described above demonstrates the character of processes that support computerized critiquing. These programs respond to interventions chosen by the physician by analyzing the order and, if appropriate, suggesting reasons to alter the therapeutic plan.

The process used by the blood-ordering program is different from that used in the alerting application in that it involves a dialogue with the user. As a result, the critique can provide a series of informational responses designed to assure that the user is fully aware of the status of the patient as well as of accepted guidelines governing blood product usage.

Historically, physician use of generalized computerized order entry programs has been limited. However, since the Centers for Medicare and Medicaid Services (CMS) have developed the Meaningful Use initiative to encourage EHR use, there has been increased interest in modern order entry programs. A part of the potential value of Computerized Physician Order Entry programs (CPOE) is the ability of these programs to critique orders. Physicians often appreciate the ability of an automated ordering system to give feedback on proper dosing and accepted care protocols as they make their interventional decisions. Opportunities for a constructive interaction between the computer and the clinician are clearly growing, and applications that critique medical decisions can contribute to this growth.

14.5 Suggestion Systems

The third category of computer applications designed to support medical decision making is potentially the most interactive. This subgroup of CDS processes is designed to react to requests (either direct or implied) for assistance. These processes respond by making concrete suggestions concerning which actions should be taken next.

Unlike alerts, action-oriented messages from these systems are expected. Clinicians would typically call up a computer screen, enter requested data, and wait for suggestions from these systems before instituting a new therapy. Unlike critiquing systems, the physician need not commit to an order before the program applies its stored medical logic. Instead, the program conducts an interactive session with the user during which a suggestion concerning a specific therapeutic decision is sought. The system then reviews relevant data, including data that has been requested from the user, and formulates a suggestion for an intervention based on the medical knowledge stored in its knowledge base.

14.5.1 Ventilator Management

The example below is, in many ways, typical of suggestion systems. It functions in the realm of ventilator therapy and has been implemented in increasingly sophisticated forms in intensive care settings at Intermountain's tertiary care hospitals since

1987. A variety of ventilator management protocols continue to function in these settings to this day.

Tertiary care settings typically see large numbers of patients with respiratory failure. One of the more difficult of these problems is that of Adult Respiratory Distress Syndrome (ARDS). This disease can complicate a number of other conditions, including trauma, infectious disease, and shock. The usual therapy includes respiratory support while the underlying pulmonary injury heals. Unfortunately, in the 1980s overall mortality for ARDS had remained at about 50 % for many years. For the subset of ARDS patients who manifest severe hypoxemia, the mortality had been approximately 90 %.

The study of computer protocols for delivering care to ARDS patients was a side effect of research into the effectiveness of a new therapeutic intervention for this difficult disease. In the early 1980s, research began to suggest that external membrane devices that bypassed the lungs to remove carbon dioxide (CO_2) directly from a patient's body might improve survival in the most severely ill ARDS patients. Physicians at the LDS Hospital wanted to study this new approach in a rigorously controlled clinical trial. They chose to do an experiment with a test group that received the external lung treatment and a control group that did not receive the treatment. However, the researchers were aware that the management of ARDS tended to differ from patient to patient, depending on the course the disease followed, and the training and previous experience of the physicians and staff caring for the patient. For this reason, they decided to standardize care by strict adherence to predetermined treatment protocols.

At first, they developed a set of paper protocols. As the protocols became more complex, it became clear that they would be difficult to follow manually. Therefore, it was decided to computerize them. The result was a set of computerized rules that were designed to direct, in detail, the management of patients in both the test and control branches of a study of extracorporeal CO_2 removal ($ECCO_2R$) [47–50]. While the rules were designed initially for this research, they were soon made general enough that they could be used in the management of other patients requiring ventilator support.

These protocols were created by a group of physicians, nurses, respiratory therapists, and specialists in medical informatics. The initial $ECCO_2R$ study period was to be 18 months. Subsequent development concentrated on first eliminating errors in protocol logic, second on extending the scope of these tools, and finally on reworking behavioral patterns in the intensive care setting so that the protocols could be effectively implemented.

The protocol system devised was used successfully during the $ECCO_2R$ study. The study was terminated after 40 patients were treated, 21 with $ECCO_2R$ and 19 with conventional therapy. At that time, there were eight survivors in the conventional therapy group (42 %) and seven in the $ECCO_2R$ group (33 %) [33]. The study team concluded that there was no significant difference between $ECCO_2R$ and conventional treatment of severe ARDS. However, the 42 % survival in the control group was unexpected. Reported survivals in these severely ill patients were less than 15 %. The results led the researchers to suspect that the quality and uniformity of care provided through the use of computerized protocols had resulted in an important improvement in patient outcomes.

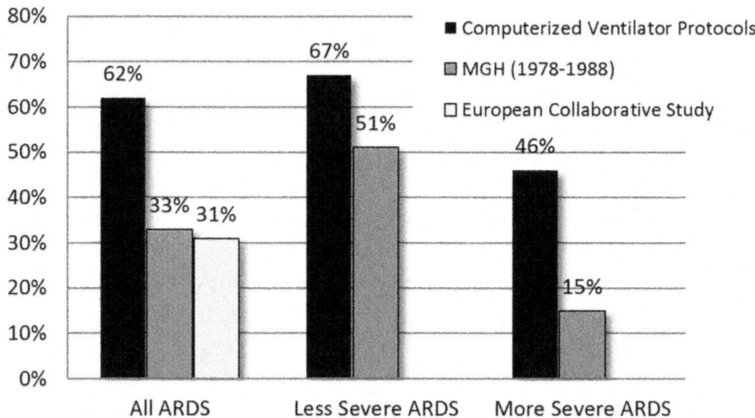

Fig. 14.3 Comparative results for groups managing ARDS patients

As a consequence, development and study of these protocols has continued. Figure 14.3 summarizes the results of their use in 111 LDS Hospital patients, and compares these results to those of two other groups, one from Massachusetts General Hospital (MGH) and a group in Europe (the European Collaborative Study), who have been interested in the problem of treating ARDS. As time went on, it became increasingly clear that the standardization of complex ventilator care decision-making using computers had a pronounced benefit for patients.

It should be noted that here we have focused the definition of systems for suggesting therapeutic interventions quite narrowly. We have limited our example to systems that respond with a suggestion when the clinician has explicitly or implicitly requested one. This type of computerized decision support process represents an area in which we are continuing to explore better ways to interact with clinicians and better ways to capture and encode protocol knowledge.

14.6 Diagnostic Decision Support in the HELP System

The examples above have stressed different approaches to the activation of medical decision support logic and to the delivery of the resulting decisions to the computer user. Below, we change our focus to consider applications that "diagnose".

One of the greatest challenges for a computerized medical decision support system is to participate usefully in the diagnostic process. Diagnostic decision support systems (DDSS) differ from the CDSS described above. Typical decision support systems can draw attention to specific data elements and/or derive therapeutic suggestions from these elements. Such applications offer assistance in the basic recognition process and can identify patients based on data suggesting underlying pathology. On the other hand, the diagnostic process is a preliminary step to suggesting therapeutic interventions. Computerized diagnostic decisions are generally involved with different goals, interfaces, and decision algorithms than the applications previously described.

Two types of diagnostic applications are described below. They differ in the degree with which the developers have solved the problem of providing a clinically useful service. The first type represents a group of applications that, using a set of raw clinical data, target key diagnostic categorizations that impact discrete therapeutic decisions. Four HELP System examples are discussed.

The second group of diagnostic processes described comes from the family of applications that attempt to simulate the more extensive and flexible diagnostic behavior of physicians. Those discussed here represent research applications whose clinical applicability remains to be determined. The behavior of these applications in terms of preliminary data and of experience gleaned in a research and development environment are described.

14.7 Diagnostic Applications

A number of applications residing in the HELP system can, through the use of various diagnostic strategies, affect patient care. Below we describe four of these applications. The first 3 are alerting systems that invoke a diagnostic process to detect clinical conditions; they intercede by alerting appropriate caregivers to the proposed diagnosis. They include an application that evaluates patient data to detect adverse drug events, a tool that recognizes nosocomial infections, and a diagnostic system running in the Emergency Department that encourages the enrollment of pneumonia patients into a detailed therapeutic protocol. The fourth application described is a computerized assistant that informs and advises physicians as they undertake the complex task of determining how to treat a patient with a possible or proven infection. This CDSS interacts with its users to provide detailed clinical suggestions for antibiotic therapy in the context of the suspected infectious condition.

14.7.1 Adverse Drug Events

Adverse drug events (ADEs) are defined by the World Health Organization as "any response to a drug which is noxious, unintended, and which occurs at doses normally used in man for the prophylaxis, diagnosis, or therapy of disease" [51]. ADEs can range in severity from drowsiness or nausea to anaphylaxis and death. In 1995, it was estimated that in the United States drug-related morbidity and mortality cost more than $136 billion per year [52]. This cost has been shown to increase with time [53].

The process of recognizing ADEs differs from that of drug monitoring at the time of drug dispensing; this latter process has become a standard part of computerized pharmacy systems. The alerting systems embedded in modern-day pharmacy dispensing systems typically evaluate ordered medications against a list of contraindications based on known allergies, expected reactions with other patient medications, or information from the clinical laboratory that can be expected to affect the drugs given or the dosage of those medications. In contrast, the goal of an ADE detection system is to diagnose the existence of a drug reaction from the patient data collected during the routine documentation of patient care.

An ADE recognition subsystem was implemented in the HELP system in the late 1980s [54, 55]. This ADE subsystem continuously monitors patients for the occurrence of an ADE. The system does so by inspecting the patient data entered at the bedside for signs of rash, changes in respiratory rate, heart rate, hearing, mental status, seizure, anaphylaxis, diarrhea, and fever. In addition, data from the clinical lab, the pharmacy, and the medication charting applications are analyzed to determine possible ADEs.

The system evaluates all of the patients in the hospital and generates a daily computer report indicating which patients have possible ADEs. Clinical pharmacists can then follows up on these patients and complete the evaluation using a verification program. This program provides a consistent method of completing the diagnostic process. A scoring system (the Naranjo method) is used to score the ADEs as definite (score ≥9), probable (score 5–8), possible (score 1–4), or unlikely (score 0) [56]. The physicians caring for each patient are notified of confirmed ADEs by the pharmacist who does the evaluation.

The existence of an application for the diagnosis of ADEs substantially increased the frequency with which these events were recognized and documented in the hospital setting. Using a voluntary reporting method, nine ADEs were recorded in the 1-year period from May 1, 1988 to May 1, 1989. In the period from May 1, 1989 to May 1, 1990, while the program was initially used, 401 adverse drug events were identified.

An additional effect of this program appears to be a reduction in the number of severe ADEs seen. During the year beginning in January of 1990, 41 ADEs occurred. In this time frame, physicians were notified of verified ADEs only if they were classified as severe or life threatening. In two subsequent periods (the year of 1991 and the year of 1992) early notification of physicians was practiced for all severities of ADE. Numbers of severe ADEs decreased to 12 and 15 during the follow-up time periods ($p<0.001$).

In an effort to understand the impact of the drug reactions that were the target of this application, the costs of ADEs were examined. In studies that used the computer tools described above, investigators found that length of hospital stay for patients with ADEs was increased by 1.91 days and that costs resulting from the increased stay were $2,262. The increased risk of death among patients experiencing ADEs was 1.88 times [57]. Thus, the cost savings and impact on quality of care in reducing ADEs was substantial.

These tools, with modest modifications, are used to this day. They leverage the fact that the majority of the data necessary for their function is available in the HELP system's integrated database. They illustrate the potential for computerized diagnostic applications to impact patient care not just by assisting with the choice of interventions, but also by focusing clinical attention on those cases where the interventions chosen have put the patient at risk.

14.7.2 Nosocomial Infections

In the previous example, a rule-based system was used to suggest the diagnosis of adverse drug events for a group of patients undergoing therapy in the hospital. Another application which originated at the LDS Hospital was designed to recognize nosocomial, or hospital-acquired infections [58]. The program served a need recognized by the Joint Commission that required ongoing surveillance for hospital-acquired infections.

The process of detecting nosocomial hospital infections serves a recognized clinical purpose. Control measures based on this information are believed to be important in interrupting the spread of hospital-acquired infections. Evidence suggests that intensive surveillance programs may be linked to reduced rates of infection. However, the process can be expensive. Traditional techniques require infection control personnel to manually screen all appropriate patients on a routine basis.

The computerized surveillance system described here relies on data from a variety of sources to diagnose nosocomial infections. Information from the microbiology laboratory, nurse charting, the chemistry laboratory, the admitting office, surgery, pharmacy, radiology, and respiratory therapy are used. Once each day, a report is produced detailing the computer's findings. This report can be used to follow up on the patients for whom there is evidence of nosocomial infection.

In the initial studies done in 1986 to compare the computer-based surveillance of nosocomial infections to the traditional, manual approach, 217 patients were determined to be possible victims of hospital-acquired infection (out of 4,679 patients discharged in a 2-month period). This included 182 patients identified by the computer and an overlapping 145 patients recognized by traditional means. Of these patients, 155 were confirmed to have nosocomial infections.

For the group of 155 patients, the computer's sensitivity was 90 % with a false positive rate of 23 %; at the same time, the infection control practitioners demonstrated a sensitivity of 76 % and a false positive rate of 19 %. When the hours required to use each approach were estimated, the computer-based approach was more than twice as efficient as the entirely manual technique.

The nosocomial infection tool, like the ADE recognition system, uses Boolean logic in its diagnostic process (see Chap. 2). In an effort to extend the process of managing hospital-acquired infections, an extension to the infection control system has been developed. The goal of the enhancement was to predict which patients were likely to contract a nosocomial infection in the hospital in the future. The tool is based on different decision algorithms. Data from patients with infections acquired in the hospital were combined with data from a control set of patients, and a group of statistical programs was used to identify risk factors. Logistic regression using these risk factors was used in the development of tools that could estimate the risk of hospital-acquired infection for inpatients. The resulting system has been shown capable of predicting these infections in 63 % of the population who are ultimately affected [59]. It has been maintained and updated for more than 20 years and continues to provide service in numerous clinical settings.

14.8 Detecting Pneumonia in the Emergency Department

Pneumonia remains a common clinical problem seen in outpatient settings and emergency departments across the country. The disease is often divided into Community-Acquired Pneumonia (CAP) and Healthcare-Associated Pneumonia (HCAP). The latter illness may be associated with a higher risk of antibiotic-resistant bacteria and therefore, needs to be recognized and approached with an altered therapeutic plan.

In 2011 researchers at Intermountain Healthcare introduced a system for diagnosing pneumonia into four emergency departments (EDs) in the Salt Lake City area in Utah [60]. The diagnostic process in three other local emergency departments was unchanged.

The pneumonia detection system was coupled with an electronic protocol for treating both CAP and HCAP [61]. The goal of the diagnostic tool was to identify potential pneumonia patients and bring their condition to the attention of the emergency department physicians in a timely fashion. By then enrolling the patient in the electronic protocol, the physician could take advantage of a decision support tool that (1) collected and displayed data relevant to the diagnosis and treatment of pneumonia, (2) calculated an individualized risk score for each patient (based on the 30-day, all-cause mortality experienced by similar pneumonia patients), and (3) used this information to suggest a patient treatment strategy. For each patient, the strategy included a suggestion for disposition (treat at home, admit to acute care bed, or admit to ICU), suggestions for appropriate labs and cultures, and individualized suggestions for antibiotic treatment.

The pneumonia detection system is implemented using a tool called the "screening framework". This application is designed to function in the background. It watches the flow of data into the EHR and captures those data elements appropriate to the diagnostic process. In the case of pneumonia, these include vital signs, laboratory results, elements from the patient history and physical examination, and information extracted from chest x-ray reports using a natural language processing application. This information is passed to a Bayesian network developed specifically to compute the probability of pneumonia for emergency department patients. For patients whose probability exceeds 40 %, a "P" is placed on the departmental tracking board to alert clinicians of the likelihood of pneumonia. Clicking on this

P takes a physician to the pneumonia protocol which provides evidence-based suggestions for continued patient care.

The diagnostic tool's accuracy was tuned with the goal of delivering a reasonable positive predictive value at an acceptable sensitivity. We believe that a system with too many false positives will invariably be ignored by busy clinicians. The resulting system had a sensitivity of 40.9 %, a specificity of 96.6 %, and a positive predictive value of 50.9 %.

The premise behind using a diagnostic system in this way is that regular, reasonably accurate, pneumonia alerts will encourage use of the electronic protocol. This premise appears to be substantiated in that use of this electronic guideline increased steadily over the course of the study period. Moreover, an analysis of the effects of the protocol demonstrated a change in 30-day all-cause mortality. While there was no difference when considering all pneumonia patients, an analysis of the community-acquired pneumonia patients treated in the intervention EDs demonstrated a significantly lower mortality when the protocol was in use (Odds Ratio: 0.53).

In this study, the diagnostic system functioned as a prompt and reminder to use an electronic treatment protocol. Physicians can use the protocol without the diagnostic reminder and can ignore the protocol even when reminded by the diagnostic alert. While the pneumonia diagnostic system may help to determine the diagnosis for some patients, its clearest value is as a reminder for busy physicians of the availability of a tool that supports and standardizes therapeutic interventions. This may be a profitable way to think about the potential contribution of diagnostic systems to real-world, clinical workflows.

14.8.1 Antibiotic Assistant

The fourth application in this group is an example of a multipronged approach to the task of supporting medical decision making. As a part of research into the use of computers in medical care, the Infectious Disease Department at LDS Hospital developed a tool to help clinicians make informed decisions concerning the administration of antibiotics [62, 63]. The "Antibiotic Assistant" application was designed to provide three basic services. First, it assembled relevant data for the physicians so they could determine whether a specific patient was infected and what sorts of interventions might be appropriate. Information such as the most recent temperature, renal function, and allergies were presented. Second, the system suggested a course of therapy appropriate to that patient's condition. Finally, the program allowed the clinician to review hospital experience with infections for the past 6 months and the past 5 years. One of the options of the program allowed the clinician to review the logic behind the computer's suggestions while another presented brief monographs on the appropriate use of each antibiotic in the hospital formulary.

The diagnostic processes embedded in this application were derived from data extracted from the HELP system and analyzed on a monthly basis. The goal of the analysis was to define the probability of each potential pathogen as a causative agent for a certain class of patient. Six clinical variables were used in this process. These variables were identified through a statistical analysis of 23 proposed data elements. They included the site of infection, the patient's status (inpatient or outpatient), the mode of transmission (community- or hospital-acquired), the patient's hospital service, the patient's age, and the patient's sex.

The result of this monthly analysis was an assessment of the likelihood of each pathogen for every combination of the patient-related variables. For example, once the analysis was complete, the percentage of hospital-acquired bacteremias due to *Escherichia coli* in male patients age 50 or less who were on the cardiovascular service would be stored in the program's knowledge base. The analytic programs also evaluated susceptibility data to determine which antibiotics were likely to cover the most probable pathogens for each combination of patient variables.

This probabilistic knowledge was then filtered through a set of rules created by infectious disease experts. These rules adjust the output of the first phase to include criteria representing basic tenets of antibacterial therapy. For example, the susceptibility information garnered from the historical data would be updated to indicate that amikacin should be used only for infections due to gram-negative organisms.

The resulting knowledge base has been used by the antibiotic assistant program to make presumptive diagnoses of infectious organisms and to suggest treatments appropriate to these organisms. By offering the monographs and explanations mentioned above and by allowing the clinicians to browse its knowledge base, it provided large amounts of information in addition to its suggestions.

In recent years, antibiotic stewardship programs have become available that provide some of the functionality of the Antibiotic Assistant. However, a number of its capabilities remain unique and it continues to provide service in a variety of clinical settings.

14.9 Research into Complex Peri-diagnostic Applications

The systems described above have had a measurable effect on improving health care provided in the hospital setting. The dream of even more sophisticated and inclusive systems was presented more than 50 years ago. In 1959, Ledley and Lusted described the application of methods from the realm of symbolic logic and statistical pattern recognition to problems in medicine [64]. They proposed that these tools be used to assist in the diagnostic process and in other problems involving medical decision making. Computer systems were the enabling technology that was predicted to bring these tools to the bedside.

A variety of researchers have accepted the challenge of Ledley and Lusted and produced experimental systems designed to diagnose a variety of illnesses. The pneumonia diagnostic system described above is one example. However, as researchers consider other ways to use the information embedded in these applications, a recurring question has to do with the activities that a diagnostic system can support *beyond diagnosis*.

An important portion of the value of computerized diagnostic tools lies in the development of well-designed models of the diagnostic process to assist in the complex clinical decision-making tasks. Physicians clearly exercise their diagnostic knowledge not only when they assign a diagnostic label to a patient, but also during processes as diverse as reading medical reports and critiquing the clinical behavior of their peers. Below, we provide two examples of experimental systems that use diagnostic knowledge to support these types of cognitive processes. These examples illustrate systems that can (1) assist with data collection; and (2) help assess the quality of medical reports.

The applications described below benefit from a long-standing interest in Bayesian techniques for probability revision among researchers using the HELP system. For more than 35 years, the HELP system has contained frame-based decision support subsystems capable of expressing and employing Bayes' equation to assess probabilistically the support for diagnoses provided by various combinations of clinical data [14].

14.9.1 Assisting Data Collection

Efforts to use diagnostic models to direct data collection in the HELP system have concentrated on the patient history. The goal has been to identify tools that could effectively collect a medical history appropriate for use in diagnostic decision support applications. While earlier efforts focused on history appropriate to a wide variety of diseases [65], subsequent efforts have focused on acquiring data bearing principally on pulmonary diseases [66, 67].

To conduct this experiment, three techniques for collecting the history were developed. The first was a simple branching questionnaire. This approach takes full advantage of the hierarchical relationship between more and less specific questions. For instance, if the question "Have you had chest pain with this illness?" was answered "Yes," then more specific questions such as "Is your chest pain brought on by exertion?" were asked. Alternately, if the answer to the first question was "No", the more specific questions would not be asked.

The second technique has been called decision-driven data acquisition (DDA). With this technique, a frame-based, Bayesian expert system analyzes all data available at any point in the patient interview. The individual disease frames determine which additional information is needed to evaluate the likelihood of the particular disease. Each frame proposes one or more questions. From this list, a supervisory program selects a group of five questions, which are then presented to the patient. The system passes through this cycle multiple times until criteria are met indicating that no additional data are needed.

A third approach has also been tested. It is similar to the DDA method except that it was adapted for use in a setting where the patient was not present at a computer terminal. The approach begins when a paper questionnaire containing screening questions is presented to a patient. Staff members enter the answers into the computer, and the patient's data are compared to the diagnostic frames. The questions

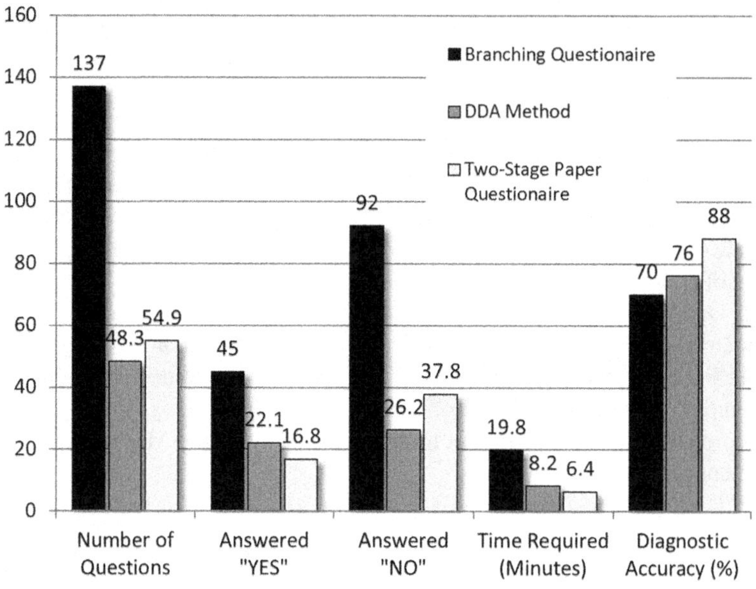

Fig. 14.4 A comparison of techniques for collecting the patient history

are scored in a filtering process, and then from 0 to 40 additional questions are printed for the patient to answer. After the patient answers these additional questions, the answers are entered into the computer and the process is completed.

The branching questionnaire mode of data collection and the DDA mode were tested on inpatients at the LDS Hospital. Fifty patients took a DDA managed history and 23 received a history managed by the branching questionnaire program. Figure 14.4 illustrates the results.

On average, the DDA mode took a significantly ($p<0.05$) shorter time to run (8.2 min) and asked significantly fewer questions (48.8 questions) than did the branching questionnaire (19.2 min and 137 questions, respectively). The two-stage, paper questionnaire was tested separately on patients coming to the X-ray department for chest X-rays. It appeared to perform similarly to the interactive DDA mode. It should be noted that there was no significant difference between the techniques in terms of diagnostic accuracy. Using history alone, all three succeeded in placing the patient's correct disease in a five-member differential diagnostic list from 70 to 88 % of the time.

14.9.2 Assessing the Quality of Medical Reports

A second example of an alternative use of diagnostic knowledge comes from a study of result reporting in the radiology department. The central goal of this project was to develop a technique for measuring the quality of X-ray reporting without requiring the review of radiographs by multiple radiologists. This is in contradistinction to typical approaches for evaluating the accuracy of radiologists. Historically, audit procedures in the radiology department require multiple readings of a select set of X-rays [68–72] . The results of the repeated readings are used to define a "gold standard" for the films. Then the individual radiologists are compared to the gold standard.

The technique developed as a part of this project was based on a simple premise. Each examination was a test of the radiologist's accuracy. Instead of comparing the abnormalities reported to a standard formulated through multiple readings, the description in the report was evaluated in comparison to the patient's overall diagnostic outcome. In the case of chest X-rays, the standard was the list of final diagnoses (ICD-9 codes) written into the patient's record at the time of discharge. The report generated by the radiologist was successful to the extent that it supported the process that led to one of the discharge diagnoses.

While a variety of algorithms can be used to link the findings represented in the X-ray report to the final diagnosis, we have demonstrated the success of a variation on Shannon Information Content in discriminating among physicians reading chest X-rays. Shannon Information Content [73] is a mathematical formalism for assessing the informational value of messages. For this project, we modified it to provide a measure of the information produced by the radiologists as each of them interpret x-rays. The assumption inherent in this usage is that the information contained in an X-ray report can be expected to alter the likelihood of the various diseases that a patient might have. Information Content is calculated from the change in probability of these diseases.

For this technique to work, a diagnostic system was required that was capable of discriminating among diseases producing abnormalities on the chest radiograph. The information content was calculated from the change in disease probability induced by the findings recorded in the chest X-ray report. A Bayesian system provided the required probabilities.

Our evidence for the success of this technique came from two studies. In the first, we used expert systems technologies to demonstrate discrimination in a controlled experiment [74]. In this experiment, five X-ray readers read an identical set of 100 films. The assessment produced by the diagnostic logic program gave results consistent with the differing expertise of the readers and similar to the results of a more standard audit procedure.

In a second study of this audit technique, we tested a group of radiologists following their standard procedure for interpreting radiographs [75]. Each chest X-ray was reviewed, the report dictated and transcribed only once, as is typical with most radiologists' daily work. The goal of the study was to test the ability of a knowledge-based approach to measure the quality of X-ray reporting, without requiring repeated reading of the radiographs.

This technique used a modified version of the Shannon Information Content measure, and was designed to assess both the positive information contributed by X-ray findings relevant to a patient's disease, and the negative information contributed by findings which do not apply to any of the patient's illnesses. X-ray readers were compared based on the *bits* of information produced. We used 651 chest X-ray reports, generated by a group of radiologists, which were compared to the patients' discharge diagnoses using a measure of information content. The radiologists were grouped according to whether they had received additional (post residency) training in chest radiology. The "trained" radiologists produced 11 % more information than the "untrained" radiologists (0.664 bits as opposed to 0.589 bits, significant at $p<0.005$).

The average information content calculated successfully discriminated these groups. However, it is an overall measure. Examination of the interaction between the groups of radiologists and disease subgroups indicates that the score can also discriminate at the level of different diseases ($p<0.05$). This suggests that the technique might not only discriminate overall quality of X-ray interpretation, but it might also be of use for pinpointing the specific diseases for which an individual radiologist may be failing to generate effective information.

14.10 Summary

In this chapter, we have reviewed a collection of hospital-based applications that provide medical decision support at the patient bedside. These applications can be categorized in a variety of different ways. We have found it profitable to characterize these systems in terms of their relationship to the data, and of their approach to communicating with their users. These foci may be helpful to future system developers and implementers, as they reflect on the environment required for the success of decision support applications.

We have also attempted to emphasize the range of sophistication that can be found in clinically operational CDSS. Applications using simple logic contribute a great deal to the quality of care provided in clinical settings. Programs that use more complex techniques and that strive to provide the more sophisticated decisions associated with disease recognition can also contribute. Among the diagnostic applications currently functioning in hospital settings, those that focus on specific, limited, diagnostic goals with a recognizable target audience have been more successful. General-purpose diagnostic programs, while capable of producing interesting results, have yet to find an audience for which they can routinely provide a valued support function.

The lessons learned from the information systems used in hospitals are diffusing rapidly into the outpatient setting. Less expensive hardware, more flexible software, and an environment that increasingly values the efficiencies that computers can offer are encouraging the development of systems for a wide range of clinical settings. The federal government is actively encouraging this shift. As this process occurs, the lessons garnered by developers of CDSS in hospital settings provide a springboard for the decision support applications of the future. These systems will embody, in their behavior and approach, computing models derived from experiments conducted in environments like the HELP system.

As new CDSS incorporate the infrastructure and decision models developed in the past, these next-generation systems will also incorporate approaches to knowledge engineering, knowledge maintenance, and system implementation that have evolved as a part of the research described above. The practices described reflect a philosophy of development and critical review whose activities are shared by communities of caregivers. Teams composed of informaticists, software developers, and clinicians are essential to an environment that can develop and iteratively refine sophisticated decision support applications.

A priority for these communities is the thoughtful evaluation of the success of CDS interventions. Assessment of the outcomes associated with these applications is important to their users. A key goal is to measure both the effect of these systems on the workflow of busy clinicians and the impact of these systems on quality, cost, and overall efficiency. Adherence to this approach will do much to reduce the challenges associated with implementing potentially disruptive CDS technologies by involving the medical community in their creation, evaluation, and growth.

References

1. Kohn LT, Corrigan JM, Donaldson MS, editors. To err is human. Washington, DC: National Academy Press; 1999.
2. Bates DW, Leape LL, Cullen DJ, et al. Effect of computerized physician order entry and a team intervention on prevention of serious medication errors. JAMA. 1998;280:1311–6.
3. Bates DW, Teich JM, Lee J, et al. The impact of computerized physician order entry on medication error prevention. J Am Med Inform Assoc. 1999;6:313–21.
4. Hunt DL, Haynes RB, Hanna SE, Smith K. Effects of computer-based clinical decision support systems on physician performance and patient outcomes. JAMA. 1998;280:1339–46.
5. Bates DW, Kuperman GJ, Wang S, et al. Ten commandments for effective clinical decision support: making the practice of evidence-based medicine a reality. J Am Med Inform Assoc. 2003;10:523–30.
6. Bleich HL. The computer as a consultant. N Engl J Med. 1971;284:141–7.
7. McDonald CJ. Protocol-based computer reminders, the quality of care and the non-perfectibility of medicine. N Engl J Med. 1976;295:1351–5.
8. Tierney WM, Overhage JM, McDonald CJ. Toward electronic records that improve care. Ann Intern Med. 1995;122:725–6.
9. Clayton PD, Sideli RV, Sengupta S. Open architecture and integrated information at Columbia-Presbyterian medical center. MD Comput. 1992;9:297–303.
10. Safran C, Herrmann F, Rind D, Kowaloff HB, Bleich HL, Slack WV. Computer-based support of clinical decision making. MD Comput. 1990;9:319–22.
11. Kuperman GJ, Gardner RM, Pryor TA. HELP: a dynamic hospital information system. New York: Springer; 1991.
12. Teich JM, Geisler MA, Cimmermann DE, Frank AD, Glaser JP. Design considerations in the BWH ambulatory medical record: features for maximum acceptance by clinicians. 14th Annual Symposium on Computer Applications in Medical Care; Washington, DC (USA); 4–7 Nov 1990. p. 735–9.
13. Geissbuhler A, Miller RA. A new approach to the implementation of direct care-provider order entry. Proc AMIA Annu Fall Symp. 1996:689–93.
14. Pryor TA, Clayton PD, Haug PJ, Wigertz O. Design of a knowledge driven HIS. Proc Annu Symp Comput Appl Med Care. 1987;11:60–3.

15. Gardner RM, Cannon GH, Morris AH, Olsen KR, Price G. Computerized blood gas interpretation and reporting system. IEEE Comput. 1975;8:39–45.
16. Gardner RM. Computerized data management and decision making in critical care. Surg Clin N Am. 1985;65:1041–51.
17. Hulse RK, Clark SJ, Jackson JC, Warner HR, Gardner RM. Computerized medication monitoring system. Am J Hosp Pharm. 1976;33:1061–4.
18. Haug PJ, Gardner RM, Tate KE, et al. Decision support in medicine: examples from the HELP system. Comput Biomed Res. 1994;27:396–418.
19. Wheeler LA, Brecher G, Sheiner LB. Clinical laboratory use in the evaluation of anemia. JAMA. 1977;238:2709–14.
20. Olsen DM, Kane RL, Proctor PH. A controlled trial of multiphasic screening. N Engl J Med. 1976;294:925–30.
21. Bradshaw KE, Gardner RM, Pryor TA. Development of a computerized laboratory alerting system. Comput Biomed Res. 1989;22:575–87.
22. Tate KE, Gardner RM, Weaver LK. A computer laboratory alerting system. MD Comput. 1990;7:296–301.
23. Tate KE, Gardner RM. Computers, quality and the clinical laboratory: a look at critical value reporting. Proc Annu Symp Comput Appl Med Care. 1993:193–7.
24. Tate KE, Gardner RM, Scherting K. Nurses, pagers, and patient-specific criteria: three keys to improved critical value reporting. Proc Annu Symp Comput Appl Med Care. 1995:164–8.
25. Johnson DS, Ranzenberger J, Herbert RD, Gardner RM, Clemmer TP. A computerized alert program for acutely ill patients. J Nurs Adm. 1980;10:26–35.
26. Kuperman GJ, Teich JM, Bates DW, et al. Detecting alerts, notifying the physician, and offering action items: a comprehensive alerting system. Proc Annu Symp Comput Appl Med Care. 1996;20:704–8.
27. Evans RS, Johnson KV, Flint VB, Kinder AT, Lyon CR, Hawley WL, Vawdrey DK, Thomsen GE. Enhanced notification of critical ventilator events. J Am Med Assoc. 2005;12:589–95.
28. Bell MB, Konrad D, Granath F, Ekbom A, Martling CR. Prevalence and sensitivity of MET-criteria in a Scandinavian University Hospital. Resuscitation. 2006;70(1):66–73.
29. McFarlan SJ, Hensley S. Implementation and outcomes of a rapid response team. J Nurs Care Qual. 2007;22(4):307–13.
30. Goldhill DR, White SA, Sumner A. Physiological values and procedures in the 24 h before ICU admission from the ward. Anaesthesia. 1999;54(6):529–34.
31. Hillman KM, Bristow PJ, Chey T, Daffurn K, Jacques T, Norman SL, et al. Antecedents to hospital deaths. Intern Med J. 2001;31(6):343–8.
32. Hillman KM, Bristow PJ, Chey T, Daffurn K, Jacques T, Norman SL, et al. Duration of life-threatening antecedents prior to intensive care admission. Intensive Care Med. 2002;28(11):1629–34.
33. Schein RM, Hazday N, Pena M, Ruben BH, Sprung CL. Clinical antecedents to in-hospital cardiopulmonary arrest. Chest. 1990;98(6):1388–92.
34. Buist MD, Jarmolowski E, Burton PR, Bernard SA, Waxman BP, Anderson J. Recognising clinical instability in hospital patients before cardiac arrest or unplanned admission to intensive care. A pilot study in a tertiary-care hospital. Med J Aust. 1999;171(1):22–5.
35. Buist M. The rapid response team paradox: why doesn't anyone call for help? Crit Care Med. 2008;36(2):634–6.
36. Kause J, Smith G, Prytherch D, Parr M, Flabouris A, Hillman K, et al. A comparison of antecedents to cardiac arrests, deaths and emergency intensive care admissions in Australia and New Zealand, and the United Kingdom – the ACADEMIA study. Resuscitation. 2004;62(3):275–82.
37. Cioffi J. Recognition of patients who require emergency assistance: a descriptive study. Heart Lung J Acute Crit Care. 2000;29(4):262–8.

38. Ott LK, Pinsky MR, Hoffman LA, Clarke SP, Clark S, Ren D, et al. Medical emergency team calls in the radiology department: patient characteristics and outcomes. BMJ Qual Saf. 2012;21(6):509–18.
39. Bruckel J. Evidence-based medicine and rapid response team implementation. McGill J Med Int Forum Adv Med Sci Stud. 2006;9(1):5–7.
40. Kumar A, Roberts D, Wood KE, Light B, Parrillo JE, Sharma S, et al. Duration of hypotension before initiation of effective antimicrobial therapy is the critical determinant of survival in human septic shock. Crit Care Med. 2006;34(6):1589–96.
41. Chan PS, Krumholz HM, Nichol G, Nallamothu BK. American heart association national registry of cardiopulmonary resuscitation I. Delayed time to defibrillation after in-hospital cardiac arrest. N Engl J Med. 2008;358(1):9–17.
42. Devita MA, Bellomo R, Hillman K, Kellum J, Rotondi A, Teres D, et al. Findings of the first consensus conference on medical emergency teams. Crit Care Med. 2006;34(9):2463–78.
43. Evans RS, Kuttler KG, Simpson KJ, Howe S, Crossno PF, Johnson KV, et al. Automated detection of physiologic deterioration in hospitalized patients. J Am Med Inform Assoc: JAMIA. 2015;22(2):350–60.
44. Gardner RM, Golubjatnikov OK, Laub RM, Jacobson JT, Evans RS. Computer-critiqued blood ordering using the HELP System. Comput Biomed Res. 1990;23:514–28.
45. Lepage EF, Gardner RM, Laub RM, Golubjatnikov OK. Improving blood transfusion practice: role of a computerized hospital information system. Transfusion. 1992;32:253–9.
46. Gardner RM, Christiansen PD, Tate KE, Laub MB, Holmes SR. Computerized continuous quality improvement methods used to optimize blood transfusions. Proc Annu Symp Comput Appl Med Care. 1993;17:166–70.
47. Sittig DF, Pace NL, Gardner RM, Beck E, Morris AH. Implementation of a computerized patient advise system using the HELP clinical information system. Comput Biomed Res. 1989;22:474–87.
48. East TD, Henderson S, Morris AH, Gardner RM. Implementation issues and challenges for computerized clinical protocols for management of mechanical ventilation in ARDS patients. Proc Annu Symp Comput Appl Med Care. 1989;13:583–7.
49. Henderson S, East TD, Morris AH, et al. Performance evaluation of computerized clinical protocols for management of arterial hypoxemia in ARDS patients. Proc Annu Symp Comput Appl Med Care. 1989;13:588–92.
50. Morris AH, Wallace CJ, Menlove RL, et al. A randomized clinical trial of pressure-controlled inverse ratio ventilation and extracorporeal CO2 removal for adult respiratory distress syndrome. Am J Respir Crit Care Med. 1994;149:295–305.
51. International drug monitoring. The role of the hospital. World Health Organ Tech Rep Ser. 1969;425:5–24.
52. Johnson JA, Bootman HL. Drug-related morbidity and mortality: a cost of illness model. Arch Intern Med. 1995;155:1949–56.
53. Ernst FR, Grizzle AJ. Drug-related morbidity and mortality: updating the cost-of-illness model. J Am Pharm Assoc (Wash). 2001;41(2):192–9.
54. Classen DC, Pestotnik SL, Evans RS, Burke JP. Computerized surveillance of adverse drug events in hospital patients. JAMA. 1991;266:2847–51.
55. Evans RS, Pestotnik SL, Classen DC, et al. Development of a computerized adverse drug event monitor. Proc Annu Symp Comput Appl Med Care. 1991:23–7.
56. Naranjo CA, Busto U, Sellers EM, et al. A method for estimating the probability of adverse drug reactions. Clin Pharmacol Ther. 1981;30:239–45.
57. Classen DC, Pestotnik SL, Evans RS, Llyod JF, Burke JP. Adverse drug events in hospitalized patients: excess length of stay, extra costs, and attributable mortality. JAMA. 1997;277:301–6.
58. Evans RS, Larsen RA, Burke JP, et al. Computer surveillance of hospital-acquired infections and antibiotic use. JAMA. 1986;256:1007–11.

59. Evans RS, Burke JP, Pestotnik SL, Classen DC, Menlove RL, Gardner RM. Prediction of hospital infections and selection of antibiotics using an automated hospital data base. Proc Annu Symp Comput Appl Med Care. 1990:663–7.
60. Dean NC, Jones BE, Ferraro JP, Vines CG, Haug PJ. Performance and utilization of an emergency department electronic screening tool for pneumonia. JAMA Intern Med. 2013;173(8):699–701.
61. Dean NC, Jones BE, Jones JP, Ferraro JP, Post HB, Vines CG, Allen TL, Haug PJ. Impact of an electronic clinical decision support tool for emergency department patients with pneumonia. Ann Emerg Med. 2015;66(5):511–20.
62. Evans RS, Classen DC, Pestotnik SL, Clemmer TP, Weaver LK, Burke JP. A decision support tool for antibiotic therapy. Proc Annu Symp Comput Appl Med Care. 1995:651–5.
63. Evans RS, Pestotnik SL, Classen DC, et al. A computer-assisted management program for antibiotics and other antiinfective agents. N Engl J Med. 1998;338:232–8.
64. Ledley RS, Lusted LB. Reasoning foundations of medical diagnosis. Science. 1959;130:9–21.
65. Warner HR, Rutherford BD, Houtchens B. A sequential Bayesian approach to history taking and diagnosis. Comput Biomed Res. 1972;5:256–62.
66. Haug PJ, Warner HR, Clayton PD, et al. A decision-driven system to collect the patient history. Comput Biomed Res. 1987;20:193–207.
67. Haug PJ, Rowe KG, Rich T, et al. A comparison of computer-administered histories. Proc Am Assoc Med Syst Inf Annu Conf. 1988:21–5.
68. Herman PG, Gerson DE, Hessel SJ, et al. Disagreements in chest roentgen interpretation. Chest. 1975;68:278–82.
69. Yerushalmy J. Reliability of chest radiology in the diagnosis of pulmonary lesions. Am J Surg. 1955;89:231–40.
70. Koran LM. The reliability of clinical methods, data, and judgments (second of two parts). N Engl J Med. 1975;293:695–701.
71. Rhea JT, Potsaid MS, DeLuca SA. Errors of interpretation as elicited by a quality audit of an emergency radiology facility. Radiology. 1979;132:277–80.
72. Raines CJ, McFarlane DV, Wall C. Audit procedures in the national breast screening study: mammography interpretation. J Can Assoc Radiol. 1986;37:256–60.
73. Shannon CE, Weaver W. The mathematical theory of communication. Urbana: University of Illinois Press; 1949.
74. Haug PJ, Clayton PD, Tocino I, et al. Chest radiography: a tool for the audit of report quality. Radiology. 1991;180:271–6.
75. Haug PJ, Pryor TA, Frederick PR. Integrating radiology and hospital information systems: the advantage of shared data. Proc Annu Symp Comput Appl Med Care. 1992;187–91.

Chapter 15
Decision Support During Inpatient Care Provider Order Entry: Vanderbilt's WizOrder Experience

Randolph A. Miller, Lemuel Russell Waitman, and S. Trent Rosenbloom

Abstract In this chapter, the authors describe a pragmatic approach to the introduction of clinical decision support at the point of care, based on more than a decade of experience in developing and evolving Vanderbilt's inpatient "WizOrder" care provider order entry (CPOE) system. The authors have developed a generic model for decision support within inpatient CPOE systems. The model is based on characteristics of end-user workflows and on decision support considerations that are common to a variety of inpatient settings and CPOE systems. The specific approach to implementing a given clinical decision support feature should involve evaluation along three axes: what type of intervention to create (four categories); when to introduce the intervention into the user's workflow (seven categories), and how disruptive, during use of the system, the intervention might be to end-users' workflows (six categories). Framing decision support in this manner may help both

---

This chapter includes an adaptation of portions of an article from the Journal of Biomedical Informatics: Miller RA, Waitman LR, Chen S, Rosenbloom ST. The anatomy of decision support during in patient care provider order entry (CPOE): Empirical observations from a decade of CPOE experience at Vanderbilt, 2005; 38:469–485, reprinted with permission from Elsevier. Vanderbilt licensed the WizOrder CPOE system to McKesson Corporation, which marketed it as Horizon Expert Orders until 2014. This article describes the WizOrder, pre-commercialization, academic version of the system as it was deployed at Vanderbilt from 1995 to 2015. The authors acknowledge the contributions of Dr. Sutin Chen to the previous version of this chapter and of Antoine Geissbuhler, MD, as the primary author of the WizOrder system from 1994 to 1999.

R.A. Miller, M.D. (✉)
Department of Biomedical Informatics, Vanderbilt University Medical Center,
2525 West End Avenue, Ste 1475, Nashville, TN 37203, USA
e-mail: randolph.a.miller@vanderbilt.edu

L.R. Waitman, Ph.D.
Internal Medicine, University of Kansas Medical Center,
3901 Rainbow Blvd, Mail Stop 3065, Kansas City, KS 66160, USA
e-mail: russ.waitman@gmail.com

S.T. Rosenbloom, M.D., M.P.H.
Department of Biomedical Informatics, Vanderbilt University Medical Center,
2525 West End Avenue, Suite #14112, Nashville, TN 37203, USA
e-mail: trent.rosenbloom@vanderbilt.edu

E.S. Berner (ed.), *Clinical Decision Support Systems*, Health Informatics,
DOI 10.1007/978-3-319-31913-1_15

developers and clinical end-users plan future alterations to their systems when needs for new decision support features arise.

Keywords CPOE systems • Care provider order entry systems • Computerized physician order entry systems • Vanderbilt • Inpatient care

Practitioners have yearned for clinical decision support systems for at least 2,500 years. Hippocrates noted "Life is short, the art long, opportunity fleeting, experience treacherous, *judgment difficult*." (*Aphorisms*, sec. I, ca. 460–400 BC). While the basis for clinical decision support has been recognized throughout the ages, careful studies in the recent medical literature document those needs specifically [1–14].

The pioneers developing early care provider order entry (CPOE) systems – e.g., McDonald, Tierney, and their colleagues at the Regenstrief Medical Institute [15–25], Warner, Pryor, Gardner and their colleagues at LDS Hospital [26–28] (see Chap. 14), and many other groups – have confirmed, through controlled studies, the initial report of Shakespeare in 1597: "If to do were as easy as to know what were good to do, chapels had been churches, and poor men's cottages princes' palaces. . . . I can easier teach twenty what were good to be done than to be one of the twenty to follow my own teaching" (*The Merchant of Venice*, Act I, Scene ii). Busy health-care providers have so many diverse tasks to perform that they are constantly distracted from being able to accomplish what they understand to be good medical practice. "Men are men; the best sometimes forget" (Shakespeare, *Othello*, 1605; Act II, Scene iii). Reminding systems and other forms of clinical decision support have been shown to be effective in overcoming such lapses of memory in a number of clinical situations [15–40]. However, the success of even the best-designed CPOE systems is not guaranteed. The socio-technical (people, workflows, and human factors) aspects of system implementation are critically important. Many clinical informatics systems (not all documented in the literature) implemented with good intentions have been met with anger and resentment [41–44]. Providing decision-support capabilities in a timely and convenient manner can add value to otherwise lackluster or marginal systems, and improve quality of care and reduce costs [15–40].

This chapter addresses the following questions: (1) What steps or stages in CPOE represent appropriate breakpoints (both computationally and with respect to end-user workflows) at which one can introduce clinical decision support? (2) What categories of decision support are relevant during CPOE sessions? and (3) What methods for workflow interruption should one consider when implementing decision-support interventions based on balancing end-user tolerance and clinical urgency?

The authors have used the Vanderbilt WizOrder CPOE system as the primary context for discussing decision support interventions, primarily because it provides a convenient example with which they are familiar. Through longstanding partnerships with clinician end-users, Vanderbilt Biomedical Informatics faculty members, fellows, and Informatics Center staff developed a CPOE system (WizOrder) in 1994–1995, implemented it on the wards of an academic teaching hospital, and evolved it in response to ongoing feedback (1995–2015) [45–55]. The approach to decision support described in this chapter was derived through generalization from that experience. While the authors have drawn heavily on their Vanderbilt past, the above questions and their answers are sufficiently generic that other developers in both academic and commercial settings may find value in the ensuing discussion. Further, the description of WizOrder functionality here serves as a historical reference as the landscape of order entry systems evolves in an increasingly vendor-based environment.

The authors describe herein the pre-commercial, academic version of WizOrder at Vanderbilt. The WizOrder CPOE system was commercialized in June of 2001. At that time, Vanderbilt University entered into a marketing agreement with McKesson to sell and distribute the WizOrder Care Provider Order Entry System commercially. McKesson rewrote large portions of the WizOrder code, adapted it to run on their preferred computer platforms, to share a common database with their nurse charting system (Horizon Expert Documentation), and recast it as Horizon Expert Orders in McKesson's product line. In early 2015, McKesson announced that it would discontinue the Horizon product line, including Horizon Expert Orders. The authors have herein refer to the system by its name at Vanderbilt, WizOrder. All descriptions are of system components developed at Vanderbilt University Medical Center and not by the commercial vendor.

15.1 Basic Care Provider Order Entry System Functionality

Order entry within many CPOE systems was initially designed to parallel traditional, manual paper chart-based order creation. Manual ordering involves: (1) physically locating the patient's chart; (2) finding the topmost blank order page; (3) handwriting a series of new orders as a block; (4) signing the orders to assert authorship and validation, thereby making them legal; (5) after setting a flag indicating presence of new orders, placing the chart where clerical unit staff expect to find charts with new orders; and (6) finding and verbally informing unit staff (patient's nurse, others) when life-critical or extremely urgent orders have been written. For the corresponding order entry performed in a typical CPOE system, the user, in some sequence: (1) authenticates with user name and password; (2) invokes the CPOE application; (3) selects a patient; (4) enters and modifies orders, using an electronic scratchpad (buffer) that holds orders but does not deliver them to ancillary departments (e.g., lab or pharmacy) for immediate action; (5) indicates when he or she is ready to finalize the set of orders on the scratchpad to send them out for processing; and (6) reviews and edits orders on the scratchpad before they are signed electronically and dispatched to be carried out. Unlike paper-based order entry, providers using CPOE can enter orders from sites remote from the patient location, without the need to have a physical chart. This may occur away from supporting

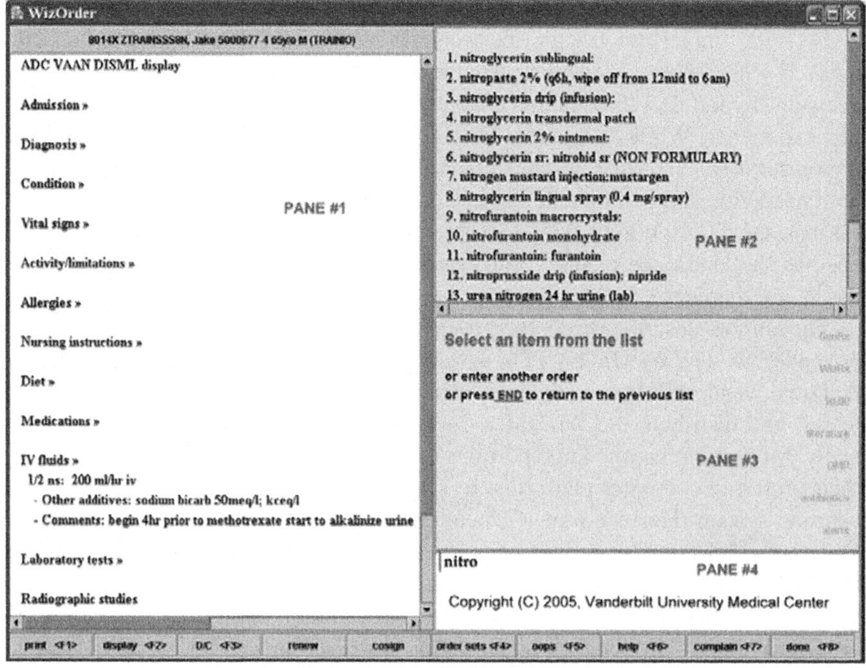

Fig. 15.1 WizOrder primary user interface screen panes: PANE #1, current and recent orders display; PANE #2, selectable "pick list" display; PANE #3, in-context instructions; PANE #4, user input text entry area. User had previously typed "nitro" into completer in PANE #4; PANE #2 shows results

staff, such as nurses. As a result, electronic CPOE without manual, person-to-person follow up may impair communication of life-critical, or otherwise very urgent, orders and thereby introduce patient safety concerns.

The panes of Fig. 15.1 present the WizOrder approach to implementing key components of an order entry interface. During initial WizOrder development, Vanderbilt beta-test users strongly recommended that the CPOE system interface should have "geographical consistency"- i.e., a given type of clinical information should always appear in the same location on the screen. This also implies that pop-up windows and pull-down menus that might obscure display of clinically important information should rarely appear. WizOrder's left-sided window displays currently active orders (and those expired in the previous 24 h) for the current CPOE patient (PANE #1). The upper right window presents context-dependent pick lists of options available for order creation or modification (PANE #2). The middle right window represents a context-sensitive help window that instructs the user on available next actions (PANE #3). The bottom right window contains a text input region (PANE #4).

15.1.1 Creating Orders

A key CPOE system design consideration involves how clinicians specify what they want to order. Many CPOE systems [56–59] use a hierarchical organization of orders, illustrated by the following example (bold font indicates hypothetical selection made at each level):

. . . *Orderable Pick List Level 1*: *Pharmacy*, ***Laboratory***, *Radiology*, *Dietary*, *Nursing* [*orders*], . . .
. . . *Orderable Pick List Level 2*: ***Hematology Tests***, *Serum Chemistry Tests*, *Urinalysis*, . . .
. . . *Orderable Pick List Level 3*: ***Complete blood count*** (***CBC***), *platelet count*, *blood Rh type*, . . .

CPOE systems also commonly have a "completer" or search engine function that allows the clinician-user to type shorthand word fragments derived from the desired order name (or its synonyms). The completer then searches for potentially matching orderable items from the system's dictionary, and provides the user with a pick list of those that the user can select. For example, typing "nitro" into a CPOE completer (Fig. 15.1, PANE #4) would result in the CPOE presenting a pick list (PANE #2) of orderable items' names, with "nitroglycerin sublingual" at or near the top of the list, and lesser/partial/wordier matches (e.g., nitrogen mustard, urea nitrogen blood) farther down the list. Vanderbilt users typically specify new orders using the completer function, and only rarely use WizOrder's hierarchies for order entry, usually when they do not know the specific name for the item they want to order. Users can also select pre-configured "order sets" using the completer function to find the grouping, and then clicking on individual orders within the group to select them.

After selecting the orderable item itself, users must then specify (enter) its component information (e.g., dose, route, frequency, etc, for a medication order). Many CPOE systems formally define orderables and their components using a data dictionary with structured templates that specify necessary and optional fields required to fully create an individual order. Figure 15.2 illustrates WizOrder sequential prompts for building an order for sublingual nitroglycerin (based on stored templates), and Fig. 15.3 indicates how the order, once fully specified for WizOrder, transfers to the left-sided active orders area (PANE #1). Another mechanism for generating new orders (used often, but less than half the time at Vanderbilt) is order sets – groupings of diagnosis or procedure-related selectable orders often with preset component information (e.g., vital signs q4h) [60]. If the user selects an order set name from a completer pick list or from the WizOrder order set hierarchy, the order set's component orders are retrieved and displayed as selectable items in the upper right pick list window (Fig. 15.4, PANE #2).

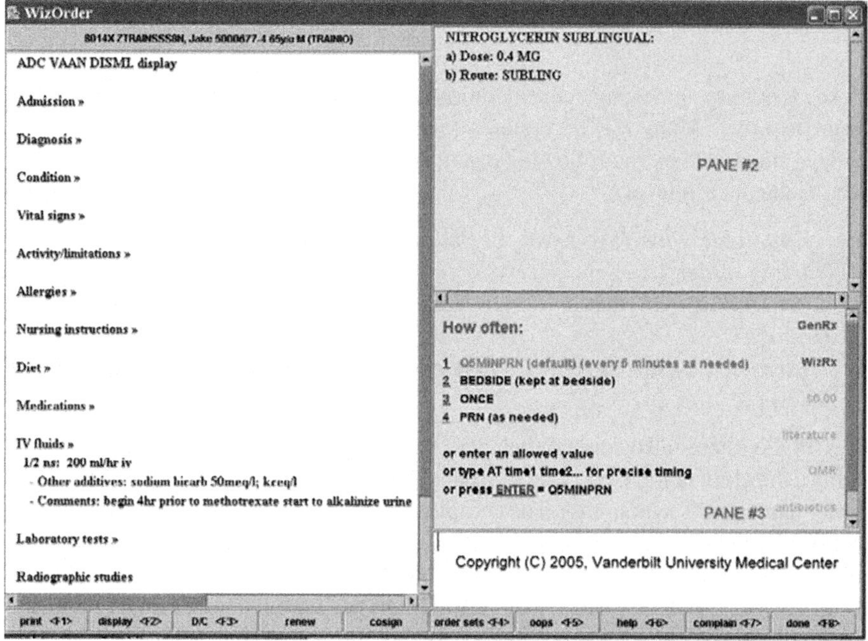

Fig. 15.2 Frequency prompts (medication-specific) for "nitroglycerin sublingual" orderable, after dose already specified by similar process

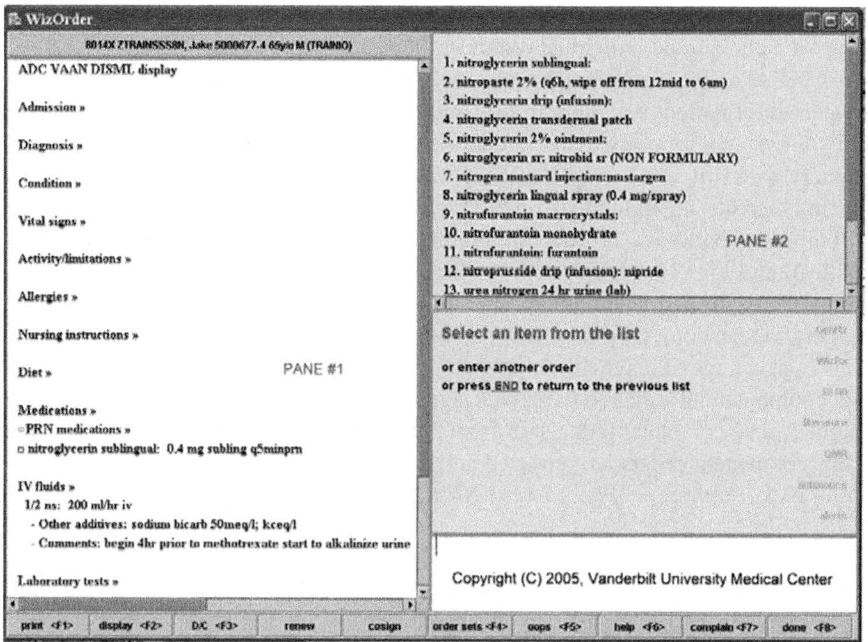

Fig. 15.3 Order for "nitroglycerin" moves to *left* window (PANE #1) once fully completed

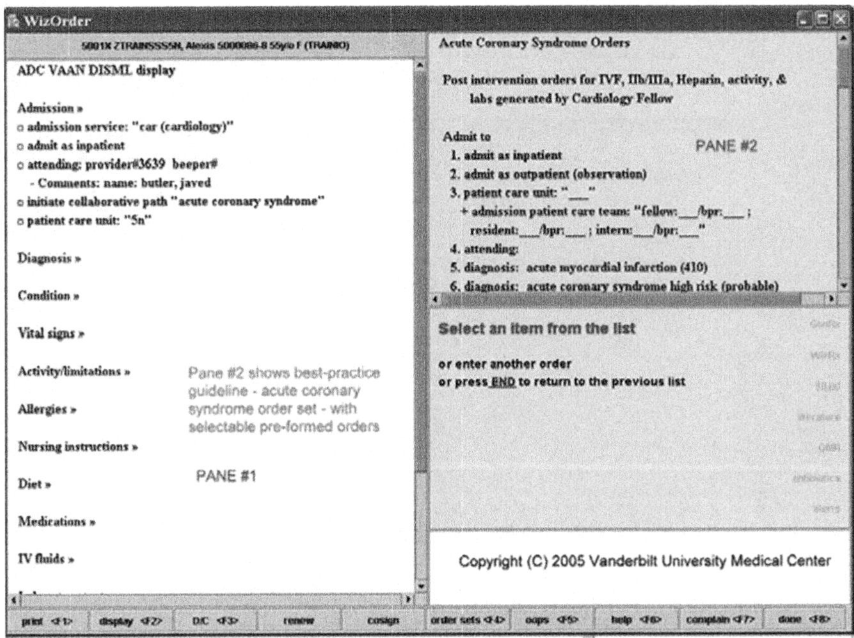

Fig. 15.4 First six orders in the acute coronary syndrome order set

15.1.2 Displaying Active Orders

Most CPOE user interfaces manage the display of currently active orders. In complex patient cases, active order counts can exceed 100. Therefore, simply listing all such orders in a display panel (sorted, e.g., alphabetically by order name) will not be helpful to clinicians unfamiliar with the patient's case, since locating an arbitrarily named specific order within a long list is difficult. Early during WizOrder development, end users requested that a display of active orders follow a grouping sequence based on the ADC VAAN DISML acronym that is familiar to physicians – **A**dmission, **D**iagnosis, **C**ondition, **V**ital signs, **A**ctivity, **A**llergies, and so on (Fig. 15.1, PANE #1). Many CPOE systems use similar methods to segment the active orders display into clinically useful buckets, and some facilitate electronic rearrangements of the active orders display to accommodate different users' typical workflows (e.g., nurses, attending physicians) as well as providing reverse chronological views to display the most recent new or changed orders. For example, Vanderbilt's specialized intensive care units and the emergency department required location-specific specialized views of active orders. As WizOrder displays active orders, it also displays recently expired orders (within the past 24 h) with a special symbol in the left margin to indicate those orders that have expired; a different left-margin symbol indicates orders soon to expire.

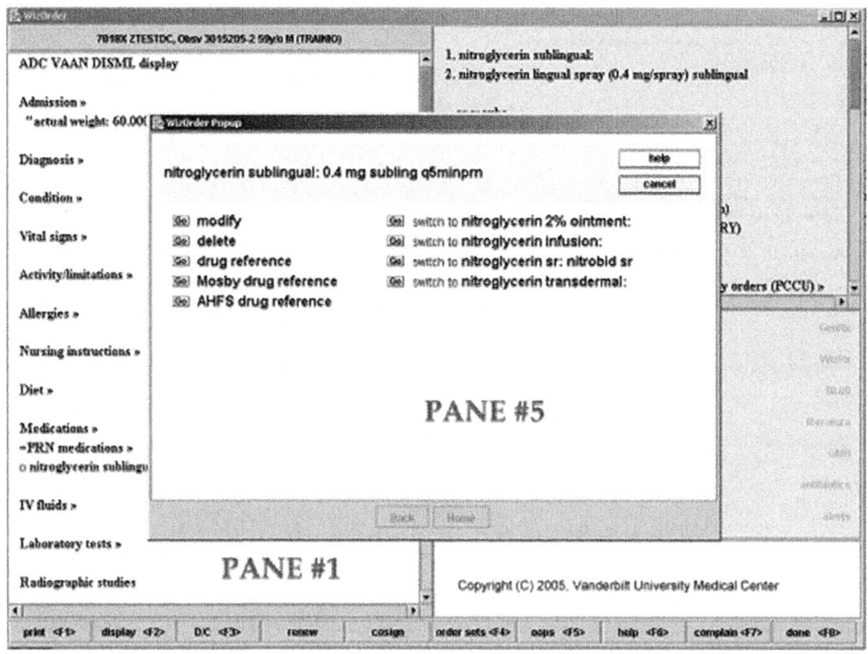

Fig. 15.5 "Pop-up" options (PANE #5) after selecting nitroglycerin order from PANE #1

15.1.3 Modifying and Finalizing Orders

Figure 15.5 illustrates the result of a mouse click on an order in the left WizOrder pane. WizOrder displays a series of options listing what the user can do to the order at that point (modify, discontinue, renew, etc.) When the WizOrder user completes generating or modifying orders during a session, clicking a designated button on the CPOE screen transfers the user to a final accept screen (see Fig. 15.6). This screen gives users a last chance to verify (or to change) their orders from the current ordering session. Once final-accepted, the orders are sent to the appropriate ancillary systems for action and committed to a relational database for archiving. Similar features are available in most CPOE systems.

15.1.4 Displaying Information and Providing Complex Decision Support

A final WizOrder component consists of an intermittently displayed, popup window that contains an internal HTML browser (labeled "PANE #5" in various figures). The WizOrder program uses this capability to display static Web documents with educational content or dynamically generated CPOE-related pages that provide complex, patient-specific decision support capabilities [49, 50].

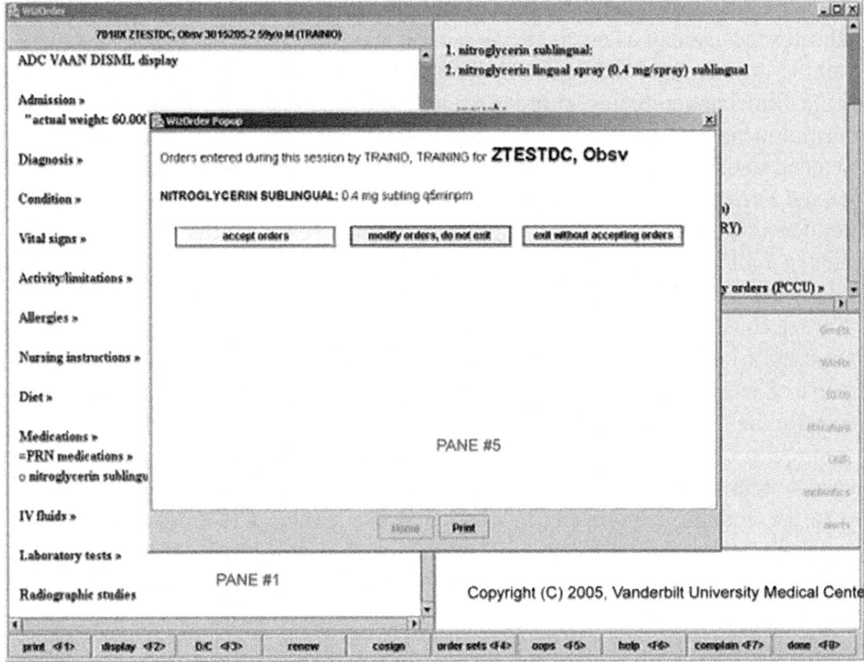

Fig. 15.6 Final accept screen (PANE #5) allows user to verify orders at end of ordering session

15.2 Philosophy Underlying Decision Support During Care Provider Order Entry

Use of a CPOE system during patient care provides a unique opportunity to interject decision support features that improve clinical workflows, provide focused relevant educational materials, and influence how healthcare providers make decisions about patient care. It is somewhat of an art to be able to provide clinical decision support that is well accepted and used widely. Key considerations in the approach to providing decision support include: what content to provide; when to intervene in the clinical workflow process; and how to intervene, in terms of both degree of disruption of workflows and mechanism of interruption. A major goal of decision support is to guide healthcare providers' decision-making as it takes place, rather than to identify errors after the fact. These considerations are addressed later in this chapter.

The nature of each clinical specialty determines what specific types of decision-support content to provide. In addition, the timing of each decision support intervention in a user's workflow is critical. For example, a decision support system should not allow a clinician to spend 1–2 min constructing an intricate medication order, only to then inform the clinician that the medication is contraindicated due to a known allergy. Allergy warnings should occur at the time the clinician first indicates the name of a new medication order. Conversely, delivering an interruptive warning to order a partial thromboplastin time (PTT) monitoring test, immediately as the clinician completes an order for unfractionated heparin, would likely cause frustration and a lost sense of autonomy – especially when that is what the clinician intended to order next. Rather, during an order entry session in which the clinician ordered intravenous unfractionated heparin, the system should check whether PTT monitoring was ordered at the end of an order entry session, after the user has indicated that all intended orders have been issued. Oppenheim et al. observed that permitting the physician to enter an order with feedback provided only at the conclusion of order construction, and then only if the order is possibly incorrect, serves dual purposes [61]. First, delayed warnings make clinicians first commit to a preferred course of action, thus discouraging reliance on CPOE systems to make clinical decisions for the users. Second, delayed warnings give the clinician user the opportunity to correct problems they detect spontaneously, whereas early warnings may impart negative reinforcement by underscoring clinicians' errors [61].

In the authors' experience, busy clinical users value CPOE system accuracy, responsiveness and intuitiveness. A key aspect of responsiveness involves creating orders at an appropriate clinical level (both for users' levels of training and for their knowledge of their patients). The physicians and nurses entering orders into a CPOE system typically have a different mindset than individuals who will carry out the orders in ancillary areas (e.g., pharmacy, radiology, and dietary departments). Problems in creating CPOE system orderable item names can occur when the technical terms used in ancillary departments are carried forward as the orderable items vocabulary for clinicians. So while radiology billing clerks might think in terms of "chest X-ray 2 views" and "knee X-ray 3 views", clinicians are more comfortable ordering "chest X-ray PA and lateral" and "knee X-ray AP, lateral and oblique." Similarly, if the CPOE system asks the physician ordering a chest X-ray how the patient should be transported to the radiology department, the physician is unlikely to give an optimal response because physicians are rarely involved in determining a patient's transport. Thus, CPOE systems should not ask clinicians to perform tasks that fall outside of their usual job responsibilities, or about which they have little knowledge. Structuring orderable items with the clinician in mind helps to overcome major barriers to adoption and can prevent errors.

Intelligent system interfaces can dramatically decrease the burden of ancillary departments in dealing with CPOE system-generated orders. For example, pharmacists use the pharmacy system to fill and dispense the clinical orders specified within the CPOE system. When a physician issues a high-level clinical order, such as gentamicin 70 mg IV, the pharmacist and pharmacy system convert the order into its dispensable form (e.g., one 80 mg ampule of injectable gentamicin) with administration instructions – e.g., draw 7/8 of ampule (70 mg) into syringe for administration. An intelligent decision support interface – provided within the CPOE or pharmacy system – can evaluate both the pharmacy's electronic formulary and the database detailing the floor stock inventory on the patient's unit, and then automatically determine the correct dispensable within the pharmacy system (done at the time of order transmission to the pharmacy, with no need for physician review). Currently, the intelligent pharmacy interface within WizOrder guesses the correct pharmacy-level dispensable item over 90 % of the time. This allows the pharmacist to devote more time to evaluating each order's clinical validity, safety, and efficacy.

An institution's CPOE system determines the workflows that will capture providers' intentions as they generate key clinical instructions. As a result, CPOE may become a target for administrators and researchers wishing to capture additional information from providers at the point of care. System administrators must avoid overburdening clinicians with requests that interrupt their workflows. In situations that require capturing extra information, the system should only ask clinicians for information about which they are the definitive source. For example, at Vanderbilt, upon patient admission, the name of the attending physician of record was originally entered into the admission, discharge, transfer (ADT) system by an admitting clerk. However, the admitting clerks were not always informed of the specifics of physician group coverage schedules, and often did not know the correct name to enter. The problem was addressed by finding a more definitive data source – the admitting house staff team, who must discuss each admission with the attending physician. Having the house staff enter the attending name into the CPOE system improved accuracy. Conversely, if one wants to record whether a patient received aspirin in the emergency department just prior to admission, asking an intern who is entering discharge orders for the patient several days later (and who did not admit the patient) could be viewed as a nuisance, and cause lower-than-optimal data quality.

While some decision support functions not directly related to order entry can be delivered during an order entry session, they will not be discussed in this chapter: for example, a laboratory system that generates alerts whenever abnormal patient results occur might notify clinicians responsible for the patient's care either by paging them or via e-mail or an asynchronous pop-up alarm that occurs when the clinician is currently logged into the CPOE application [62]. Such alerts originate outside of the CPOE session context. Many CPOE systems, including WizOrder, display permanent taskbars, comprising an array of useful links, continuously during the order entry session; [45, 59, 63–65] however, such taskbars rarely provide context-specific decision support of the sort described here. Instead, they allow the user to access common CPOE functions. For instance, the mid-1990s to early 2000s BICS (Brigham Integrated Computer System, in Boston) toolbar allowed the clinician to quickly view orders and search for patients, among other functions [64, 66].

15.3 Roles for Decision Support Within Care Provider Order Entry: Categories of Interventions

15.3.1 Creating Legible, Complete, Correct, Rapidly Actionable Orders

A CPOE system can avert problems previously associated with handwritten order creation [67], for example, illegibility, incompleteness, and incorrectness. Improved legibility not only reduces errors, but also saves staff time because nurses, pharmacists, and medical technicians need not spend time and energy as they decipher the meaning of ambiguous handwritten orders and they no longer make phone calls to clarify what was meant. Complete orders contain all the necessary parameters to make an order actionable (order name, start date and time, duration, frequency, etc.). Correct orders have parameter values that meet requirements for safe, prudent patient care (e.g., drug doses are appropriate for the patient's age, weight, and renal function). Most CPOE system interfaces ensure completeness and promote correctness of orders [67–69].

15.3.2 Providing Patient-Specific Clinical Decision Support

An important CPOE system capability is generation of decision support recommendations customized to individual patients' specific conditions. A CPOE system can provide a safety net through behind-the-scenes reconciliation of patient-specific information (laboratory results, age, allergies, current medications [70]) with stored best practice rules. For example, most CPOE systems screen patient orders against safe dosing rules and drug interaction references to reduce medication prescribing errors [53, 66, 71–74]. A CPOE system can also facilitate clinical care improvement by promoting use of evidence-based clinical practice guidelines [58, 75, 76] through end-user order generation via diagnosis or procedure-specific order sets [56, 59, 65, 70, 76] or via computer-based advisors [58, 64, 73, 77, 78], as detailed below.

15.3.3 Optimizing Clinical Care (Improved Workflow, More Cost-Effective and Regulatory-Compliant)

End-users of complex software systems learn to combine sequences of steps into a higher-level "programming language" to make the system do things that system developers neither foresaw nor intended. Clinicians regularly using a CPOE system begin to make suggestions about how to modify it to make their work easier and more effective. For example, early CPOE users at Vanderbilt requested printed rounding reports to facilitate patient care during work rounds and attending (teaching) rounds. The rounding reports concisely summarize, on the front and back of an 8.5×11 in. piece of paper, both the patient's active orders and all laboratory results reported in the prior 72 h with highlight markers next to significant (e.g., abnormal) results. In another instance, to improve workflows, several surgical services at Vanderbilt encouraged WizOrder developers to create "registry" orders. Such orders placed patients into a local, CPOE-associated registry database that allowed clinicians to track diagnoses and procedures performed on registry patients (e.g., patients on the neurosurgery service). At the same time, registries enabled efficient transfer of appropriate information to the registry's specialty-related billing office, relieving physicians of that responsibility.

After several years of CPOE implementation, the institution's administration began to view the system as a tool to implement quality of care, cost containment, and compliance initiatives [52–54]. Institution-wide CPOE interventions, if implemented with the minimal degree of disruption required (see details below), can: discourage the ordering of inappropriate, recurring tests; [20, 52, 79] advise against costly tests or require further justification before allowing them to proceed; [22, 55, 80] display formulary information; [55, 57] and help the ordering clinician to enter requisite third party payer compliance codes (e.g., ICD-10 or CPT) for diagnostic tests. Clinicians are not always familiar with compliance rules, and they tend to write reasons for tests based on suspected diagnoses (e.g., "rule out MI" for an electrocardiogram, or "possible pneumonia" for a chest X-ray) rather than indications for testing approved by third party payers. Orders that require specific reasons for compliance can be made to trigger the WizOrder internal Web browser to display and capture order-specific compliance-related reasons for testing. This can increase the rate of third party payer reimbursements for those tests due to more accurate, complete capture of compliant reasons.

Clinical decision support features within CPOE systems can also promote implementation and enforcement of local hospital policies. The Regenstrief Medical Record System (RMRS), successfully used computer reminders circa 1997 to increase discussion about, and completion of, advanced directives (end-of-life, "do not resuscitate" related orders) [81]. Previous studies had indicated that too few patients completed advance directives [82]. In Boston in the mid-1990s, the BICS was modified in order to prevent the appearance of vancomycin-resistant microorganisms by requiring clinicians ordering vancomycin to enter a reason for using the antibiotic [83].

The challenge for CPOE system developers is to honor the care improvement goals while keeping the system responsive and intuitive. Developers must strike a proper balance between clinical improvements versus cost containment. At times, both goals may be achieved in a single intervention – judiciously ordering fewer tests does not mandate a lower quality of care [52]. However, care improvement interventions may themselves have unintended consequences that require continuous monitoring and feedback for optimal results [54].

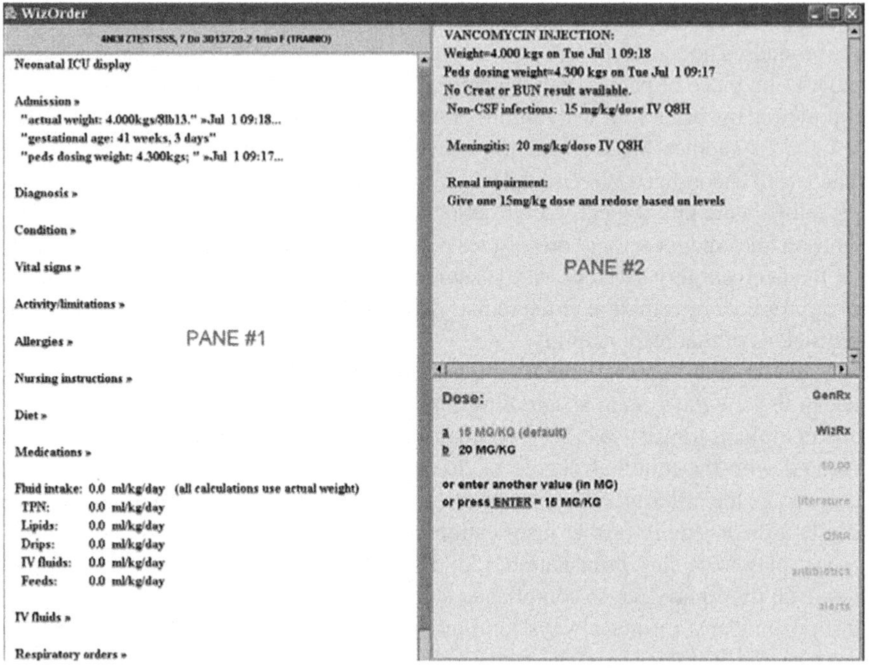

Fig. 15.7 In-line recommendations for dosing vancomycin in NICU include: (**a**) PANE #2, suggested doses for regular use, for meningitis, and for renal impairment; (**b**) PANE #1, passive display of weight, dosing weight, and gestational age; and (**c**) PANE #2, display of renal function test results (not available for training patient in this example)

15.3.4 Providing Just-in-Time, Focused Education Relevant to Patient Care

Many CPOE systems provide relevant prompts for educational materials targeting system users. Often, the materials are fairly terse, with hyperlinks to more detailed educational information resources [55]. Educational prompts can be introduced as in-line summaries that appear while prescribing a medication. Figure 15.7 shows in the upper right WizOrder panel in-line suggestions for vancomycin dosing adjustments in neonates with meningitis or with renal impairment. An embedded CPOE Web browser content can also provide effective educational information, for example, presenting a summary of disease-specific national guidelines, links to educational monographs, or a summary of indications and contra-indications for a specific therapy. Educational links can assist clinician users to perform complex ordering, such as for total parenteral nutrition (TPN) in a neonatal intensive care unit. The design of a CPOE system user interface can significantly influence the rate at which users follow educational links and read the related materials. Simply having an option for decision support may not be sufficient to command users' attention, and stronger cues, such as different visual displays as to the relevance of the information, may be needed [55].

15.4 Critical Points at Which to Implement Decision Support Within Care Provider Order Entry

Each stage of use of a CPOE system permits a focused repertoire of decision support interventions, both in terms of user community affected, patients affected, and appropriateness of the intervention for the task the end user intends to perform. For example, as the CPOE system is launched from a clinical workstation desktop, system-wide messages may appear, but patient-specific advice should not (since, typically, the user has not yet selected a patient). Below, authors discuss the type of decision support that is appropriate and feasible for each stage of order entry.

15.4.1 Stage of Care Provider Order Entry Session Initiation

Upon launching a typical CPOE application, the system will know the identity of the clinician user, but not of the patient. As a result, patient-specific decision support is inappropriate here. Rather, at this stage, the system can advise users about new CPOE system features, e.g., on a once-only basis for this user. Such interventions should appear sparingly. One-time announcements of general interest to all users might appear, e.g., describing a new method to enter a specific group of commonly used orders. Once the alert is displayed, the system removes the current user from the list of users who still must see that message. At launch, the CPOE system can also inform users of information related to their personal use of the system, such as the number of old orders (and number of patients) requiring their countersignature, and provide a link to facilitate completing the task.

15.4.2 Stage of Selecting Care Provider Order Entry Patient from Hospital Ward Census

After CPOE system launch, users typically select an individual patient for order entry. A number of alerts can occur at the stage of displaying the census of available patients for CPOE. Similar to the 1990s BICS system in Boston (and other CPOE systems), WizOrder provided, via the patient census screen, an inpatient, unit-wide view of the status of recently issued orders (see Fig. 15.8). A map view of the given hospital ward shows all beds and uses color coding to indicate which beds have new unacknowledged, urgent (i.e, STAT) orders and which beds have unacknowledged routine orders. A care provider wishing to enter new orders (or acknowledge recent orders) can click on a bed on the display screen to initiate an order entry session for that particular patient.

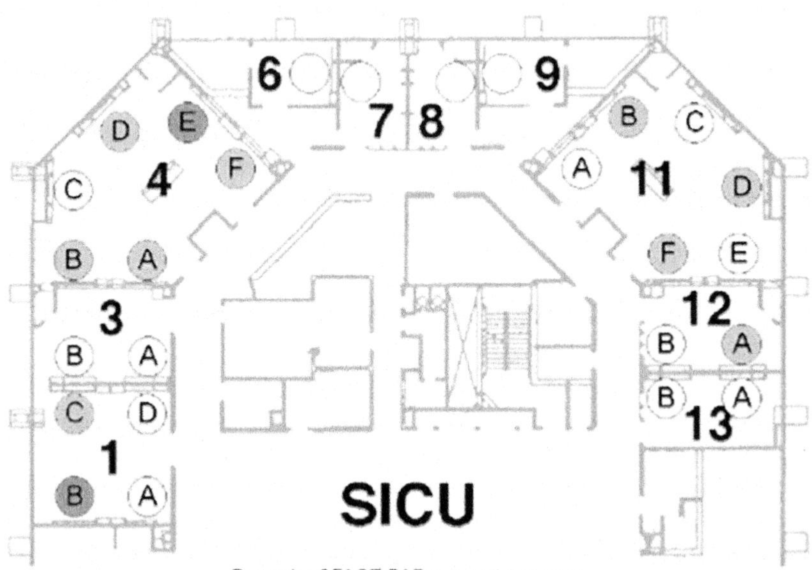

Fig. 15.8 CPOE "map" view of hospital ward. *Map* indicates beds (*circles*) with different shading to indicate new, urgent "stat" orders or those with new "routine" orders; *right border shading* indicates highest priority of new orders not yet acknowledged (across all beds) by nursing staff

An alternative to the map view of a hospital unit census is a list view that includes patients on the unit, and that can be sorted by patient name or by ascending bed number. In WizOrder, icons located beside patients' names in the list view provide useful information (Fig. 15.9). Using a similar list census screen, the 1990s BICS system presented a renewal reminder next to the patient's name when a medication order for a given patient nears expiration [84].

15.4.3 Stage of Individual Patient Session Initiation

Once the user has selected an individual patient and the order entry session focuses on that patient, several additional types of decision-support related events become feasible. In WizOrder, once the patient is identified, the system retrieves all relevant past (active and inactive) orders for the patient, and previously stored patient-specific information such as weight, height, coded allergies, and active protocols (with dates of each protocol initiation). As the user waits for the initial patient-specific CPOE screen to appear, WizOrder queries the patient data repository. The

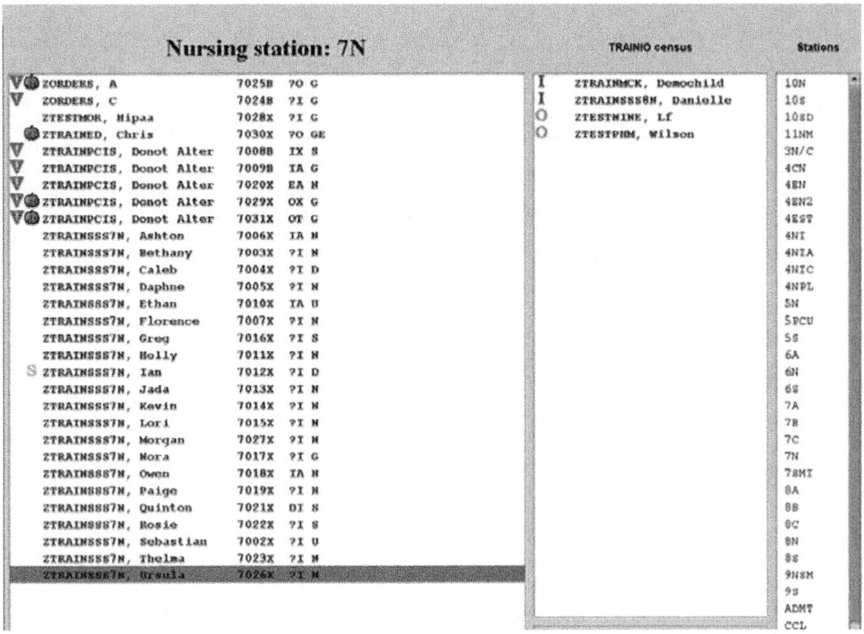

Fig. 15.9 "Patient list" view of CPOE ward census. Several graphical "icon" alerts (*left* margin next to patient name) provide useful information regarding ward census at a glance. The *inverted triangles* provide duplicate last name warnings; "S" indicates patients for whom medical students have entered orders that must be reviewed by a licensed medical doctor to become "activated;" and pumpkins indicate patients who have been bedded as outpatients long enough that conversion to inpatient status (or discharge to home) should be considered

system, to prepare to assist with subsequent CPOE decision support requirements, uses this "delay" to obtain the patient's recent laboratory results for common important tests.

Ability to recover from an interrupted CPOE session without loss of work (time and effort) is critical to busy clinicians' acceptance of such systems. Lost sessions can occur due to system bugs (such as the users' workstation crashing), environmental factors (such as network outages or power failures), and user factors (such as abandoning a workstation during a medical emergency, with a subsequent session timeout). Figure 15.10 shows the alert that occurs upon initiation of a patient-specific CPOE session for a patient with a previously interrupted session. The user is then given the option to play back and recover the orders from the previously interrupted session.

Among the many other types of alerts that can occur at the stage of initiating a patient-specific CPOE session are: presentation of a summary of past alerts and warnings related to the patient's orders – e.g., allergies and drug interactions; notification of medications about to expire; display of the names of active protocols for the patient (e.g., "Deep Venous Thrombosis prophylaxis protocol"); and promotion, via reminders, of new protocols for which the patient is eligible. Figure 15.11

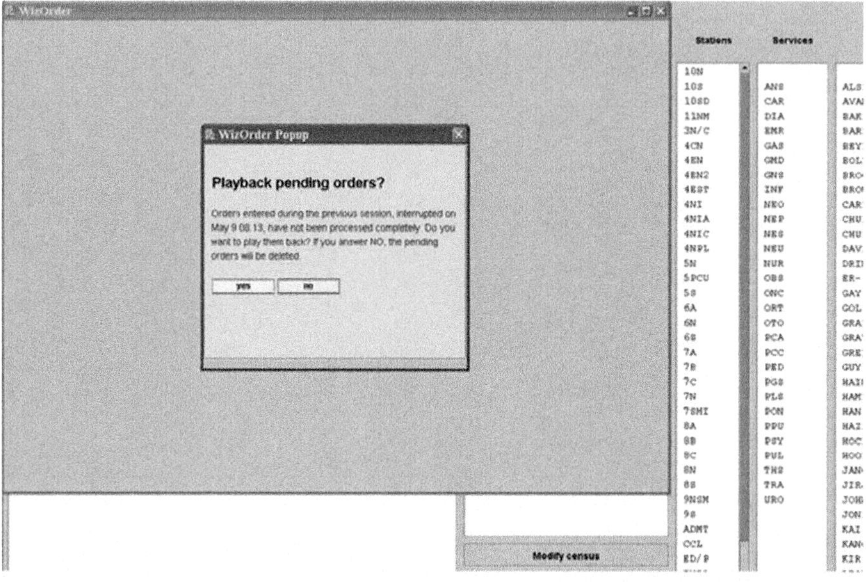

Fig. 15.10 Interrupted/incomplete previous WizOrder CPOE session warning. Allows user to recover from previously interrupted ordering session

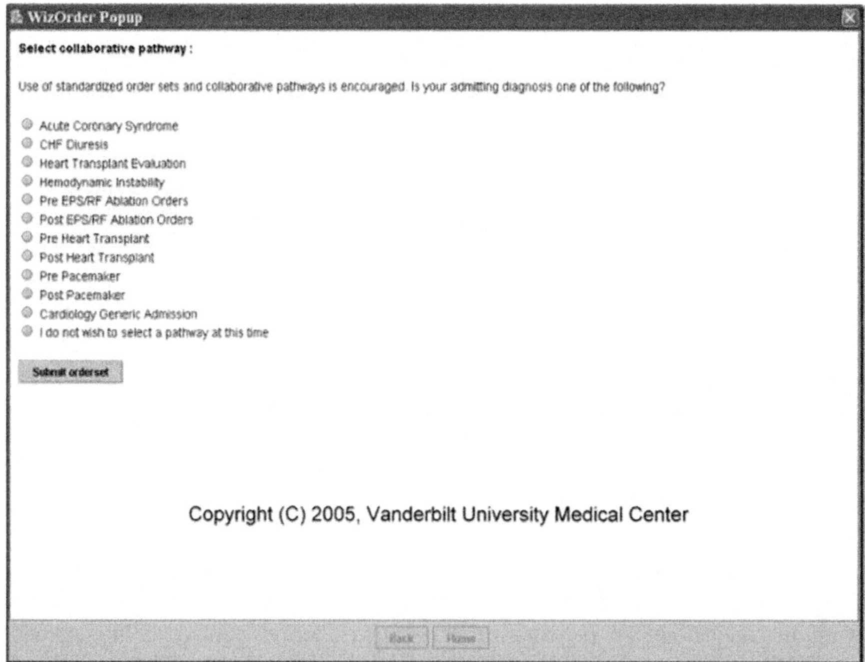

Fig. 15.11 Admission Wizard prompts user to select evidence-based protocol for patient when relevant to case

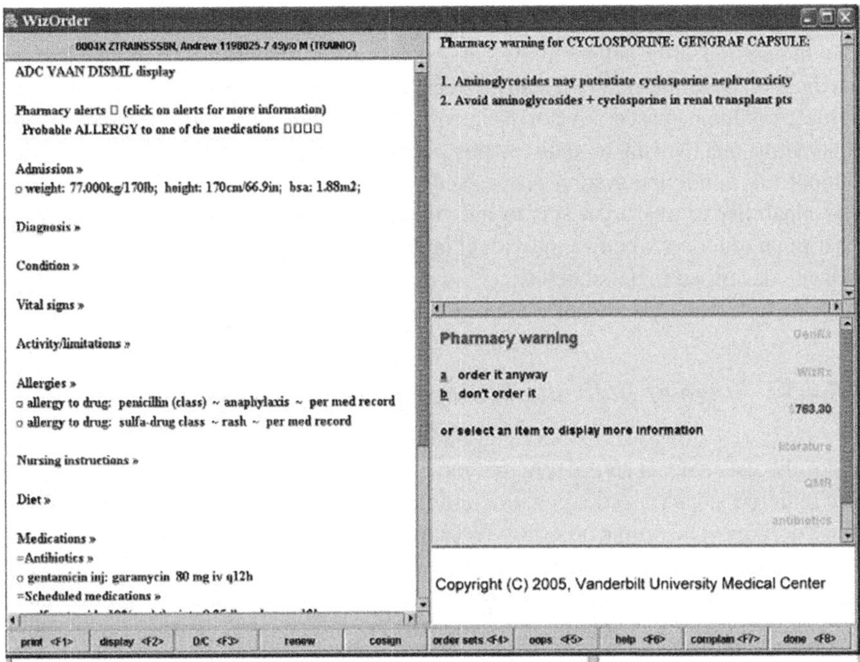

Fig. 15.12 Drug-drug interaction warning after entry of new medication name

illustrates an admission wizard that indicates to the user, for the ward on which the patient is bedded (e.g., Cardiology), the commonly used, evidence-based best-of-care order sets that are available within the system (e.g., acute coronary syndrome), and it encourages the user to select one for use on the patient, if applicable. The structure of such an order set, once selected, is shown in Fig. 15.4 in the upper right window (acute coronary syndrome, PANE #2).

15.4.4 Stage of Individual (Single) Order Selection

Upon selecting a specific CPOE orderable item, and before the user specifies the exact details of the order, certain types of decision support checks become appropriate. For example, at the time the user indicates the next order is a drug, CPOE-based allergy and drug-drug interaction checking should display any relevant warnings. These alerts should appear before the user can specify any details of the drug order (dose, route, frequency, etc) – to avoid wasting the user's time. Figure 15.12 illustrates the latter category of WizOrder warnings, after entry of a new medication name.

Individual order selection can also trigger protocol-based interventions such as recommending drug substitutions (suggesting a less expensive or more effective medication than the one originally selected). Similarly, single order selection can initiate computer-based advisors related to the specific order (Fig. 15.13a, b). An analogous mechanism to redirect physician workflow existed circa 2000 in the BloodLink-Guideline system in the Netherlands [58]. Many CPOE systems offer the capability to link order sets to individual selectable orders (i.e., to transfer the user to an order set when an individual order is selected) [56, 59, 65, 70, 76]. Order sets are described in detail below.

15.4.5 Stage of Individual (Single) Order Construction

Once the user selects an order name, the CPOE system assists the user in completing required steps for order construction (see Fig. 15.14 for an example of instructions during cyclosporine ordering). WizOrder guides medication order construction by highlighting recommended drug doses and common drug administration frequencies; it also presents alerts for potentially incorrect decisions. This is similar to what is described in the literature for the BICS system implemented in Boston circa 2000 [66, 73]. Many CPOE systems also provide computer-based advisors to enforce compliance with established, evidence-based guidelines [58, 77]. As described in Chap. 14, the antibiotic assistant system at LDS Hospital in Salt Lake City recommends therapy options for critically ill patients based on patient vital signs and serology, microbiology, pathology, and radiology results [77].

Based on their research, Bates et al. observed that clinicians generally take the path of least resistance when multiple options are available during decision-making [73, 85, 86]. Providing effective decision support involves not only alerting the provider about a potential error, but providing a correct alternative option as well. For instance, in the BICS system, if meperidine hydrochloride is prescribed for a patient whose creatinine clearance (a measure of renal function), is significantly impaired, an alert notifies the user that the drug might possibly promote seizures in this patient, and suggests a substitute medication rather than stop the user outright. [84] Similar approaches have been used to guide geriatric medication dosing and substitutions.

15.4.6 Stage of Individual Order Completion

Once an individual order's components have been fully specified (and any allergy or other alerts that might have prevented order construction have been dealt with), a number of decision-support functions related to the order as a whole become appropriate. Upon completed order construction, many CPOE systems suggest corollary orders – follow-up tasks clinically indicated after certain orders [73, 84, 87, 88]. For

a
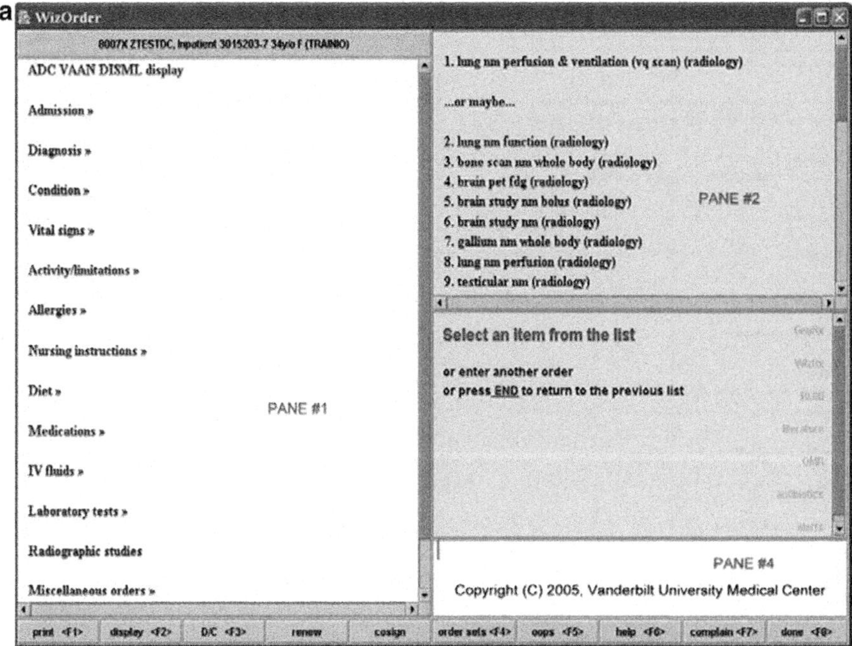

b
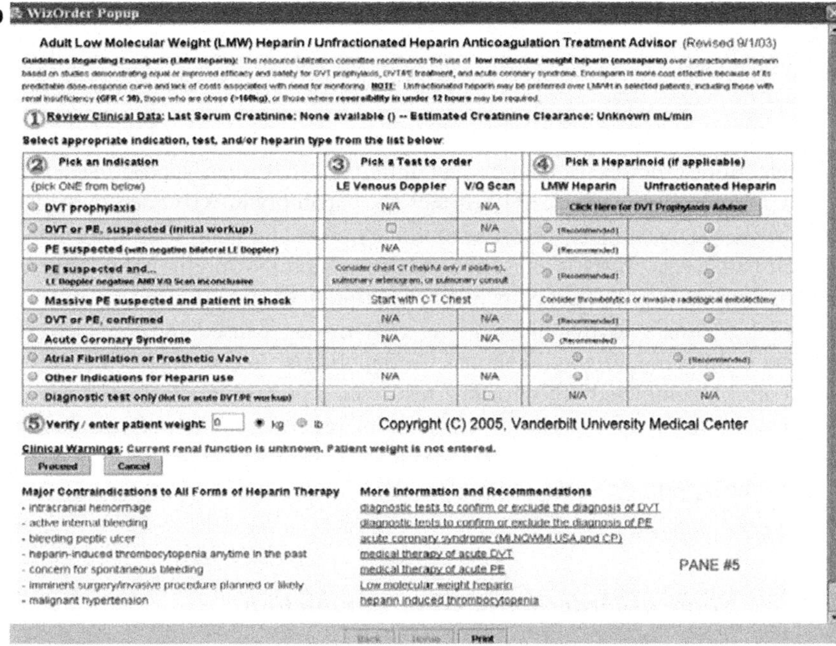

Fig. 15.13 (**a**) Clinician-user initially attempted to order "VQ scan" of lung for pulmonary embolism, and WizOrder completer maps to official name of test (item 1 in PANE #2), which user then selects by typing choice in PANE #4. (**b**) Selecting lung scan order from A launches anticoagulation adviser in WizOrder, helps clinician select appropriate diagnostic workup, and therapy for suspected or confirmed deep venous thrombosis (DVT) or pulmonary embolism (as well as DVT prophylaxis and therapy for other disorders such as acute coronary syndrome)

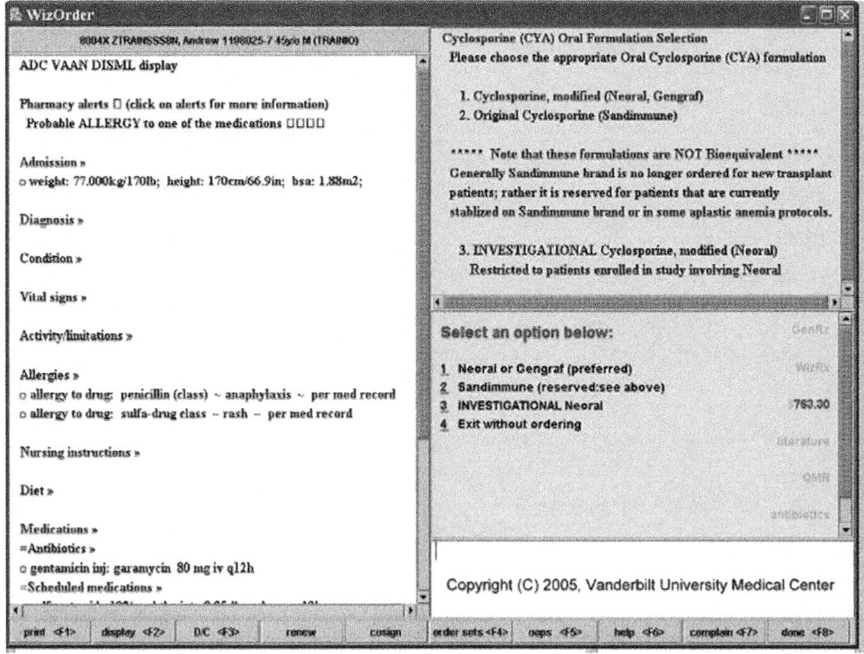

Fig. 15.14 "In-line", patient-specific, interactive advice for clinician while attempting to prescribe cyclosporine for patient; developed by experts in the pharmacy to guide clinician to best choice

example, after ordering gentamicin, an antibiotic, it is often appropriate to order serum drug levels. Figure 15.15 illustrates this capability in WizOrder. In the 1990s the RMRS system similarly presented corollary orders for many drug-drug monitoring test pairs (e.g., warfarin prescriptions and related INR/prothrombin time tests) and for drug-drug side effect pairs (e.g., prescription of class II narcotics and orders for stool softeners to treat/prevent the constipation caused by narcotics) [87]. Another example is offering clinicians the opportunity to order heparin (to prevent DVT) after a completed order for bed rest (which predisposes to DVT); however, this may be more appropriate at the stage of ordering session completion [84]. Research has shown more effective ordering and improved outcomes as a result of such systems [89].

15.4.7 Stage of Ordering Session Completion

Once the user has specified all individual new (or modified) orders and wishes to finalize the ordering session, various decision-support related exit checks are appropriate. As noted above, recurring reminders to do what the clinician user already

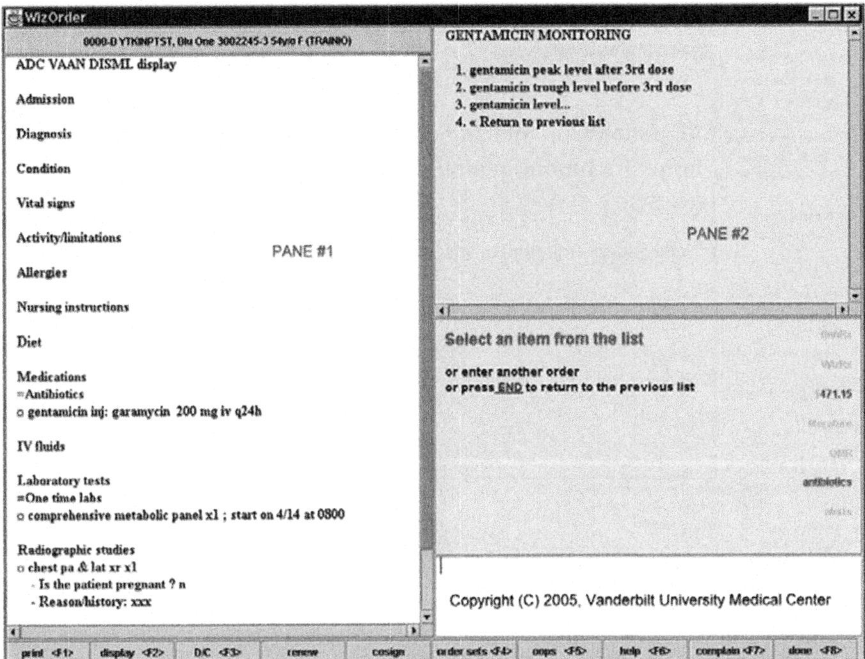

Fig. 15.15 After completing gentamicin order (seen in PANE #1), system offers selectable gentamicin monitoring orders (in PANE #2) as "one click away" for convenience (suggesting best practice, but not requiring it)

intended to do are not well tolerated. Instead of using automatically generated ("corollary") orders to prompt PTT and INR monitoring after orders for heparin and warfarin, respectively, WizOrder waits until the user indicates that the ordering session is complete. At that point, it becomes fair game to issue warnings if appropriate monitoring tests have not been issued. Also at that point, if a recent monitoring test indicates that the prescribed anticoagulant dose is suboptimal or excessive with respect to national guidelines, the system can issue an alert. Conversely, if during a given ordering session, a clinician discontinues either the heparin infusion or the PTT monitoring tests but not the other item of the pair, it is appropriate to use an ordering session exit check that warns the clinician that parallel actions to discontinue both are usually needed. Figures 15.16 and 15.17 illustrate the two-part WizOrder exit check for ordering or updating the Richmond Agitation and Sedation Scale (RASS) target score whenever pain medications or sedatives are ordered for a patient in an ICU.

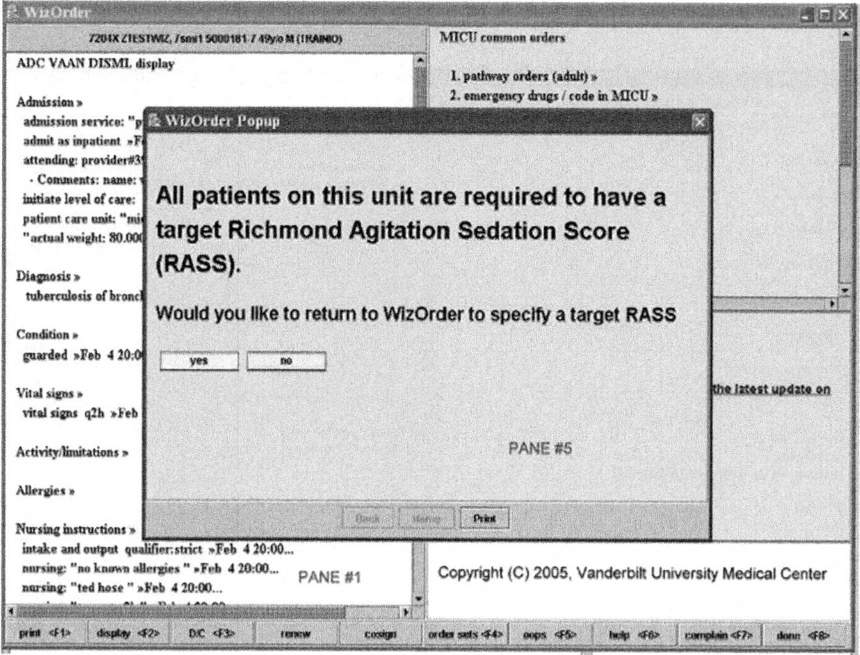

Fig. 15.16 WizOrder "exit check." On completing admission orders on an ICU patient, if the clinician-user has not specified a target RASS (Richmond Agitation Sedation Scale) score, the system uses a pop-up alert to remind the clinician that it is ICU policy to do so

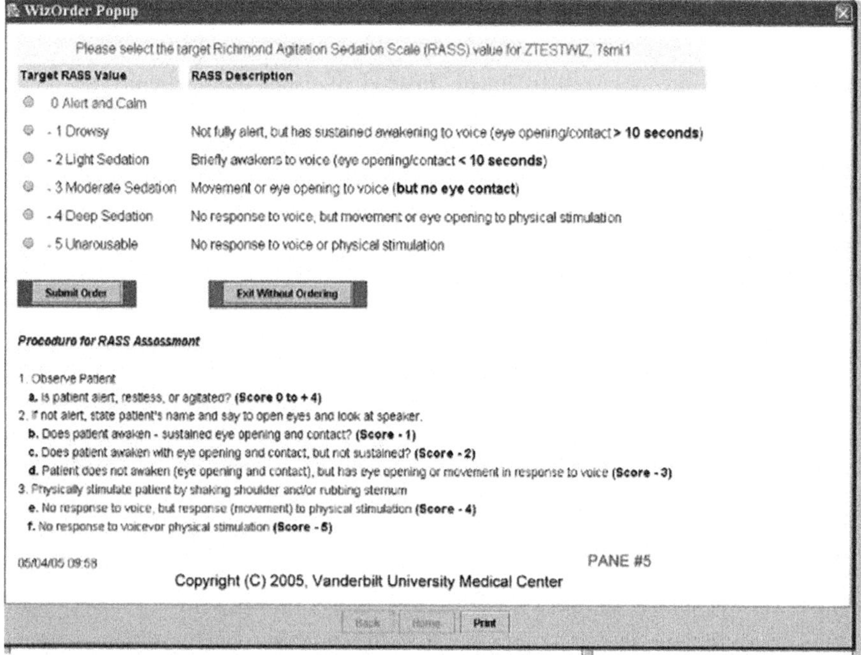

Fig. 15.17 User (from Fig. 15.16) requests assistance in specifying RASS score; web-based advisor assists user with data collection and score calculation

15.5 Care Provider Order Entry Intervention Approaches: From Subtle to Intrusive

While the interfaces of successful CPOE systems are rarely seamless, users adapt to their styles of workflow after training and repeated use. Once acclimated to the CPOE system workflows, users do not appreciate interruptions that deter them from the previously noted path of least resistance [86]. Determining whether, how, and when to disrupt clinician workflows to provide appropriate decision support is critical to end-user acceptance of both the decision support and the CPOE system overall. Below, we describe a number of approaches to introducing decision support, from non-disruptive to very disruptive, and give examples of where each may appropriate. The sections below describe how and when to interrupt workflows.

15.5.1 Incidental Display of Relevant Information

Presentation of additional viewable text on a portion of the usual application screen allows the user direct access to relevant information with minimal interruption to workflow. Because no user input (e.g., acknowledgment of the information) is required, and no additional information is available (e.g., the user cannot click on or select the displayed information to learn more), the clinician is free to read or to ignore the displayed information. WizOrder displays the most recent results of serum electrolyte tests during ordering of intravenous fluid therapy. WizOrder also displays relevant dosing information for prescribing medications, for example, on pediatric units, the patient's actual weight, dosing weight, and pharmacy-recommended dosing guidelines (see Fig. 15.7). When relevant, the system may also display information related to the patient's renal function, or to the medication costs.

15.5.2 Incidental Display of Linked Educational Opportunities

A CPOE system may have order-related educational information that is too voluminous to include in the usual order entry screen. Under such circumstances, the CPOE system can present links for users to select (click on). These lead to a separate screen/window providing the relevant textual information. Examples include links to relevant drug guidelines and formulary information [59]. The Vanderbilt Patient Care Provider Order Entry with Integrated Tactical Support study, [55] provided links to pharmacotherapy-related information (illustrated by the "GenRx" and "WizRx" links on the right margin of PANE #3, Fig. 15.2), and reference material for diagnosis in internal medicine. Figure 15.18 provides an example, in PANE #5, of displaying an evidence-based summary of what is known about a specific

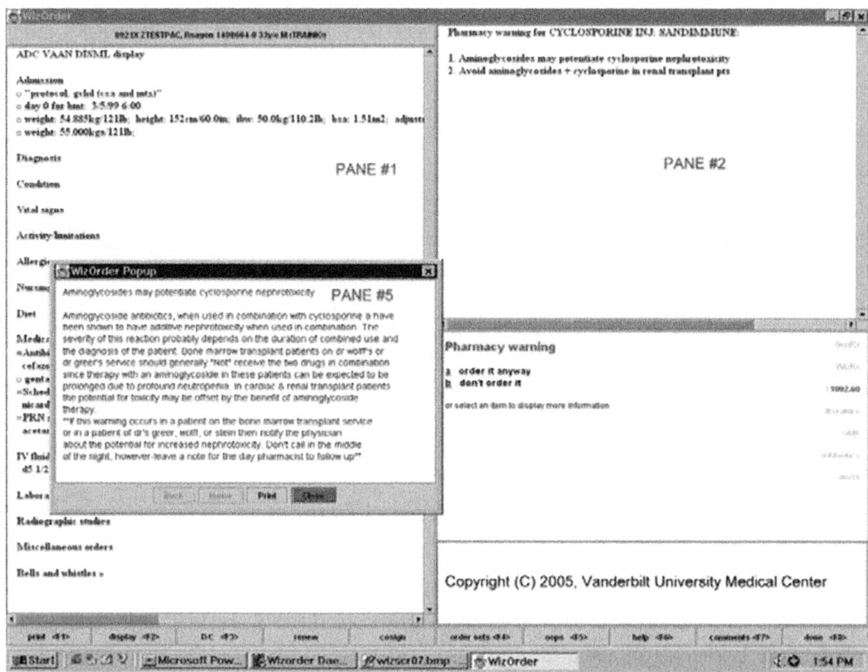

Fig. 15.18 Clinician prescribed cyclosporine while a currently active order for gentamicin was in place. Following a drug interaction alert (PANE #2), user clicks on item 1 to request evidence basis for what is known about the drug interaction (displayed in pop-up window, PANE #5)

drug interaction (selected by the user from the drug interaction warnings list of Fig. 15.18, PANE #2). In other systems, as clinicians review recommended drug doses for patients with renal impairment, they can display the data used to calculate creatinine clearance using a keyboard shortcut link [64].

15.5.3 *Interactive Sequential Advice for User-Directed Clinical Activity*

By presenting stepwise instructions in context, CPOE systems help users to carry out discrete tasks. Figure 15.2 presents the default minimum type of advice that WizOrder provides for order construction; Fig. 15.14 provides a more complex example whereby the user is sequentially prompted, through questions and answers, to order the most appropriate form of cyclosporine for the patient. Another system, the circa 2000 BloodLink Guideline system [58] directed blood test ordering decisions by first having the clinician select the appropriate guideline, then presenting a menu of related indications, and, finally, presenting a menu of relevant tests for a selected indication.

15.5.4 *Recallable Best Practice Guidelines with Actionable Pre-formed Pick List Selections*

Order sets are pick lists containing constituent individual pre-specified full (or partially complete) orders, often representing standardized protocols. Figure 15.4 illustrates a portion of the WizOrder order set for acute coronary syndrome. Hierarchies of order sets enable easier end-user access, organized by clinical department, [40, 59] by organ system, or by clinical diagnosis, condition, or procedure [57, 76, 90]. While users may view picking orders from order sets as foreign to, or a diversion from, the usual manner of constructing individual orders, appropriate use of order sets can often increase users' time-efficiency and promote completeness and correctness of orders [58, 60, 91]. Order sets have become a commonly used mechanism for organizations to distribute "actionable" evidence-based medicine practice guidelines across healthcare systems.

15.5.5 *Pop-Up Alerts That Interrupt Workflow and Require a Response for the User to Continue*

Pop-up alerts can present clinically important information (in a separate user interface window) that must be acknowledged by the user before resuming previous CPOE activity. Use of such interventions is typically viewed by users as disruptive, and should be reserved for only the most severe clinical indications. So called "pop-up alert fatigue" can occur when too many alerts of this type disrupt clinical workflows [92]. In WizOrder and other systems, pop-up windows alert physicians when excessive chemotherapy doses are ordered [48, 93]. Figure 15.19 illustrates how WizOrder notifies the user that the most recent laboratory test ordered will be sent out to a reference laboratory for completion. It provides advice on how to optimize ordering with respect to institutional policies regarding reimbursement for testing. This mechanism is used to display hospital-approved drug substitution regimens. Figure 15.20 shows a WizOrder drug substitution pop-up (implemented as an advisor, see section 15.5.6 below). Figure 15.16 shows how the RASS exit check was implemented as a pop-up alert in WizOrder. Figure 15.12 illustrates how WizOrder uses the pop-up method to present a drug interaction alert.

15.5.6 *Complex, Computer-Based Protocols That Interact with the User to Make Patient-Specific Calculations and Recommendations*

The most complex form of decision support is an interactive advisor that integrates patient-specific information (laboratory results, active orders, weight, allergies, etc.) with complex guidelines or protocols, and presents calculated/derived

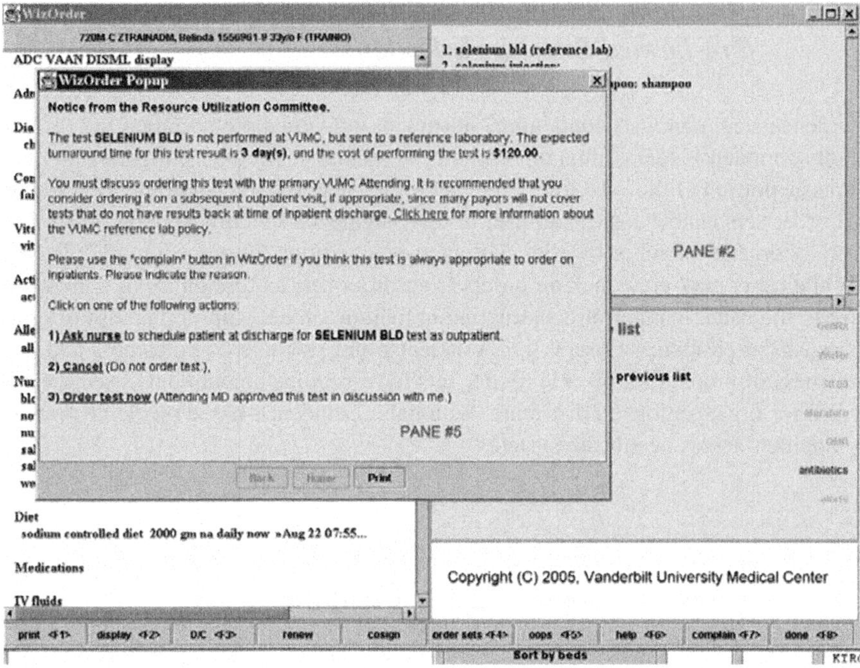

Fig. 15.19 Clinician user begins to order "selenium blood" level (PANE #2), prompting a pop-up warning (PANE #5) that stops workflow and demands attention. The pop-up explains that the test is sent to a reference laboratory and takes 3 days to perform. User is notified that reimbursement may be compromised if patient is discharged before result is known. Pop-up provides instructions for alternative ordering mechanisms (that can be selected directly from pop-up) if clinician believes that obtaining the result of the order is not urgent/emergent for the current patient

information to the user for decision making, typically involving a two-way dialogue between the application and the user. Complex advisors may combine educational advice, calculators for patient-specific dosing, and other functionality in one screen (Fig. 15.20). For example, the Antibiotic Assistant system at LDS Hospital in Salt Lake City is described in Chap. 14. The LDS Antibiotic Assistant analyzes patient data and laboratory results in order to determine likely pathogens, and then determines the optimal treatment for the patient, including factors such as patient allergies and local patterns of antimicrobial functions into its assessment. Using a different but analogous mechanism, WizOrder employs locally scripted Web browser pop-up windows to dynamically generate patient-specific advisory content [49, 50]. Figure 15.21 illustrates the WizOrder TPN ordering advisor for the neonatal intensive care unit (NICU).

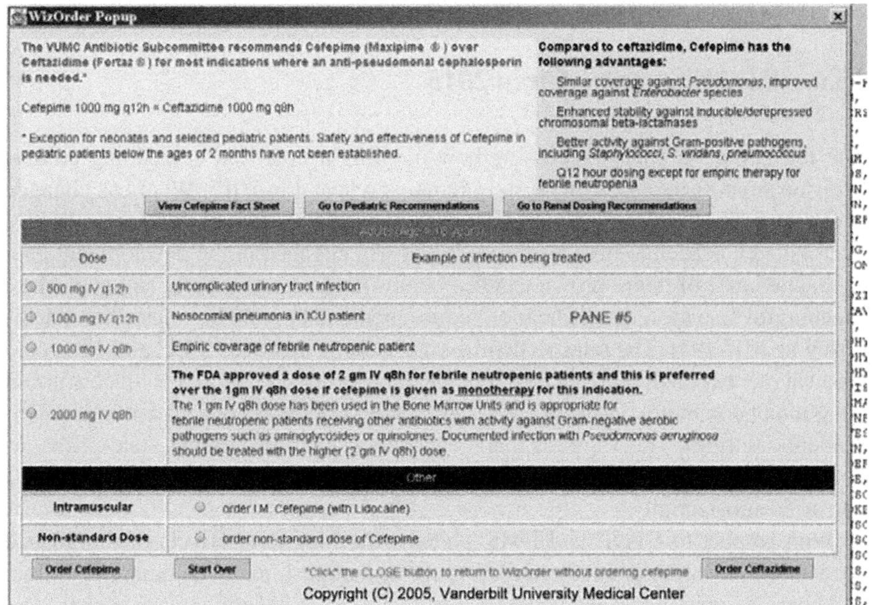

Fig. 15.20 User ordered an antibiotic for which the Pharmaceuticals and Therapeutics (P&T) Committee had recommended a substitution. A variant pop-up, this educational advisor guides the clinician through ordering an alternative antibiotic. Links to "package inserts" (via buttons) detail how to prescribe the recommended drug under various circumstances. A physician who knows little about the recommended drug could learn enough to prescribe it appropriately

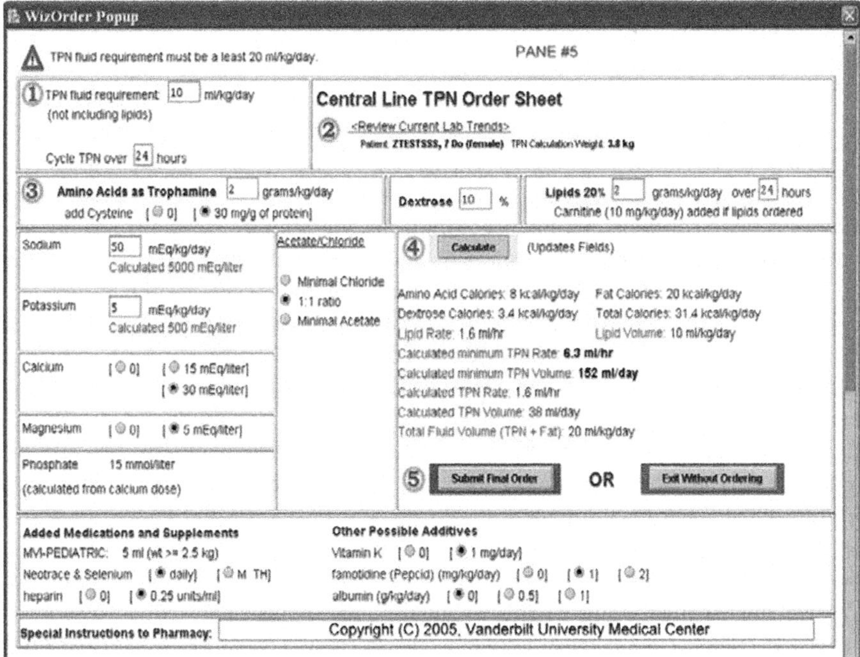

Fig. 15.21 NICU total parenteral nutrition (TPN) advisor provides complex interactive advice and performs various calculations

15.6 CPOE Systems Circa 2015

The foregoing summary discussing how one might approach embedding clinical decision support into a CPOE system remains relevant in 2015. What has changed in the past decade is the likely recipients of such advice. Two to three decades ago, over a dozen academic institutions were actively engaged in the development and/or maintenance of home-grown CPOE systems [94]. Due to several factors such as Meaningful Use system certification requirements, that number is less than a half-dozen in 2015 [95]. The relative demise of academic de novo CPOE and electronic medical record (EMR) system development has occurred in parallel with concurrent adoption of commercial vendor CPOE and EMR systems in both academic and non-academic settings. This suggests that the gap between more flexible, state-of-the-art home-grown academic CPOE and EMR systems and commercial systems may have narrowed substantially.

With respect to CPOE and EMR systems the long-term effects of diminished academic innovation is uncertain. Up to the recent past, many commercial system technologies were patterned after, or licensed from, pioneering academic systems [94]. In the near-term future, responsibility for innovation will increasingly fall to the vendor community. If so, it is unclear if vendors can develop as nimbly and flexibly as previous academic developers. Academic innovation took place in the setting of a single medical center populated by clinician end-users who were faculty colleagues of the developers. In academic settings, the end-user community was immediately available to provide unabashed, frank feedback regarding proposed system changes and their effects once implemented. Academic settings also enabled rapid deployment cycles (new releases of the "live" system every few days or every few weeks). Whether vendors can develop at a similar rate and in a similar manner is yet to be determined. A more deliberate development process is to some extent necessary, as vendors must safely support broad customer bases and maintain meaningful use certification. Additionally, many current high-ranking officers of current CPOE vendor companies learned their trade in academic settings before being recruited to the vendor community. Similarly, the abilities of academic clinical informatics units to teach their trainees how to develop and socio-technically implement innovative clinical systems may diminish. Optimal decision support development requires a deep understanding of clinical practice and of clinical workflows in myriads of care providing settings. Ready access to practicing clinicians who can quickly provide first-hand knowledge about how healthcare providers think and what information they require to make decisions may become less accessible to future developers. The relative decline of academic development may diminish the pipelines that have historically provided innovative technologies and accomplished leaders to the vendor community.

If a small number of future vendors provide the majority of systems to the academic community, benefits not possible with home-grown, one-of-a-kind academic systems may accrue. To the extent that vendors provide open systems, consortia of academic end-user informatics groups using the same vendor system (or the same open-source standards adopted by different systems) may be able to collaborate across institutions. They could develop sharable CPOE and EMR functionality, as well as data-sharing modules, which add capabilities to the base vendor systems. A current example of such activity is the i2b2 consortium work [96–98] pioneered by Kohane and colleagues at Boston Children's Hospital and the emerging SMART and FHIR interoperability standards [99]. Similarly, vendor systems that incorporate programmable external decision support modules may also enable collaborative decision support module development across academic sites. Whether such generic systems can tightly integrate physician-centric decision-making environments into the CPOE systems in the manner illustrated in the discussion and figures above is uncertain.

15.7 Conclusion

System developers, the technologists maintaining the system, and clinical experts must collaborate in managing clinical systems development and implementation. Integrating decision-support capabilities within clinical systems requires an understanding of the clinical significance of a proposed intervention, detailed knowledge of the intervention itself, and a good understanding of the workflows of the clinicians who will be affected by the intervention. The authors have described multiple mechanisms for delivering decision support within the context of CPOE systems using Vanderbilt's WizOrder system for illustration. There are three important axes to consider: the role of decision support, when to intervene, and the method of intervention. Framing decision support in this manner may help both developers and clinical end users to understand how to tailor the system whenever new decision-support needs arise. This framework may also be useful when evaluating and reviewing decision support within CPOE systems.

Offering decision support within a CPOE system provides both clinical end users and institutional administrators with the opportunity to substantially change the way that an institution carries out its work, and to improve patient care processes in terms of quality and safety.

References

1. Kassirer JP, Gorry GA. Clinical problem solving: a behavioral analysis. Ann Intern Med. 1978;89:245–55.
2. Covell DG, Uman GC, Manning PR. Information needs in office practice: are they being met? Ann Intern Med. 1985;103:596–9.
3. Kassirer JP, Kopelman RI. Knowledge and clinical expertise. Hosp Pract (Off Ed). 1988;23:46, 53, 57 passim.
4. Jelovsek FR, Rittwage J, Pearse WH, Visscher HC. Information management needs of the obstetrician-gynecologist – a survey. Obstet Gynecol. 1989;73(3 Pt 1):395–9.

5. Williamson JW, German PS, Weiss R, Skinner EA, Bowes 3rd F. Health science information management and continuing education of physicians. A survey of U.S. primary care practitioners and their opinion leaders. Ann Intern Med. 1989;110:151–60.
6. Timpka T, Arborelius E. The GP's dilemmas: a study of knowledge need and use during health care consultations. Methods Inf Med. 1990;29:23–9.
7. Berner ES, Shugerman AA. Needs assessment for diagnostic decision support systems (DDSS). Proc Annu Symp Comput Appl Med Care 1991:605–8.
8. Osheroff JA, Forsythe DE, Buchanan BG, Bankowitz RA, Blumenfeld BH, Miller RA. Physicians' information needs: analysis of questions posed during clinical teaching. Ann Intern Med. 1991;114:576–81.
9. Forsythe DE, Buchanan BG, Osheroff JA, Miller RA. Expanding the concept of medical information: an observational study of physicians' information needs. Comput Biomed Res. 1992;25:181–200.
10. Bowden VM, Kromer ME, Tobia RC. Assessment of physicians' information needs in five Texas counties. Bull Med Libr Assoc. 1994;82:189–96.
11. Gorman PN, Ash J, Wykoff L. Can primary care physicians' questions be answered using the medical journal literature? Bull Med Libr Assoc. 1994;82:140–6.
12. Lundeen GW, Tenopir C, Wermager P. Information needs of rural health care practitioners in Hawaii. Bull Med Libr Assoc. 1994;82:197–205.
13. Wildemuth BM, de Bliek R, Friedman CP, Miya TS. Information-seeking behaviors of medical students: a classification of questions asked of librarians and physicians. Bull Med Libr Assoc. 1994;82:295–304.
14. Verhoeven AA, Boerma EJ, Meyboom-de Jong B. Use of information sources by family physicians: a literature survey. Bull Med Libr Assoc. 1995;83:85–90.
15. McDonald CJ. Protocol-based computer reminders, the quality of care and the nonperfectability of man. N Engl J Med. 1976;295:1351–5.
16. McDonald CJ, Wilson GA, McCabe Jr GP. Physician response to computer reminders. JAMA. 1980;244:1579–81.
17. Tierney WM, Hui SL, McDonald CJ. Delayed feedback of physician performance versus immediate reminders to perform preventive care. Effects on physician compliance. Med Care. 1986;24:659–66.
18. Tierney WM, McDonald CJ, Martin DK, Rogers MP. Computerized display of past test results. Effect on outpatient testing. Ann Intern Med. 1987;107:569–74.
19. McDonald CJ, Tierney WM. Computer-stored medical records. Their future role in medical practice. JAMA. 1988;259:3433–40.
20. Tierney WM, McDonald CJ, Hui SL, Martin DK. Computer predictions of abnormal test results. Effects on outpatient testing. JAMA. 1988;259:1194–8.
21. McDonald CJ. Computers. JAMA. 1989;261:2834–6.
22. Tierney WM, Miller ME, McDonald CJ. The effect on test ordering of informing physicians of the charges for outpatient diagnostic tests. N Engl J Med. 1990;322:1499–504.
23. McDonald CJ, Tierney WM, Overhage JM, Martin DK, Wilson GA. The Regenstrief Medical Record System: 20 years of experience in hospitals, clinics, and neighborhood health centers. MD Comput. 1992;9:206–17.
24. Tierney WM, Miller ME, Overhage JM, McDonald CJ. Physician inpatient order writing on microcomputer workstations. Effects on resource utilization. JAMA. 1993;269:379–83.
25. McDonald CJ, Overhage JM. Guidelines you can follow and can trust. An ideal and an example [editorial; comment]. JAMA. 1994;271:872–3.
26. Warner HR, Olmsted CM, Rutherford BD. HELP – a program for medical decision-making. Comput Biomed Res. 1972;5:65–74.
27. Evans RS, Larsen RA, Burke JP, et al. Computer surveillance of hospital acquired infections and antibiotic use. JAMA. 1986;256:1007–111.
28. Larsen RA, Evans RS, Burke JP, Pestotnik SL, Gardner RM, Classen DC. Improved perioperative antibiotic use and reduced surgical wound infections through use of computer decision analysis. Infect Control Hosp Epidemiol. 1989;10:316–20.

29. Gardner RM, Golubjatnikov OK, Laub RM, Jacobson JT, Evans RS. Computer critiqued blood ordering using the HELP system. Comput Biomed Res. 1990;23:514–28.
30. Pestotnik SL, Evans RS, Burke JP, Gardner RM, Classen DC. Therapeutic antibiotic monitoring: surveillance using a computerized expert system. Am J Med. 1990;88:43–8.
31. Evans RS, Pestotnik SL, Classen DC, et al. Development of a computerized adverse drug event monitor. Proc Annu Symp Comput Appl Med Care. 1991;15:23–7. PMID: 1807594.
32. Lepage EF, Gardner RM, Laub RM, Jacobson JT. Assessing the effectiveness of a computerized blood order "consultation" system. Proc Annu Symp Comput Appl Med Care. 1991:33–7.
33. Classen DC, Evans RS, Pestotnik SL, Horn SD, Menlove RL, Burke JP. The timing of prophylactic administration of antibiotics and the risk of surgical wound infection [see comments]. N Engl J Med. 1992;326:281–6.
34. Evans RS, Pestotnik SL, Classen DC, Bass SB, Burke JP. Prevention of adverse drug events through computerized surveillance. Proc Annu Symp Comput Appl Med Care. 1992:437–41. PMID: 1482913.
35. Hales JW, Gardner RM, Huff SM. Integration of a stand-alone expert system with a hospital information system. Proc Annu Symp Comput Appl Med Care. 1992:427–31.
36. Evans RS, Classen DC, Stevens LE, et al. Using a hospital information system to assess the effects of adverse drug events. Proc Annu Symp Comput Appl Med Care. 1993:161–5. PMID: 8130454.
37. Gardner RM, Christiansen PD, Tate KE, Laub MB, Holmes SR. Computerized continuous quality improvement methods used to optimize blood transfusions. Proc Annu Symp Comput Appl Med Care. 1993:166–70.
38. Evans RS, Classen DC, Pestotnik SL, Lundsgaarde HP, Burke JP. Improving empiric antibiotic selection using computer decision support. Arch Intern Med. 1994;154:878–84.
39. White KS, Lindsay A, Pryor TA, Brown WF, Walsh K. Application of a computerized medical decision-making process to the problem of digoxin intoxication. J Am Coll Cardiol. 1984;4:571–6.
40. Halpern NA, Thompson RE, Greenstein RJ. A computerized intensive care unit order-writing protocol. Ann Pharmacother. 1992;26:251–4.
41. Dambro MR, Weiss BD, McClure CL, Vuturo AF. An unsuccessful experience with computerized medical records in an academic medical center. J Med Educ. 1988;63:617–23.
42. Williams LS. Microchips versus stethoscopes: Calgary hospital, MDs face off over controversial computer system. CMAJ. 1992;147:1534–40. 1543–1544, 1547.
43. Massaro TA. Introducing physician order entry at a major academic medical center: II. Impact on medical education. Acad Med. 1993;68:25–30.
44. Massaro TA. Introducing physician order entry at a major academic medical center: I. Impact on organizational culture and behavior. Acad Med. 1993;68:20–5.
45. Geissbuhler A, Miller RA. A new approach to the implementation of direct care-provider order entry. Proc AMIA Annu Fall Symp. 1996:689–93. PMID: 8947753.
46. Stead WW, Borden R, Bourne J, et al. The Vanderbilt University fast track to IAIMS: transition from planning to implementation. J Am Med Inform Assoc. 1996;3:308–17.
47. Geissbuhler A, Grande JF, Bates RA, Miller RA, Stead WW. Design of a general clinical notification system based on the publish-subscribe paradigm. Proc AMIA Annu Fall Symp 1997;126–30. PMID: 9357602.
48. Geissbuhler A, Miller RA, Stead WW. The clinical spectrum of decision-support in oncology with a case report of a real world system. In: Keravnou ET, Garbay C, et al., editors. Artificial intelligence medicine, 6th conference on artificial intelligence in medicine in Europe, AIME'97, Grenoble, France, March 23–26, 1997, Proceedings. Lecture Notes in Computer Science 1211 Springer 1997.
49. Heusinkveld J, Geissbuhler A, Sheshelidze D, Miller R. A programmable rules engine to provide clinical decision support using HTML forms. Proc AMIA Symp 1999;800–3.
50. Starmer JM, Talbert DA, Miller RA. Experience using a programmable rules engine to implement a complex medical protocol during order entry. Proc AMIA Symp 2000;829–32.

51. Stead WW, Bates RA, Byrd J, Giuse DA, Miller RA, Shultz EK. Case study: the Vanderbilt University Medical Center information management architecture. In: Van De Velde R, Degoulet P, editors. Clinical information systems: a component-based approach. New York: Springer; 2003.
52. Neilson EG, Johnson KB, Rosenbloom ST, et al. The impact of peer management on test-ordering behavior. Ann Intern Med. 2004;141:196–204.
53. Potts AL, Barr FE, Gregory DF, Wright L, Patel NR. Computerized physician order entry and medication errors in a pediatric critical care unit. Pediatrics. 2004;113(1 Pt 1):59–63.
54. Rosenbloom ST, Chiu KW, Byrne DW, Talbert DA, Neilson EG, Miller RA. Interventions to regulate ordering of serum magnesium levels: an unintended consequence of decision support. J Am Med Inform Assoc. 2005;12:546–53.
55. Rosenbloom ST, Geissbuhler AJ, Dupont WD, et al. Effect of CPOE user interface design on user-initiated access to educational and patient information during clinical care. J Am Med Inform Assoc. 2005;12:458–73.
56. Teich JM, Spurr CD, Schmiz JL, O'Connell EM, Thomas D. Enhancement of clinician workflow with computer order entry. Proc Annu Symp Comput Appl Med Care 1995;459–63. PMID: 8563324.
57. McDonald CJ, Overhage JM, Tierney WM, et al. The Regenstrief Medical Record System: a quarter century experience. Int J Med Inform. 1999;54:225–53.
58. van Wijk MA, van der Lei J, Mosseveld M, Bohnen AM, van Bemmel JH. Assessment of decision support for blood test ordering in primary care. A randomized trial. Ann Intern Med. 2001;134:274–81.
59. Kalmeijer MD, Holtzer W, van Dongen R, Guchelaar HJ. Implementation of a computerized physician medication order entry system at the Academic Medical Centre in Amsterdam. Pharm World Sci. 2003;25:88–93.
60. Payne TH, Hoey PJ, Nichol P, Lovis C. Preparation and use of preconstructed orders, order sets, and order menus in a computerized provider order entry system. J Am Med Inform Assoc. 2003;10:322–9.
61. Oppenheim MI, Vidal C, Velasco FT, et al. Impact of a computerized alert during physician order entry on medication dosing in patients with renal impairment. Proc AMIA Symp. 2002:577–81.
62. Kuperman GJ, Teich JM, Tanasijevic MJ, et al. Improving response to critical laboratory results with automation: results of a randomized controlled trial. J Am Med Inform Assoc. 1999;6:512–22.
63. Stead WW, Miller RA, Musen MA, Hersh WR. Integration and beyond: linking information from disparate sources and into workflow. J Am Med Inform Assoc. 2000;7:135–45.
64. Chertow GM, Lee J, Kuperman GJ, et al. Guided medication dosing for inpatients with renal insufficiency. JAMA. 2001;286:2839–44.
65. Murff HJ, Kannry J. Physician satisfaction with two order entry systems. J Am Med Inform Assoc. 2001;8:499–509.
66. Kuperman GJ, Teich JM, Gandhi TK, Bates DW. Patient safety and computerized medication ordering at Brigham and Women's Hospital. Jt Comm J Qual Improv. 2001;27:509–21.
67. Bizovi KE, Beckley BE, McDade MC, et al. The effect of computer-assisted prescription writing on emergency department prescription errors. Acad Emerg Med. 2002;9:1168–75.
68. Barlow IW, Flynn NA, Britton JM. The Basingstoke Orthopaedic Database: a high quality accurate information system for audit. Ann R Coll Surg Engl. 1994;76(6 Suppl):285–7.
69. Apkon M, Singhaviranon P. Impact of an electronic information system on physician workflow and data collection in the intensive care unit. Intensive Care Med. 2001;27:122–30.
70. Teich JM, Glaser JP, Beckley RF, et al. The Brigham integrated computing system (BICS): advanced clinical systems in an academic hospital environment. Int J Med Inform. 1999;54:197–208.
71. Bates DW, Kuperman G, Teich JM. Computerized physician order entry and quality of care. Qual Manag Health Care. 1994;2:18–27.

72. Bates DW. Using information technology to reduce rates of medication errors in hospitals. BMJ. 2000;320:788–91.
73. Teich JM, Merchia PR, Schmiz JL, Kuperman GJ, Spurr CD, Bates DW. Effects of computerized physician order entry on prescribing practices. Arch Intern Med. 2000;160:2741–7.
74. Bates DW, Cohen M, Leape LL, Overhage JM, Shabot MM, Sheridan T. Reducing the frequency of errors in medicine using information technology. J Am Med Inform Assoc. 2001;8:299–308.
75. Tierney WM, Overhage JM, McDonald CJ. Computerizing guidelines: factors for success. Proc AMIA Annu Fall Symp. 1996:459–62. PMID: 8947708.
76. Chin HL, Wallace P. Embedding guidelines into direct physician order entry: simple methods, powerful results. Proc AMIA Symp. 1999:221–5.
77. Evans RS, Pestotnik SL, Classen DC, et al. A computer-assisted management program for antibiotics and other antiinfective agents. N Engl J Med. 1998;338:232–8.
78. Maviglia SM, Zielstorff RD, Paterno M, Teich JM, Bates DW, Kuperman GJ. Automating complex guidelines for chronic disease: lessons learned. J Am Med Inform Assoc. 2003;10:154–65.
79. Bates DW, Kuperman GJ, Rittenberg E, et al. A randomized trial of a computerbased intervention to reduce utilization of redundant laboratory tests. Am J Med. 1999;106:144–50.
80. Bates DW, Kuperman GJ, Jha A, et al. Does the computerized display of charges affect inpatient ancillary test utilization? Arch Intern Med. 1997;157:2501–8.
81. Dexter PR, Wolinsky FD, Gramelspacher GP, et al. Effectiveness of computer generated reminders for increasing discussions about advance directives and completion of advance directive forms. A randomized, controlled trial. Ann Intern Med. 1998;128:102–10.
82. Gamble ER, McDonald PJ, Lichstein PR. Knowledge, attitudes, and behavior of elderly persons regarding living wills. Arch Intern Med. 1991;151:277–80.
83. Shojania KG, Yokoe D, Platt R, Fiskio J, Ma'luf N, Bates DW. Reducing vancomycin use utilizing a computer guideline: results of a randomized controlled trial. J Am Med Inform Assoc. 1998;5:554–62.
84. Fischer MA, Solomon DH, Teich JM, Avorn J. Conversion from intravenous to oral medications: assessment of a computerized intervention for hospitalized patients. Arch Intern Med. 2003;163:2585–258.
85. Harpole LH, Khorasani R, Fiskio J, Kuperman GJ, Bates DW. Automated evidence-based critiquing of orders for abdominal radiographs: impact on utilization and appropriateness. J Am Med Inform Assoc. 1997;4:511–21.
86. Bates DW, Kuperman GJ, Wang S, et al. Ten commandments for effective clinical decision support: making the practice of evidence-based medicine a reality. J Am Med Inform Assoc. 2003;10:523–30.
87. Overhage JM, Tierney WM, Zhou XH, McDonald CJ. A randomized trial of "corollary orders" to prevent errors of omission. J Am Med Inform Assoc. 1997;4:364–75.
88. Horsky J, Kaufman DR, Patel VL. Computer-based drug ordering: evaluation of interaction with a decision-support system. Medinfo. 2004;11(Pt 2):1063–7.
89. Kucher N, Koo S, Quiroz R, et al. Electronic alerts to prevent venous thromboembolism among hospitalized patient. N Engl J Med. 2005;352:969–77.
90. Payne TH. The transition to automated practitioner order entry in a teaching hospital: the VA Puget Sound experience. Proc AMIA Symp. 1999:589–93. PMID: 10566427.
91. Lovis C, Chapko MK, Martin DP, et al. Evaluation of a command-line parser based order entry pathway for the Department of Veterans Affairs electronic patient record. J Am Med Inform Assoc. 2001;8:486–98.
92. Ash JS, Berg M, Coiera E. Some unintended consequences of information technology in health care: the nature of patient care information system-related errors. J Am Med Inform Assoc. 2004;11:104–12.
93. Gainer A, Pancheri K, Zhang J. Improving the human computer interface design for a physician order entry system. AMIA Annu Symp Proc. 2003:847

94. Collen MF, Ball MJ, editors. The history of medical informatics in the United States. Chapter 6: the early history of hospital information systems. New York: Springer; 2016.
95. Mitchell JA, Gerdin U, Lindberg DA, Lovis C, Martin-Sanchez FJ, Miller RA, Shortliffe EH, Leong TY. 50 years of informatics research on decision support: what's next. Methods Inf Med. 2011;50(6):525–35.
96. Murphy SN, Weber G, Mendis M, Gainer V, Chueh HC, Churchill S, Kohane I. Serving the enterprise and beyond with informatics for integrating biology and the bedside (i2b2). J Am Med Inform Assoc. 2010;17(2):124–30.
97. Weber GM, Murphy SN, McMurry AJ, Macfadden D, Nigrin DJ, Churchill S, Kohane IS. The Shared Health Research Information Network (SHRINE): a prototype federated query tool for clinical data repositories. J Am Med Inform Assoc. 2009;16(5):624–30.
98. Murphy SN, Mendis M, Hackett K, Kuttan R, Pan W, Phillips LC, Gainer V, Berkowicz D, Glaser JP, Kohane I, Chueh HC. Architecture of the open-source clinical research chart from Informatics for Integrating Biology and the Bedside. AMIA Annu Symp Proc. 2007;11:548–52.
99. Alterovitz G, Warner J, Zhang P, Chen Y, Ullman-Cullere M, Kreda D, Kohane IS. SMART on FHIR genomics: facilitating standardized clinico-genomic apps. J Am Med Inform Assoc. 2015;22(6):1173–8. doi:10.1093/jamia/ocv045. pii: ocv045.

Index

A
Accountability, 140, 141
Adverse drug events (ADEs), 5, 7, 158, 159, 210, 217, 232, 249, 261–263
Agency for Healthcare Research and Quality (AHRQ), 73, 111, 113, 115, 122, 127, 128, 150–152, 168, 201, 215
Alert fatigue, 38, 70, 73, 74, 106, 117, 127, 237
Antibiotic assistant, 265–266

B
Bayes' theorem, 28–30, 190
Big Data analytics, 61, 64–65
Bioethics, 131, 134, 135
Brigham and Women's Hospital, 93, 246

C
Care Provider Order Entry System, 277–279
Centers for Medicare and Medicaid Services (CMS), 2, 111, 115–117, 122–124, 127, 128, 258
Clinical decision support system (CDSS), 1–14, 19, 20, 24–26, 30–40, 47–48, 62, 64, 65, 69–75, 77–79, 81, 83, 87–95, 99–108, 111–113, 115–119, 122, 123, 125–128, 132, 136–140, 142–143, 147–160, 202, 210–224, 228–241, 246–271, 276, 283, 286, 287, 304
Clinical outcomes, 60, 148–152, 160, 166, 193, 230
Clinical reminders, 238
Computerized physician order entry (CPOE) systems, 2, 4, 6, 240, 258, 276–279, 281–289, 294, 299, 300, 304–305
Cost-effectiveness, 150, 216, 240

D
Data mining, 2, 45–65
Decision aids, 164, 167–169, 171, 172
Decision support, 2, 6, 8–10, 12, 19, 35, 38, 39, 46, 77, 102, 103, 105, 117, 125, 126, 128, 131–144, 151–153, 160, 163–175, 216–218, 224, 229, 232–233, 239, 241, 246, 247, 249, 250, 252, 255, 260, 264, 267, 270, 271, 276–305
Decision support system, 3–11, 13, 19–40, 45–65, 71, 78, 107, 132–138, 140–142, 160, 163, 175, 181–204, 211, 247, 248, 260, 270, 283
  development, 4
Decision trees, 51, 52, 139
Diagnosis, 4, 6, 25, 28, 30–32, 34–36, 40, 47, 55, 56, 58, 60, 65, 87, 103, 131–133, 135–137, 139, 141, 142, 144, 151, 164, 167–169, 182–187, 189–194, 196, 197, 200–203, 211, 239, 246, 261–266, 269, 279, 281, 286, 299, 301
Diagnostic decision support, 19, 20, 167, 189, 191, 260–261, 267

E.S. Berner (ed.), *Clinical Decision Support Systems*, Health Informatics,
DOI 10.1007/978-3-319-31913-1

E

Electronic health record (EHR), 2–9, 11, 19, 20, 34, 35, 38–40, 64, 65, 70, 72, 73, 78, 80, 88–91, 93, 94, 103–105, 117, 119, 124, 133, 139, 151, 152, 157, 165, 210, 215–219, 221, 222, 224, 230, 237, 239–241, 246, 247, 256, 258, 264
Empowerment, 165–166
Error, 1, 4–6, 8–13, 49, 54, 57, 58, 63, 70, 73, 75, 78–80, 132, 134–136, 141, 144, 185, 187, 190, 196, 197, 201, 224, 230, 232, 246, 259, 283, 284, 286, 294
Ethics, 131, 133, 142–144
Evaluation, 5, 6, 20, 38, 47, 56–58, 61, 71, 76, 79–81, 91, 94, 101, 105, 107, 113, 114, 134, 137, 144, 147–160, 169, 175, 184, 185, 190, 193, 195–200, 202, 228, 231, 235, 238, 240, 241, 250, 255, 262, 271
  methodology, 148

F

Federal health policy, 112–113, 121, 125
Formative evaluation, 149, 196

G

Genetic algorithms, 5, 38, 47, 61–62, 65
Genomics, 139–140, 210–224

H

Healthcare quality, 69, 153
Health Level 7 (HL7), 91–93, 106, 114–116, 121, 153, 218, 219
HELP system, 5, 88, 246–253, 257, 260–261, 265, 267, 270
Human-computer interaction (HCI), 70, 75, 99
Human reasoning, 185–188

I

Implementation, 4, 6–8, 10, 11, 40, 71, 73, 74, 80, 81, 88–95, 99–108, 113, 115, 117, 118, 122, 123, 143, 148–150, 152, 153, 159, 184, 193, 195, 201, 212, 216, 218–221, 224, 228, 230, 233–236, 239–241, 249, 252, 271, 276, 287, 305
Inpatient care, 276–305
Intermountain healthcare, 246–271

K

Knowledge base, 2–4, 7, 11, 13–14, 30–32, 34, 36, 40, 72, 77–78, 191, 193–196, 198, 200–204, 210, 215, 219–220, 224, 232, 237, 258, 266
Knowledge-based system, 3, 5, 11, 240
Knowledge formalization, 99, 101–103
Knowledge localization, 99, 103
Knowledge maintenance, 271
Knowledge representation, 93, 102, 195
Knowledge synthesis, 99–101, 107

L

Legal issues, 10, 13, 131–144, 201
Liability, 10, 115, 140–142
Logic, 6, 11, 12, 20–27, 30–32, 35, 37, 38, 40, 63, 64, 90, 102, 103, 116, 119, 126, 189, 219, 229, 249, 251, 252, 258–260, 263, 265, 266, 269, 270

M

Mathematics, 20, 24, 38, 83
Medical information systems, 246

N

National Quality Strategy (NQS), 112, 113, 124, 128
Neural network, 5, 37, 38, 47, 48, 51, 54–55, 58, 60, 62–64, 192
Nosocomial infection, 26, 249, 261, 263–264

O

Office the National Coordinator (ONC), 6, 7, 13, 90, 94, 111, 115, 116, 119, 121–123, 125–128
Ontology, 77, 78

P

Partners Healthcare, 5, 93, 228–241, 246
Patient-centric, 239–240
Patient preferences, 100, 166, 172
Pharmacogenomics, 139, 140, 211, 212, 220, 222, 224
Pharmacology, 214
Probability, 20–23, 26–31, 34, 36, 40, 50, 52, 53, 58, 169, 185, 210, 235, 264, 266, 267, 269
Prognostic scoring systems, 138

Q

Quantum computing, 61, 63, 65

R

Randomized controlled trial, 149–151, 155, 157–160, 203
Regulation, 13, 91, 113, 117, 119, 120, 123–127, 135, 140, 142–143, 200, 201
Responsibility, 13, 14, 133, 134, 140–142, 234, 239, 287, 304

S

Safety, 2, 5, 9, 40, 70, 75, 77–82, 100, 105, 106, 113, 115, 125, 126, 143, 202, 228, 230, 235, 241, 253, 278, 285, 286, 305
Service-oriented architecture (SOA), 9, 88–92, 94, 95
Service oriented computing, 90
Service-oriented design, 91
Set theory, 20–23, 40, 64, 189, 192
Shared decision making, 137, 138, 140, 164, 165, 167–169
Software architecture, 88
Statistical pattern recognition, 3, 48, 56, 266
Study design, 149, 154, 157, 158, 160, 197, 198
Summative evaluation, 149, 154

U

Usability, 4, 7, 69–83, 107, 108, 125, 127, 128, 171–175

V

Vanderbilt, 4, 5, 212, 216, 218, 220, 246, 276–305
Ventilator management, 24, 248, 258–260

W

Workflow integration, 71, 74